I0030957

De Haan's Health of Southern Africa

12th edition

Editors:
Sharon Vasuthevan and Sindi Mthembu

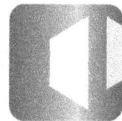

juta

De Haan's Health of Southern Africa

First published 1943 as Wright's Hygiene in South Africa
Seventh edition 1996
Eighth edition 2001
Ninth edition 2005
Tenth edition 2013
Eleventh edition 2016
Twelfth edition 2021

Juta and Company (Pty) Ltd
First floor, Sunclare building, 21 Dreyer Street, Claremont 7708
PO Box 14373, Lansdowne 7779, Cape Town, South Africa
www.juta.co.za

© 2021 Juta and Company (Pty) Ltd

978 1 48513 070 3 (Print)
978 1 48513 071 0 (WebPDF)

All rights reserved. No part of this publication may be reproduced or transmitted in any form or by any means, electronic or mechanical, including photocopying, recording, or any information storage or retrieval system, without prior permission in writing from the publisher. Subject to any applicable licensing terms and conditions in the case of electronically supplied publications, a person may engage in fair dealing with a copy of this publication for his or her personal or private use, or his or her research or private study. See section 12(1)(a) of the Copyright Act 98 of 1978.

Print production specialist: Seshni Kazadi
Editor: Inge du Plessis
Proofreader: Liesbet van Wyk
Cover designer: Drag and Drop
Typesetter: Elinye Ithuba DTP Solutions
Indexer: Lexinfo

Typeset in 9.5pt on 13pt ITC Stone Serif

The author and the publisher believe on the strength of due diligence exercised that this work does not contain any material that is the subject of copyright held by another person. In the alternative, they believe that any protected pre-existing material that may be comprised in it has been used with appropriate authority or has been used in circumstances that make such use permissible under the law.

Disclaimer

In the writing of this book, every effort has been made to present accurate and up-to-date information from the best and most reliable sources. However, the results of healthcare professionals depend on a variety of factors that are beyond the control of the authors and publishers. Therefore, neither the authors nor the publishers assume responsibility for, nor make any warranty with regards to, the outcomes achieved from the procedures described in this book.

Contents

About the Authors xi

List of Abbreviations xii

Chapter 1: Overview of health
Sindi Mthembu 1

Learning outcomes. 1
Key terms 1
Introduction: Definition of health 2
Attaining and maintaining optimal health for all 4
Health and development 10
Disease profiles. 11
Demography. 15
Conclusion. 16
Self-assessment. 16
Bibliography. 16

Chapter 2: The United Nations and the World Health Organization
Sindi Mthembu 18

Learning outcomes. 18
Key terms 18
Introduction: The United Nations (UN) 19
The World Health Organization (WHO) 22
Conclusion. 29
Self-assessment. 29
Bibliography. 29

Chapter 3: Health policy and health systems in South Africa and the southern African region
Sindi Mthembu 31

Learning outcomes. 31
Key terms 32
Introduction: The development of health policy and health systems
in South Africa 32
The Constitution of the Republic of South Africa, 1996 33
The South African health policy 35
The South African healthcare system 42
Re-engineering primary healthcare in South Africa 46

The roles and functions of primary healthcare outreach teams 50
School health nursing 51
National health insurance in South Africa 52
The National Core Standards. 56
Health policy in the Southern African Development Community. 60
Conclusion. 61
Self-assessment. 62
Bibliography. 62

Chapter 4: Promoting health through health education
Shanti Ramkilowan 64

Learning outcomes. 64
Key terms 64
Introduction. 64
Health education 66
Outcomes of health education. 67
Teaching methods 67
Teaching aids and media 68
Planning a health education session 69
Organisations promoting health through education. 69
Important principles for success in health education 70
Conclusion. 71
Self-assessment. 71
Bibliography. 71

Chapter 5: Epidemiology and health information
Shanti Ramkilowan 73

Learning outcomes. 73
Key terms 73
Introduction. 74
Using epidemiology in healthcare practice 74
Demographic data 76
Health data. 77
International Classification of Diseases 79
Using health statistics 79
Health information management systems. 80
Epidemiological research methods 81
Conclusion. 81
Self-assessment. 81
Bibliography 82

Chapter 6: Non-communicable diseases

Shanti Ramkilowan 83

Learning outcomes. 83

Key terms 83

Introduction. 84

Non-communicable diseases 85

Caring for patients with chronic NCD 87

Burden of disease 89

Conclusion. 105

Self-assessment. 105

Bibliography. 106

Chapter 7: Microbiology and the transmission of infection

Joy Cleghorn 107

Learning outcomes. 107

Key terms 107

Introduction. 108

The single-cell microorganism. 109

Living characteristics of microbes 110

Laboratory examination of microorganisms 112

Destroying pathogenic microorganisms 113

Portals of entry. 116

Classification of microorganisms. 117

Reservoirs of infection 124

Immunity. 125

Immunisation 126

Vaccine administration 128

Conclusion 130

Self-assessment. 130

Bibliography. 130

Chapter 8: Infection prevention and control

Joy Cleghorn 131

Learning outcomes. 131

Key terms 131

Introduction. 132

Surveillance 132

Preventing spread or 'breaking the chain' of infection. 133

Routes of infection. 133

Risk factors for healthcare-associated infections. 133

Hand hygiene. 133
Infection prevention and control: Roles and responsibilities 135
Outbreaks. 137
The importance of antimicrobial stewardship. 137
Conclusion. 137
Self-assessment. 138
Bibliography. 138

Chapter 9: Communicable diseases
Joy Cleghorn 139

Learning outcomes. 139
Key terms 139
Introduction. 140
Epidemiology of communicable diseases. 141
Communicable diseases in Africa 144
Parasitic diseases common in Africa 155
The six major communicable diseases. 159
Conclusion. 164
Self-assessment. 164
Bibliography. 164

Chapter 10: Genetic factors in health and disease
Colleen Aldous 165

Learning outcomes. 165
Key terms 165
Introduction. 165
Basic genetics concepts. 166
Chromosomal abnormalities 172
Gene defects. 173
Inheritance patterns. 174
The effect of teratogens 178
Genetic counselling and referring people who may be at risk 178
Conclusion. 180
Self-assessment. 180
Bibliography. 180

Chapter 11: Health needs through the lifespan
Sharon Vasuthevan 181

Learning outcomes. 181
Key terms 181

Introduction. 182
Maternal and child health 182
Well baby clinics 193
Adolescent health 195
Men's health. 197
Health of the elderly 197
Conclusion 204
Self-assessment. 205
Bibliography. 205

Chapter 12: Home accidents
  Sindi Mthembu 207

Learning outcomes. 207
Key terms 207
Introduction. 207
Demographic factors in home accidents 208
Types of home accidents 208
Burns 210
Poisoning 214
Drowning. 215
Choking 216
Suffocation. 217
Objects in the ear, nose and eye 219
Conclusion. 220
Self-assessment. 220
Bibliography. 220

Chapter 13: Social and mental health
  Sharon Vasuthevan 221

Learning outcomes. 221
Key terms 221
Introduction. 222
Self-destructive behaviours 222
Obesity. 227
Child abuse 230
Intimate partner violence and rape 237
Drug addiction. 240
Mental health. 240
Classification of mental conditions 241
Conclusion 246

Self-assessment. 247
Bibliography. 247

Chapter 14: Sustainable development
Sindi Mthembu 249

Learning outcomes. 249
Key terms 249
Introduction. 250
The sustainable development goals (SDGs) 252
Health and sustainable development in southern Africa 256
Organisations involved in sustainable development in Africa 257
Intersectoral collaboration in sustainable development 259
Conclusion. 261
Self-assessment. 261
Bibliography. 262

Chapter 15: Environmental sustainability
Roelien Els 263

Learning outcomes. 263
Key terms 263
Introduction. 264
Sustainable Development Goals. 265
Health effects of air pollution and inadequate ventilation 269
Ventilation 271
Housing 273
Lighting and heating 276
Climate change 279
Conclusion. 283
Self-assessment. 283
Bibliography. 283

Chapter 16: Safe water and sanitation
Roelien Els 287

Learning outcomes. 287
Key terms 287
Introduction. 288
Water 289
Common water contaminants 294
Environmental hygiene 298
Household refuse: Dry or solid refuse 299

Conclusion. 303
Self-assessment. 304
Bibliography. 304

Chapter 17: Nutrition and food safety
Roelien Els 307
Learning outcomes. 307
Key terms 307
Introduction. 308
Food groups and classifications 310
Food safety. 327
Foodborne disease 328
Biological contaminants 328
Chemical contaminants 331
The regulation of food safety. 332
Promoting food hygiene 332
Food preservation. 334
Milk 336
Food security 339
Conclusion. 340
Self-assessment. 340
Bibliography. 340

Index 345

About the Authors

The general editors

Dr Sharon Vasuthevan is currently the Group Nursing and Quality Executive for a private hospital group and has been involved in nursing education at various professional levels for many years. Dr Vasuthevan has been involved with this publication since 2005. She has published various articles and chapters on nursing education and leadership.

Dr Sindi Mthembu is Principal of the KwaZulu-Natal College of Nursing. She has lectured at various nursing education institutions, including the then Natal College of Nursing, Durban University of Technology and University of KwaZulu-Natal. She is also a member various professional organisations and has published in various journals on nursing and nursing education, community health nursing and HIV and AIDS and has contributed to other books as well.

The contributors

Professor Colleen Aldous is the Academic Leader for Research in the School of Clinical Medicine at the Nelson R. Mandela School of Medicine, University of KwaZulu-Natal. She has been involved in genetics research at the university since 2004.

Joy Cleghorn is currently the National Infection Prevention and Control Risk Manager with a private hospital group. Joy's interests lie in improving patient safety through consistent best practice of infection control procedures.

Roelien Els is a nurse educator with a private hospital group. She has a special interest in promoting quality in all aspects of the nursing profession and is a strong proponent of life-long learning.

Shanti Ramkilowan is currently Vice-principal of the KwaZulu-Natal College of Nursing and has over three decades of experience in nursing education. In addition to her qualifications in nursing education, she has a special interest in community nursing and holds a Masters of Nursing from the University of KwaZulu-Natal.

List of Abbreviations

A-SDA	African Sustainable Development Association
ABHR	alcohol-based hand rub
ANC	African National Congress
ARV	antiretroviral (therapy)
BCG	bacille Calmette-Guerin
BNG	Breaking New Ground (previously called RDP Housing Plan)
CAI	community-associated infection
CANSA	Cancer Association of South Africa
CAUTI	catheter-associated urinary tract infection
CCMDD	Centralized chronic medicine dispensing and distributing
CHC	Community Health Centres
CHW	Community Healthcare Worker
CLABSI	central line associated bloodstream infection
CNS	central nervous system
COPD	chronic obstructive pulmonary disease
COVID-19	Coronavirus Disease 2019
CUP	Cancer of Union Primary
CVA	cerebrovascular accident
CD4	cluster of differentiation
CPR	cardio-pulmonary resuscitation
DAFF	Department of Agriculture, Forestry and Fisheries
DCST	District Clinical Specialist Team
DHS	District Health System
DNA	deoxyribonucleic acid
DOTS	Directly Observed Treatment Support
DWS	Department of Water and Sanitation
EPI(SA)	Expanded Programme of Immunisation
FAO	Food and Agricultural Organization
GBD	Global Burden of Disease
GN	General Nurse
GP	General Practitioner
GPW 13	Thirteenth General Programme of Work
HAI	healthcare-associated infection
HPRS	Health Patient Registration System

HPV	Human Papillomavirus
HSDG	Human Settlement Development Grant
HSS	Health System Strengthening
ICD	International Classification of Diseases
ICLEI	International Council for Local Environmental Initiatives
ICT	Information Communication Technology
ILO	International Labour Organization
IPV	intimate partner violence
ISHP	Integrated School Health Programme
IUD	intra-uterine device
KZN	KwaZulu-Natal
MDG	Millennium Development Goal
MDT	Multidisciplinary Team
MUS	multiple use system
NAFCI	National Adolescent-friendly Clinic Initiative
NCD	non-communicable disease
NCS	National Core Standards
NHI	National Health Insurance
NICD	National Institute of Communicable Diseases
NIMART	nurse management of antiretroviral treatment
NPO	non-profit organisation
NWRS2	National Water Resource Strategy
OHSC	Office of Health Standards Compliance
PCSA	Pharmacy Council of South Africa
PHC	Primary Healthcare
PLWA	People Living with HIV and AIDS
PM	particulate matter
PMCT	prevention of mother-to-child transmission
PN	Professional Nurse
POP	persistent organic pollutants
PPP	public–private partnership
RDP	Reconstruction and Development Programme
RDSA	Rare Diseases South Africa
rPHC	re-engineering
SADC	Southern African Development Community
SANC	South African Nursing Council
SARS-Cov-2	Severe Acute Respiratory Syndrome Coronavirus 2
SDG	sustainable development goal

SHN	School Health Nurse
SN	Staff Nurse
SSI	surgical site infection
STI	sexually transmitted infection
SWELL	securing water to enhance local livelihoods
TB	tuberculosis
TDS	total dissolved solids
TOP	termination of pregnancy
UHC	Universal Health Coverage
UN	United Nations
UNAIDS	Joint United Nations Programme on HIV and AIDS
UNCED	UN Conference on Environmental Development
UNDP	United Nations Development Programme
UNEP	United Nations Environmental Programme
UNICEF	United Nations Children's Fund
UN Women	United Nations Women
UVGI	Ultraviolet Germicidal Irradiation
VAP	ventilator associated pneumonia
VCT	voluntary counseling and testing
WBPHCOT	Municipal Ward Based Primary Healthcare Outreach Team
WFP	World Food Programme
WHA	World Health Assembly
WHO	World Health Organization
WISN	Workload Indicator for Staffing Needs
WSA	water services authorities
WWSD	World Summit on Sustainable Development

Overview of health

Sindi Mthembu

1

CHAPTER

Learning outcomes

After studying this chapter, you should be able to:

- Define health and its components.
- Discuss and reflect on the various factors that can have an impact on health.
- Explain how health and development are interrelated.
- Compare the disease profile in southern Africa to that in the rest of the world.
- Explain the term demography.
- Outline the demographic composition of the South African population.
- Explain how the population's demographic composition affects its health.

Key terms

Comprehensive approach: Focuses more on coordinated and integrated forms of healthcare provision, including or dealing with all or nearly all elements or aspects of something.

Holistic approach: Characterised by the treatment of the whole person, taking into account mental and social factors, rather than just the symptoms of a disease.

Morbidity: The state of being sick or diseased/the incidence of disease.

Mortality: The death rate/the number of deaths in a unit of population occurring within a prescribed time.

Psychosocial: Pertaining to a person's psychological development in relation to his or her social environment.

Vectors: Living carriers of disease, such as flies and mosquitoes, that transmit disease-causing organisms from one host to another.

Introduction: Definition of health

In 1948, the World Health Organization (WHO) defined health as 'a state of complete physical, mental and social well-being, and not merely the absence of disease and infirmity'. Since then many definitions have been suggested, but this definition remains one of the most accepted as it acknowledges the psychosocial aspects of health. The terms 'health', 'well-being' and 'wellness' tend to be used interchangeably. Health does not just mean the physical well-being of the individual but refers inclusively to social, emotional, spiritual and cultural well-being.

With the emergence of medicine as a science over the last centuries, the *bio-medical model* of health was established. This term refers to the scientific approach to medicine, where every disease or illness is believed to have an associated cause (a disease-causing organism) for which an appropriate form of treatment has been researched and identified. This treatment is then administered to the person to rid his or her body of the ailment. In other words, the science of medicine offers technical solutions to an identified health problem. Medicine cures diseases and the person returns to health. The bio-medical model would say that the person is healthy if the body is in 'normal' working order.

However, attaining and maintaining health is not so simple. Health and disease are closely linked to the environment in which people live and work. The health status of people will be affected by where they live, the type of dwelling in which they live, the food they have access to or can afford to buy and the *environmental* conditions under which they live. *Cultural* practices, such as matters of personal hygiene, nutrition, perceptions of health and disease, traditional practices and way of life preferences, can also affect people's health. All these factors are determined by the society in which a person lives and by his or her particular position within that society. The *physical* factors that can affect health include exercise, diet, alcohol, smoking and genetic inheritance. Social divisions occur in all societies and the gap results in the underprivileged usually being more prone to disease and ill-health than those who are referred to as 'privileged'. However, the privileged often have their own health problems. A higher social and economic status often means living the 'good life', which is often accompanied by unhealthy eating habits and associated diseases, referred to as the diseases of the 'rich'. *Psychosocial* factors are the main cause of health inequalities. Such factors include negative behaviour, stress, violence, distrust, anger, dietary deprivation, drug abuse, parental problems, sexual, physical or emotional abuse, hostility, depression, anxiety and many other aspects of the social environment that have a negative impact on one's personal life. *Economic* factors include the distribution of income, wealth, influence and power to meet healthcare needs in society.

This comprehensive, holistic approach to attaining and maintaining health is referred to as the *psychosocial–environmental model* of health. The primary and secondary factors for this model are set out in Table 1.1 and Figure 1.1.

Table 1.1 Primary and secondary factors of the psychosocial–environmental model

Primary factors	Secondary factors
Economic	Cultural
Political	Environmental
	Physical
	Psychosocial

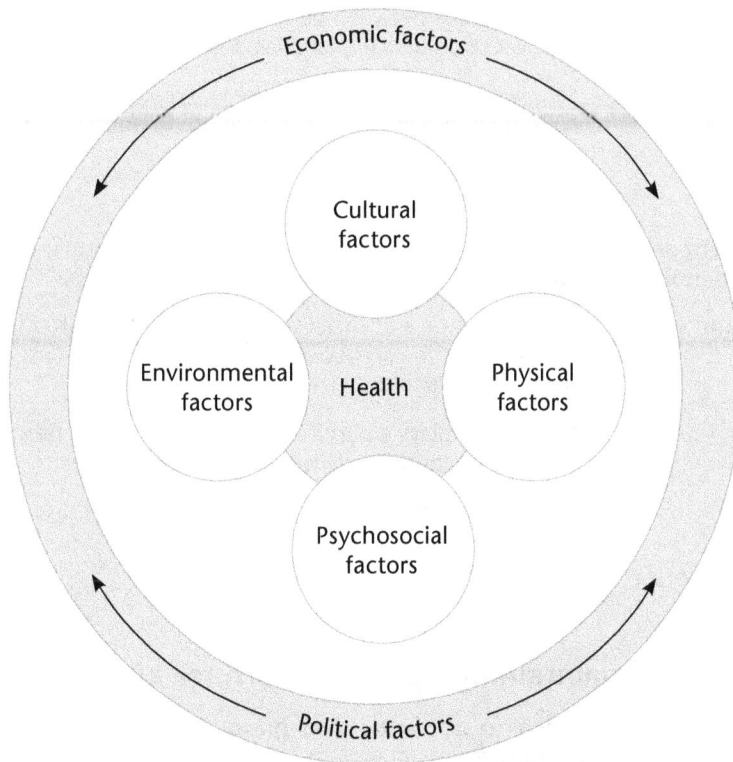

Figure 1.1 Determinants of health according to the psychosocial–environmental model

According to the WHO (2015b), there are many other factors that affect the health of individuals and communities at large. Whether people are healthy or not, is determined by their circumstances and environment. To a large extent, factors such as where we live, the state of our environment, genetics, our income and education level and our relationships with friends and family all have considerable impact on health, whereas the more commonly considered factors such as access to and use of healthcare services often have less of an impact.

The health determinants therefore include many other factors as outlined in Table 1.2.

Table 1.2 Determinants of health by the World Health Organization

Determinants	Description
Health services	Access to and use of health services influence the level of wellness and general health.
Culture	Customs, traditions and the beliefs of the family and community all affect health.
Personal behaviour and coping skills	Eating habits, level of activity, smoking, drinking, and how we deal with life's stresses and challenges all affect health.
Social support networks	There is a link between better health and strong social support structures (eg families, friends and communities).
Physical environment	Safe water and clean air, healthy workplaces, safe houses, communities and roads all contribute to good health.
Education	Low education levels are linked to poor health, more stress and lower self-confidence.
Employment and working conditions	People in employment are healthier, particularly those who have more control over their working conditions.
Income and social status	Higher income and social status are linked to better health. The greater the gap between the richest and poorest people, the greater the differences in health.
Genetics	Inheritance plays a part in determining lifespan, healthiness and the likelihood of developing certain illnesses.
Gender	Men and women suffer from different types of diseases at different ages.

Source: WHO (2015b)

Attaining and maintaining optimal health for all

A comprehensive approach to attaining and maintaining optimal health for people requires that we identify the factors that can affect health. The effect of these factors on people's health can be both positive and negative.

Treatment to attain health cannot be confined to medical treatment alone. It should be more comprehensive in nature and include improvement of the environment or the conditions in which people live, thus preventing disease conditions from occurring or from re-occurring.

This holistic approach to health forms the basis of Public Health, a health science in its own right. Public Health is the science and art of protecting and improving the health of communities through education, promotion of healthy lifestyles and research on disease and injury prevention. It helps to improve the health and well-being of people in local communities and across the globe.

It can also be said that attaining health becomes more than 'curing' or treating, and should include 'caring', which requires a more holistic approach. The most important factors affecting health can be divided into two groups:

1. Appropriate health service provision
2. Environmental and psychosocial factors.

Appropriate health service provision

Political factors: A government determines legislation or laws to outline the way it wants to govern its people. Laws reflect the government's commitment to the area or field to which the particular legislation applies. Therefore, the health legislation of a country expresses the leaders' commitment to health. However, the commitment can only be realised if the government makes the necessary resources available to implement the legislation.

In Africa, most countries are regarded as developing countries and may not have the resources to develop and implement the health services that are required to meet the health needs of the people. This is reflected in the disease profile of a region, which includes many diseases and conditions that are preventable.

Health legislation: Health legislation refers to laws that have a direct impact on health services and healthcare. Wherever necessary, *regulations* are developed to assist the people who implement these laws. Regulations give guidelines on how to implement the legislation. Appropriate laws and associated regulations are necessary as a basis on which to develop suitable healthcare policies.

The advent of good public health legislation ensures education and literacy, safe drinking water and sanitation, better housing, improved working conditions, land and food (agriculture) and healthcare. These laws drastically reduced the occurrence of communicable diseases in developed countries.

Health policies: Health policies determine the structure of the health sector and how it will operate. The policies also identify priorities and determine appropriate processes to offer and implement healthcare services geared towards improving the standard of healthcare delivery that will ensure a healthier nation. Health policies usually include measurable outcomes that can be applied to determine how successful a policy is in meeting the health needs of the people it was developed to serve.

Inequity in health: There is still a marked difference between the disease profiles of the developed and the developing world. Developing countries still have a high incidence of communicable and other preventable diseases associated with the environment in which they live, coupled with a lack of resources such as sufficient income, homes and electricity provision, and access to food, safe water and sanitation. Many of these inequities are not so evident in the developed world.

There is also inequity in health between people in rural and urban areas. In most parts of Africa, including South Africa, morbidity and mortality rates are higher in rural areas than in towns and cities. This occurs for the following reasons:

- In rural areas, standards of environmental hygiene are poor. There is a lack of available services, which results in poor sanitation and poor access to safe water. Due to this situation, gastrointestinal and parasitic infections are common in these areas.
- There is more poverty in rural areas because there are fewer educational and employment opportunities; therefore, all the diseases related to poverty, such as malnutrition and the 'deficiency' diseases, are common.
- There are fewer medical care services available in rural areas and they are often inaccessible because transport is inadequate.

Adequate health services and resources: Health services must be available in sufficient numbers and staffed by adequate numbers of personnel, who are well trained and adequately deployed, to serve both urban and rural communities.

The basic services or clinics need to be accessible to the communities they serve by being within walking distance or on transport routes. Accessibility also refers to the suitability of services for the people they serve. People using these services should be treated with respect and preferably spoken to in their own language. Services should be affordable and, especially in developing countries, there is a need for public health facilities that the poor are able to access.

In developed countries, where people can afford to choose the health services they wish to use, there should be a mixture of public and private health services. However, services can only meet the needs of the community if they have adequate supplies and resources.

Health information: For health services to be planned and developed appropriately, information on the health status of the community and the country must be collected and made available. The data are usually lacking in developing countries as statistics are not collected or are not adequately processed. This means that the limited resources available in these countries are often used inefficiently as there are no good data or sources of information on which to determine the priorities or even to plan appropriate health services.

Environmental and psychosocial factors

Socioeconomic factors: Research has shown that disease, disability and death are far more common in the lower socioeconomic groups and that rates decline steadily as people's socioeconomic situations improve. In addition, it is well known that health is not high in the value system of the economically deprived section of the community and that they are not motivated to pursue behavioural patterns that may lead to an improvement in their health status.

Growth in the economy has not matched growth in the population in sub-Saharan Africa which has resulted in more people being unemployed and an increase in the number of people living in poverty. Informal settlements have developed in urban areas as people move to the cities in search of work and a chance for a better life. Many of the informal settlements do not even have basic services, with the result that the environment does not support good health. The frustration of living in these conditions leads to behavioural problems, such as alcohol and other substance abuse, violence and crime, all of which have a negative impact on the health of communities.

The wealthy live in an environment where they often have more than they need, which can have a negative impact on health as well. They often have poor dietary habits and suffer from conditions such as obesity or over-nutrition, an increase in cardiovascular disease and some forms of cancer that result from their unhealthy lifestyles.

In many parts of Africa there has been political instability during the last century and many countries have experienced conflict and wars that have had a negative effect on the economy and environment. Poverty gets worse as a result of this situation and the general health status of the population deteriorates. Conditions associated with poverty include communicable diseases, parasitic infections and malnutrition.

Cultural factors: Culture may be defined as a way of life that includes ways of thinking, feeling, believing and behaving. Culture influences the type of clothes we wear, how and when we sleep, what we eat and how our food is prepared. It also determines how we rear our children and what languages we speak. There is, in fact, no aspect of our lives that is not influenced, in some way, by the culture to which we belong. Cultural practices also affect health. The following are a few examples of diseases that are linked to cultural practices:

- *Osteomalacia.* This is caused by a deficiency of vitamin D. The condition is common in some Muslim women, who are required to cover their bodies in public by wearing a burqa, which is a black garment that covers the entire body, leaving only a slit for the eyes. Because their skin is seldom exposed to the rays of the sun, their bodies are unable to synthesise sufficient vitamin D for their needs.

- *Cancer.* Carcinoma of the colon is associated with a so-called Western diet that is composed of highly refined foods and lacks natural fibre and roughage. Carcinoma of the stomach, which is common in Japan, is thought to be related to the large amount of polished rice that the Japanese eat. Polished rice contains traces of asbestos and has been associated with the carcinoma. There has been an escalating cancer rate in South Africa, mainly due to changing community lifestyles.

- *Tetanus neonatorum.* In some African cultures it is the custom to dress the umbilical cord of the newborn with mud. This practice has been associated with a very high incidence of tetanus neonatorum.

Environmental factors: The extent of ill-health in a community is directly related to standard of environmental hygiene. Lack of sanitation and inadequate facilities for the treatment and disposal of sewage, an insufficient and contaminated water supply and the presence of flies and insect vectors all lead to increased morbidity and mortality rates. Improvement in the standard of environmental hygiene is one of the most effective methods of improving the health of a community.

Environmental issues that impact on health are many and include any form of pollution, noise, overcrowding, rapid urbanisation, informal settlements, food-borne disease and any activity that degrades the surroundings. Certain government sectors provide services that have an impact on the environment and therefore on health. They include departments such as those responsible for housing, agriculture, roads, electricity and veterinary services. It can therefore be said that health is not the responsibility of the health department alone but rather of a number of sectors in government. Health can therefore only be attained through intersectoral collaboration of all government departments. This approach demands a multidisciplinary and interdisciplinary approach.

Geological or geochemical factors found in certain areas can also influence health. It has long been known that plants and animals can suffer from certain diseases as a direct result of either the deficiency or the presence of certain minerals in the soil. The relationship between the geochemistry of an area and the incidence of certain conditions such as kidney stones, diabetes and angina is being researched. Examples of such relationships are the incidence of simple goitre in areas where the soil and the water lack iodine, such as in Bolivia, South America and certain areas of Western Europe, as well as the higher incidence of coronary artery disease in regions of Britain where the water is said to be soft.

Educational factors: Literacy is an important factor in attaining optimal health. People must be able to make informed decisions regarding healthcare and even regarding issues of lifestyle. To do this they need to be able to read and make their own decisions. In a developing country like India, a four-year literacy campaign was run to educate women. Funding was limited and it was decided that women should be targeted as they were the group responsible for raising the new nation. The impact on health as a result of the campaign has been a drop in the infant and under-five mortality rate in the country. These and other improvements in health that occurred in India have been attributed to the educational campaign. In South Africa, such campaigns by the government are seen especially in rural areas where Adult Basic Education and Training (ABET) programmes are decentralised to the illiterate.

There is a definite relationship between health and education, and it is therefore important that educators work with health professionals to ensure that health issues are addressed as part of an educational programme. An example is HIV and AIDS prevention, where two departments (health and education) are and must continue working together if the pandemic is to be controlled.

Social welfare: According to a Chinese proverb, 'you can give a man a fish and he will eat for a day, but if you teach a man how to fish, he will eat for the rest of his life.' Where poverty is rife in a country or a community, social welfare systems often support people to ensure that they have access to food, water and shelter. These are not only the basics necessary for survival; they are also the basic elements on which health depends.

However, social welfare supports communities in many ways: government and welfare organisations assist with programmes aimed at helping people to find employment or to grow their own food. One of the objectives of such programmes is to help communities achieve optimal health.

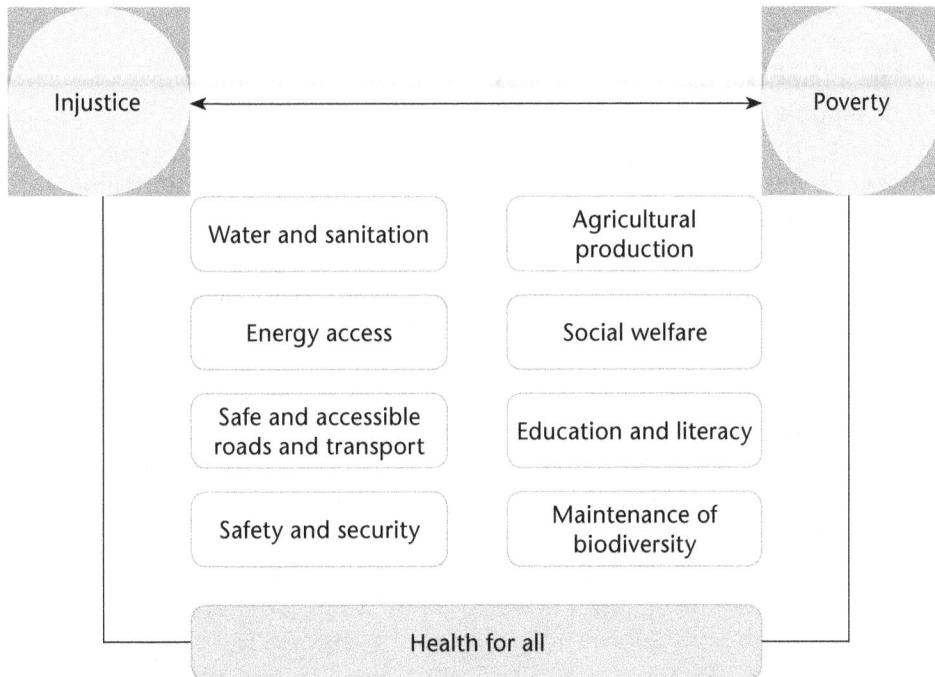

Figure 1.2 Intersectoral approach to health

For better health for all, communities must have access to:
- effective health services
- water and sanitation
- agricultural production
- energy
- maintenance of biodiversity
- social welfare services
- safe and accessible roads and transport
- safety and security
- education and literacy.

Health and development

We are living in an era of rapid change where the world is undergoing overwhelming social, economic and environmental changes. Alongside these changes we are witnessing an unequalled pace of development. This has given rise to a series of threats, not only directly to the health of people but to their physical and mental development as well. It has been estimated that one-third of the global burden of disease can be attributed to environmental factors such as polluted water and air.

In 2002, the Johannesburg Declaration on Sustainable Development was adopted at the World Summit on Sustainable Development (WSSD). This is also referred to as the Earth Summit 2002, at which the plan to implement the WSSD was agreed.

The Johannesburg Declaration was built on earlier declarations made at the Earth Summit in Rio de Janeiro in 1992. This summit also included substantial mention of the principle or belief that several nations should be cooperatively involved in the process of achieving a goal, especially nuclear disarmament, as the path forward.

In terms of the political commitment of parties, the declaration was a more general statement than the Rio Declaration. There was also agreement to focus particularly on worldwide conditions that pose severe threats to the sustainable development of the people, including chronic hunger; malnutrition; foreign occupation; armed conflict; illicit drug problems; organised crime; corruption; natural disasters; illicit arms trafficking; trafficking in persons; terrorism; intolerance and racism; ethnic, religious and other hatreds; xenophobia; and endemic, communicable and chronic diseases, in particular HIV and AIDS, malaria and tuberculosis (WHO, 2002).

In 2012 the United Nations (UN) convened the UN Conference on Sustainable Development, also known as 'Rio 2012 or Rio+20', hosted by Brazil in Rio de Janeiro, as a 20-year follow-up to the historic 1992 UN Conference on Environmental Development (UNCED) that was held in the same city. The conference was organised by the UN Department of Economic and Social Affairs.

All countries in the Johannesburg Declaration committed themselves to freeing the world of the indignity and indecency occasioned by poverty, environmental degradation and patterns of unsustainable development. Poverty increases people's vulnerability to ill-health, which leads to illnesses through economic underdevelopment, unemployment and low incomes, environmental degradation, poor agricultural production, inequitable land reform, lack of education, poor infrastructure and the oppression of women, children and physically challenged people. Even the world pandemic of HIV and AIDS spreads much more rapidly where there is poverty.

Many of the key determinants of health and disease lie outside the direct control of the health sector. This means that, in order to attain optimal health for all, a multidisciplinary and intersectoral approach to healthcare is required.

In other words, health and healthcare are not the responsibility of health professionals alone, but of a much wider group of people, including community members.

The WHO recommends that development programmes be implemented alongside health services and health programmes. Through this process the environment can be protected or changed to become supportive of health. These programmes may also enable people to develop self-reliance as they may help them to acquire both the knowledge and the skills to find employment or to generate an income that may help alleviate poverty. Even if this is not fully possible, development initiatives enable people to produce food, build houses and create an environment that might be able to give them a chance to be healthy. Community involvement and participation are important in achieving health for all. An example of such programmes, according to the WHO, is home-based community healthcare that can be done by healthcare cadres trained to take care of their communities, including people living with HIV and AIDS, who can safely and effectively provide specific HIV services both in a health facility and in the community in the context of service delivery according to the task-shifting approach (WHO, 2008).

> **Task-shifting**
>
> The concept of 'task-shifting' was first introduced by the WHO and refers to delegating tasks from doctors to nurses and from nurses to other assistants.
>
> The other programme that was aimed at countering poverty and deprivation in South Africa was the Reconstruction and Development Programme (RDP). The RDP was based on the principles of nation-building, protection of the environment and improvement of health services and making them accessible to all.

Disease profiles

There are marked differences in the disease profile of the different populations in the world. If we compare the developing countries of Africa, for example, with the disease profiles of Western Europe, we find the following:

- **Mortality rates**: These are lower in the developed (high income) countries of Western Europe than they are in Africa (low income). This is particularly noticeable if we compare infant mortality rates. In Europe the infant mortality rate varies between 1 and 6 per 1 000 live births (Slovenia has the lowest rate of 1.7 per 1 000 live births); in Africa it ranges between 9 and 89.5 per 1 000 live births. In Europe fewer than 5 children out of every 1 000 die before they reach the age of five, but in Africa almost half of all children born will die before they reach their fifth birthday. The infant mortality rate in South Africa was estimated to be about 25.77 per 1 000 live births in 2020 and 26.50 per 1 000 live births in 2019 (CIA, 2017–2018).

According to the WHO (2018), the three leading causes of mortality in lower-middle-income countries (LMIC) are ischaemic heart disease (IHD), stroke, and lower respiratory infections (LRIs), causing 111.8, 68.8, and 51.5 annual deaths per 100 000, respectively.

Top 10 causes of death in low-income countries in 2016

Crude death rate (per 100 000 population)

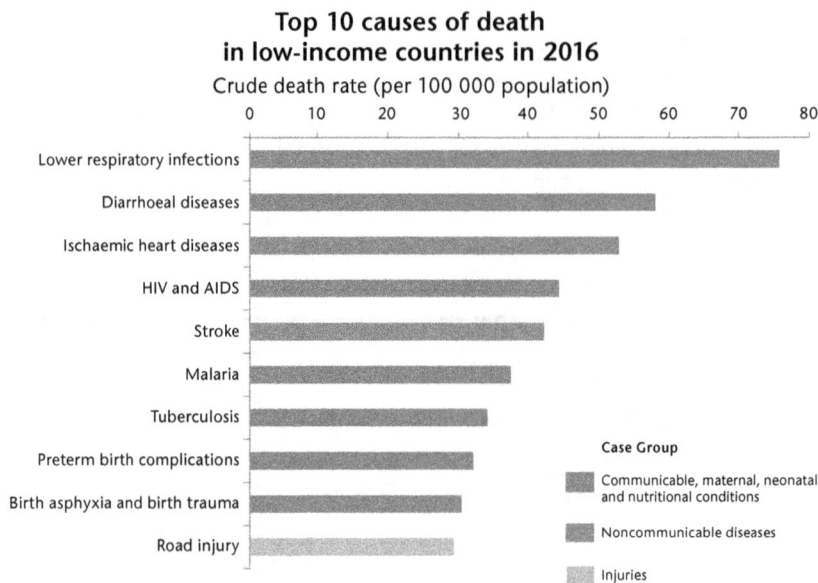

Source: Global Health Estimates 2016: Deaths by Cause, Age, Sex, by Country and by Region, 2000–2016. Geneva, World Health Organization; 2018. World Bank list of economies (June 2017). Washington, DC: The World Bank Group; 2017 (https:// datahelpdesk.worldbank.org/knowledgebase/articles/906519-world-bank-country-and-lending-groups).

Top 10 causes of death in high-income countries in 2016

Crude death rate (per 100 000 population)

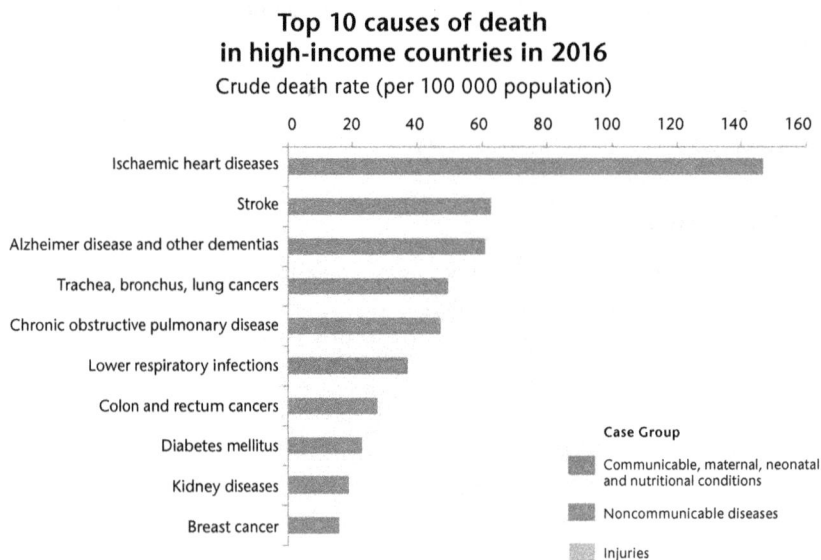

Source: Global Health Estimates 2016: Deaths by Cause, Age, Sex, by Country and by Region, 2000–2016. Geneva, World Health Organization; 2018. World Bank list of economies (June 2017). Washington, DC: The World Bank Group; 2017 (https:// datahelpdesk.worldbank.org/knowledgebase/articles/906519-world-bank-country-and-lending-groups).

Figure 1.3 Top 10 causes of death globally

Source: WHO (2018)

- **Life expectancy**: As a measure of the health of a community, life expectancy also differs greatly. In Europe the life expectancy is about 79 years for males and 84 years for females, but in many of the African nations it ranges between 52.94 and about 74.82 years. Life expectancy in South Africa is 61.5 (StatsSA, 2019). Wherever they live in the world, women live longer than men (WHO, 2014).

- **Principal causes of death**: In developed countries, these are cardiovascular disease, neoplastic diseases and chronic respiratory diseases, but in the developing countries of Africa, communicable diseases, parasitic infections and conditions associated with malnutrition account for most deaths.

- **Major causes of death**: In 2017, an estimated 56 million people died worldwide, more than half (54 per cent) of which were attributed to the top 10 causes. Ischaemic heart disease and stroke are the world's biggest killers, accounting for a combined 15.2 million deaths in 2016. These diseases have remained the leading causes of death globally in the last 15 years. Non-communicable diseases (NCDs) remain responsible for two-thirds of all deaths globally. The four main NCDs are cardiovascular diseases, cancers, diabetes and chronic lung diseases. Cardiovascular diseases are also the main cause of death throughout the world, with a total of nearly 17 million people in 2017, that is 3 in every 10 deaths. Of these, 7 million people died of ischaemic heart disease and 6.2 million from stroke.

  - Of 56.9 million global deaths in 2016, 40.5 million, or 71 per cent, were due to NCDs. The four main NCDs are cardiovascular diseases, cancers, diabetes and chronic lung diseases. The burden of these diseases is rising disproportionately among lower-income countries and populations. In 2016, over three-quarters of NCD deaths, 31.5 million, occurred in low- and middle-income countries, with about 46 per cent of deaths occurring before the age of 70 in these countries.

  - The leading causes of NCD deaths in 2016 were cardiovascular diseases (17.9 million deaths, or 44 per cent of all NCD deaths), cancers (9.0 million, or 22 per cent of all NCD deaths), and respiratory diseases, including asthma and chronic obstructive pulmonary disease (3.8 million, or 9 per cent of all NCD deaths). Diabetes caused another 1.6 million deaths.

One of the biggest challenges health systems will have to contend with in the next few decades is how to deal with the increasing number of health problems and new emerging diseases. At present, HIV and the AIDS-related diseases are causing havoc in the developing world and particularly in Africa. Associated with this are sexually transmitted infections (STIs) and tuberculosis, which are also increasing in numbers along with HIV.

Leading causes of death in South Africa

Other
- Nervous System
- Perinatal
- Other
- **26%**
- Urinary System
- Digestive System
- Blood & Immune

Cancers/ Neoplasms
- Male Genital
- Lymph
- Digestive Organs
- Breast
- **9%**
- Respiratory
- Female Genital

Accidents, Assault & External Causes
- Medical Surgical Complications
- Intentional Self Harm
- Car Accidents
- **11%**
- Assault
- Undetermined Intent
- Accidental Injury

Infectious & Parasitic Diseases
- Intestinal Infectious Diseases
- Tuberculosis
- HIV
- **18%**
- Viral Infections
- Protozoal
- Other Viral Diseases
- Other Bacterial Diseases

**2016 Deaths
456,612**

Metabolic Disorders
- Malnutrition
- **7%**
- Diabetes Mellitus
- Metabolic Disorders

Circulatory System Diseases
- **19%**
- Heart Diseases
- Hypertensive Diseases
- Cerebrovascular Diseases

Respiratory Diseases
- Chronic Lower Respiratory Diseases
- **9%**
- Influenza & Pneumonia
- Other Acute Lower Respiratory Diseases

Info from statssa.gov.za
©lifecoversouthafrica.co.za

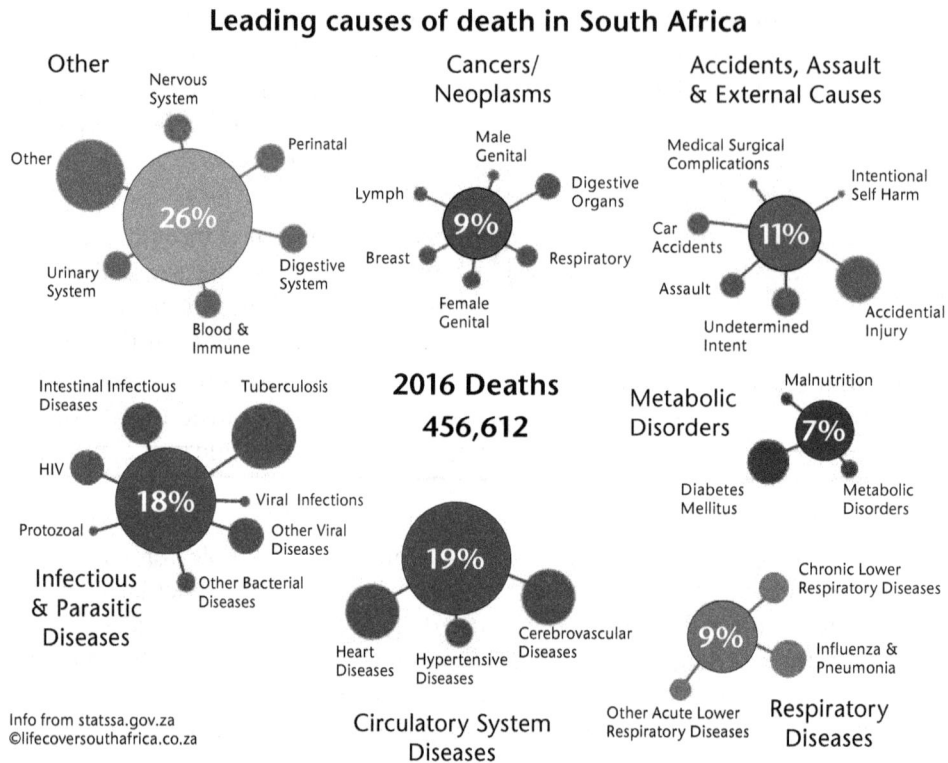

Figure 1.4 Leading causes of mortality in South Africa in 2016 (percentages averaged)
Source: Adapted from WHO Stats (2017)

In Africa, other communicable diseases like measles, malaria and diarrhoeal diseases are problematic and the incidence of these diseases, which can be relatively easily prevented, is increasing. The WHO had hoped to eradicate polio from the world, but incidences of the disease are still being diagnosed regularly in Africa, especially in West Africa. Non-communicable 'diseases of lifestyle' that are of concern in Africa include those related to:

- nutrition
- mental health
- occupational health
- maternal and women's health
- chronic diseases such as hypertension, diabetes and cancer
- disabilities and birth disorders
- intentional and unintentional injuries
- trauma from conflict/landmines
- environmental health
- substance abuse.

Causes of death in children under 5, World, 2017

Annual number of deaths by leading causes in children under 5 years old.

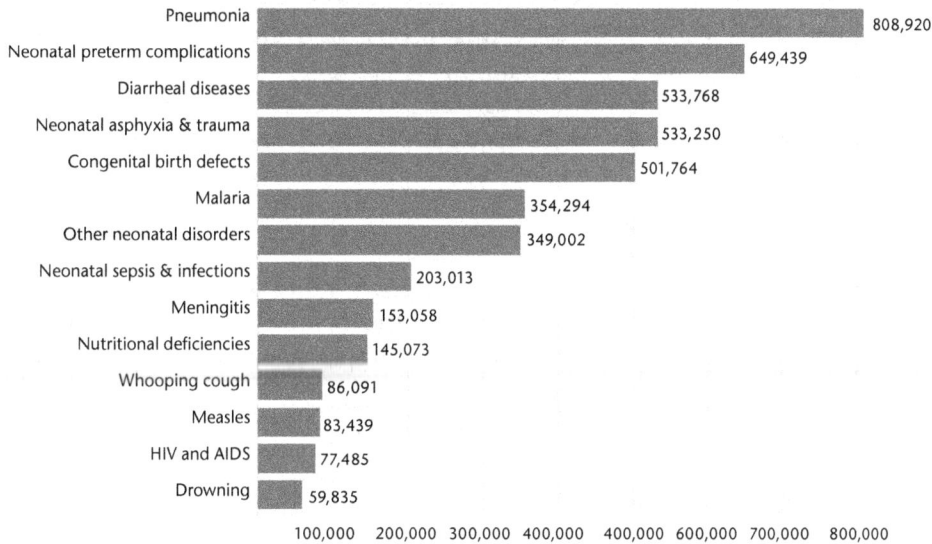

Pneumonia	808,920
Neonatal preterm complications	649,439
Diarrheal diseases	533,768
Neonatal asphyxia & trauma	533,250
Congenital birth defects	501,764
Malaria	354,294
Other neonatal disorders	349,002
Neonatal sepsis & infections	203,013
Meningitis	153,058
Nutritional deficiencies	145,073
Whooping cough	86,091
Measles	83,439
HIV and AIDS	77,485
Drowning	59,835

100,000 200,000 300,000 400,000 400,000 600,000 700,000 800,000

Source: IHME, Global Burden of Disease (GBD)
Note: Pneumonia includes deaths from lower respiratory infections, which include a range of pathogens that can cause clinical pneumonia

Figure 1.5 Major causes of death in neonates and children under five globally
Source: Adapted from WHO Stats (2017)

In 2017, 4.1 million (75 per cent) of all under-five deaths occurred within the first year of life. The risk of a child dying before completing their first year was highest in the WHO African Region (51 per 1 000 live births), over six times higher than that in the WHO European Region (8 per 1 000 live births). In South Africa, the infant mortality rate is 31 per 1 000 live births (CIA, 2017–2018).

Demography

Demography is the study of human populations. The size, gender and age composition, and the distribution of the members, have a profound effect on a population's health. In Africa, most populations are 'young', with approximately 35 per cent of the population being under the age of 20 years, and 80 per cent under 40 years. This means that a large number of women are of childbearing age in the population and therefore fertility rates are high. The crude birth rates in the region were approximately 35.67 per 1 000 of the population in 2017 (CIA, 2017–2018).

Infant mortality rates are very high in these populations because women in some areas are not motivated or permitted to limit the number of children they have. This fact, together with poverty and other factors, leads to poor child nutrition, which results in high child death rates. Conversely, we find that the populations of the developed countries are 'ageing' populations with a relatively high percentage of people over the age of 65 years, and fewer young people. This means that there are fewer women of childbearing age in these societies, fertility rates are lower and infant and child mortality rates are also low.

Due to the large number of young people and children in developing countries, infectious diseases are common and, as there are few elderly people in the society, degenerative conditions are rare. In developed countries, infectious conditions are less common, while the degenerative diseases occur frequently.

Conclusion

Ensuring good health for all cannot be the responsibility of healthcare providers and healthcare services alone. In fact, health is the joint responsibility of a number of sectors within the government as well as the responsibility of every individual. Intersectoral collaboration and community participation and involvement are some of the strategies that can assist in achieving healthy living and health for all.

Self-assessment

1. Explain the main factors that have an impact on health.
2. Describe the determinants of health, providing an example of each.
3. Provide a detailed example that clearly shows how a combination of the determinants of health can affect an individual's health.
4. How can intersectoral collaboration be facilitated among the different governmental departments?
5. Give examples of environmental factors that impact on people's health.
6. Outline the outcomes that could be measured to determine if a community is healthy.
7. List 10 non-communicable diseases that are common in African countries.
8. Explain this statement: One of the examples of task-shifting is Nurse Management of Antiretroviral Treatment (NIMART).

Bibliography

Central Intelligence Agency (CIA). 2017–2018. The World Factbook: Infant mortality rate. Available: http://cia.gov (Accessed 11 September).

Hannah, R. & Max, R. 2020. Causes of death. Available: https://ourworldindata.org/causes-of-death (Accessed 4 April 2020).

Lee, L. & Ghanime, L. 2005. Environmental sustainability in 100 millennium development goal country reports. United Nations Development Programme. Energy and Environment Group. Bureau for Development Policy.

Roth, G.A., Abate, D., Abate, K.H., Abay, S.M., Abbafati, C., Abbasi, N. & Abdollahpour, I. 2018. Global, regional, and national age-sex-specific mortality for 282 causes of death in 195 countries and territories, 1980–2017: A systematic analysis for the Global Burden of Disease Study 2017. *The Lancet*, 392(10159), 1736–1788.

Statistics South Africa (StatsSA). 2019. Life expectancy. Available: http://www.statssa.gov.za (Accessed 4 April 2020).

United Nations Children's Fund. 2014. Child mortality report. Available: www.data. unicef.org (Accessed 21 September 2020).

United Nations Development Programme (UNDP). 2013. Millennium development goals. Available: https://www.undp.org/content/undp/en/home/librarypage/mdg/the-millennium-development-goals-report-2013.html (Accessed 11 September 2020).

United Nations Educational, Scientific and Cultural Organization. 1992. The RIO declaration on environment and development. Available: http://www.unesco.org/education/nfsunesco/pdf/RIO_E.PDF (Accessed 11 September 2020).

United Nations (UN). nd. Report of the world summit on sustainable development. Available: www. un.org/jsummit/html/docs/131302_wssd_report_reissued.pdf (Accessed 11 September 2020).

World Bank. 2002. *The Environment and the Millennium Development Goals*. Washington DC: The World Bank.

World Health Organization (WHO). 2002. Johannesburg declaration on sustainable development. Available: https://www.who.int/mediacentre/events/HSD_Plaq_02.8_def1.pdf (Accessed 11 September 2020).

World Health Organization (WHO). 2008. Task shifting: Rational redistribution of tasks among health workforce teams. Global recommendations and guidelines. Available: http://www. who.int/healthsystems/TTR-TaskShifting.pdf (Accessed 11 September 2020).

World Health Organization (WHO). 2014. World health statistics: Large gains in life expectancy. Available: https://www.who.int/mediacentre/news/releases/2014/world-health-statistics-2014/en/ (Accessed 11 September 2020).

World Health Organization (WHO). 2015a. Reducing child mortality to achieve MDG 4. Available: http://www.who.int/gho/child_health/mortality/mortality_under_five/en/ (Accessed 11 September 2020).

World Health Organization (WHO). 2015b. The determinants of health: Health impact assessment (HIA). Available: https://www.who.int/health-topics/health-impact-assessment#tab=tab_1 (Accessed 11 September 2020).

World Health Organization (WHO). 2017. Life expectancy. Available: https://www.who.int/gho/publications/world_health_statistics/2017/en/ (Accessed 11 September 2020).

World Health Organization (WHO). 2018. The top 10 causes of death. Available: https://www.who.int/news-room/fact-sheets/detail/the-top-10-causes-of-death (Accessed 11 September 2020).

2

The United Nations and the World Health Organization

Sindi Mthembu

Learning outcomes

After studying this chapter, you should be able to:

- Describe the role of the United Nations in achieving peace and security in the world.
- Identify the various organisations and programmes within the United Nations that are concerned with health and health matters.
- Explain the World Health Organization's structure and how it operates.
- Discuss the role of the World Health Organization in improving and maintaining health globally.
- Outline the critical areas identified by the World Health Organization budget that received funding.
- Describe the impact of the World Health Organization strategies on healthcare programmes in South Africa.

Key terms

Grass roots: Refers to the ordinary people in a community, country, society or organisation rather than its leaders.

Humanitarian: Someone who helps people who live in poor conditions or who receive unfair treatment.

Monograph: A written statement that deals systematically with a specific subject such as a drug, a medical procedure, or the management of a specific health issue.

Multinational agency: An agency whose members consist of several different national groups.

Introduction: The United Nations (UN)

The UN is an international organisation founded in 1945 after the Second World War by 51 countries committed to maintaining international peace and security, developing friendly relations among nations and promoting social progress, better living standards and human rights. The principles of the UN as explained in the United Nations' Charter are to save future generations from war, reaffirm human rights, and establish equal rights for all persons. In addition, it aims to promote justice, freedom and social progress for the people of all of its member states. It also acknowledges that to uphold security, it is necessary to establish conditions under which justice can be maintained. Ensuring that people are given the opportunity to attain health is a condition aligned with justice, and for this reason it is recognised that a world global partnership in achieving health is an important part of the UN strategy for attaining peace and security.

The UN has 193 member countries and its main headquarters is located in New York City. Membership of the UN is by choice and is determined by the government of the country. Membership requires that countries pay an annual fee to the UN, and that they meet the criteria, as determined by the UN, that the rights of their citizens are respected and that the associated justice is maintained within the country. During the time of the previous South African government and the policy of apartheid, South Africa was suspended from the UN because it did not meet these criteria. However, since the first democratic election and the new government in 1994, South Africa was readmitted as a full member of the UN.

The main sections, often referred to as the principals, of the UN are the General Assembly, which is the plenary body, consisting of five nations, and the Security Council. These nations form permanent members of the Council and together determine the position and role that the UN will take in countries or regions where conflict, political unrest and/or natural disasters have occurred. The UN has established an international peace-keeping force, which can be used to assist in these areas, and it also undertakes numerous other activities to improve both security and justice.

Several institutions or organisations within the UN are concerned with health. These are discussed in the next section.

Specialised United Nations agencies

There are many specialised agencies in the UN, but only those that have a bearing on health will be discussed in this chapter.

1. The International Labour Organization (ILO)

The main task delegated to the ILO is to promote justice and internationally recognised human and labour rights. It also determines internationally accepted labour standards, which are given to member states as guidelines for national labour policies.

2. The Food and Agricultural Organization (FAO)

This agency leads international efforts to reduce hunger and ensure food security. It does this by serving both developed and developing countries, assisting them by supplying technical advice and information that will improve agricultural, forestry and fishery practices and thereby the production of food. It concentrates its attention on the rural areas, which are home to 70 per cent of the world's hungry people.

3. The World Health Organization (WHO)

The WHO is the directing and coordinating authority for health within the UN system. The WHO will be discussed in more detail later in this chapter.

United Nations programmes and funds

In this section we discuss some of the programmes and funds run by the UN.

1. The United Nations Environmental Programme (UNEP)

This programme provides leadership and encourages partnerships in caring for the environment by inspiring, informing and enabling nations and people to improve their quality of life without compromising the environment. Through determined strategies, it aims to identify ways to promote sustainable and equitable human development using environmentally sound management principles.

2. The United Nations Children's Fund (UNICEF)

This is one of the oldest programmes championed by the UN. It was established to ensure that children's rights are respected in times of crisis and/or war but has changed to assume a much wider function. The success of this UN programme is widely acknowledged and the need for such a programme and the services it offers remains a high priority as children, and especially girl-children and women, are still widely abused in many countries around the world. Although UNICEF programmes are adapted to meet the specific needs of the different countries, the principles remain the same and are based on:

- ensuring child protection
- encouraging the development of appropriate public policy and legislation
- ensuring appropriate basic life-skill education and equal opportunities for girls to allow them access to quality basic education
- recognising children's and women's rights in a way that supports gender equality and the development of a sustainable and just society
- ensuring a safe and protective environment for children
- securing adequate nutrition for health, including the promotion of breastfeeding

- ensuring adequate access to healthcare that includes preventative healthcare programmes such as immunisation and the prevention of HIV, as well as curative healthcare services.

A large proportion of UNICEF time is spent determining interventions in countries, with government representatives, to assist in crises that impact on the health and safety of children and women. They institute initiatives to ensure the safety and meet the immediate needs of the group. Where necessary, they help to secure the necessary funding to support and implement humanitarian programmes to help those affected by conflict, war, starvation and disease outbreaks. In sub-Saharan Africa, they are helping to care for, and support children orphaned by AIDS. UNICEF also supports research that will improve the lives of children and women and makes these findings freely available to all.

3. The United Nations Development Programme (UNDP)

The reason for the existence of this programme is to use joint expertise to share solutions that assist developing countries to overcome their problems. The focus is on poverty reduction interventions that promote socioeconomic development. To direct this process the Sustainable Development Goals (SDGs) were identified in 2015 . These are dealt with in more detail in Chapter 14.

4. The World Food Programme (WFP)

Known as the world's largest humanitarian agency, the WFP locates the world's hunger hotspots and determines ways to help those affected by supplying food and other humanitarian help. The programme also aims to determine ways to stop the global spread of hunger, which has been accomplished with only limited success.

5. The Joint United Nations Programme on HIV and AIDS (UNAIDS)

This programme has been established to deal with the rapidly increasing world pandemic of the disease. The purpose is to advocate for global action on the pandemic through promoting leadership for these programmes, supporting the people living with HIV and AIDS, and through the supply of strategic information that will assist people responsible for developing and managing programmes in the field of HIV and AIDS. The outcome is aimed at preventing the transmission of HIV, providing care and support, reducing the vulnerability of individuals and communities to HIV and AIDS, and reducing the impact of the pandemic. South Africa has adopted these guidelines in combating the HIV and AIDS pandemic.

6. United Nations Women (UN Women)

UN Women is the UN organisation dedicated to gender equality and the empowerment of women. South African, Phumzile Mlambo-Ngcuka, is the

Executive Director of UN Women. The organisation focuses its efforts on human rights and security and has the following goals:

- Reducing poverty and exclusion among women
- Ending violence against women
- Eliminating discrimination against women and girls
- Reversing the spread of HIV and AIDS among women and girls
- Supporting women's leadership in governance and post-conflict reconstruction
- Empowering women
- Achieving equality between women and men as partners and beneficiaries of development.

The main roles of UN Women are:

- to support intergovernmental bodies, such as the Commission on the Status of Women, in their formulation of policies, global standards and norms
- to help Member States to implement these standards
- to provide suitable technical and financial support to countries that request it
- to forge effective partnerships with civil society
- to hold the UN system accountable for its own commitments on gender equality, including regular monitoring of system- wide progress.

The World Health Organization (WHO)

The WHO was established in August 1948. Not the first international body concerned with health issues, it was established after the Second World War to replace the Health Section of the League of Nations. The WHO has its headquarters in Geneva, Switzerland, and has six regional offices, each serving a specific region of the world. Each regional office has a regional committee and a regional director.

Table 2.1 The six regions of the World Health Organization

	Headquarters	Notes
Africa (AFRO)	Democratic Republic of the Congo, Brazzaville	The Regional Director is Dr Matshidiso Moeti from Botswana. AFRO includes most of Africa, with the exception of Egypt, Sudan, Djibouti, Tunisia, Libya, Somalia and Morocco (all fall under the Eastern Mediterranean Regional Office (EMRO)).

	Headquarters	Notes
America (PAHO)	USA, Washington DC	The Regional Director is Dr Carissa F. Etienne from Dominica. This region is known as the Pan American Health Organization (PAHO) and covers the whole of America.
South-East Asia (SEARO)	India, New Delhi	The Regional Director is Dr Poonam Khetrapal Singh from India. India and North Korea are served by SEARO.
Europe (EURO)	Denmark, Copenhagen	The Regional Director is Dr Zsuzsanna Jakab from Hungary. EURO includes all of Europe, Israel (except Liechtenstein), and all of the former Union of Soviet Socialist Republics (USSR).
Western Pacific (WPRO)	Philippines, Manila	The Regional Director is Dr Shin Young-soo from South Korea. WPRO covers all the Asian countries not served by SEARO and EMRO, and all the countries in Oceania. South Korea is also served by WPRO.
Eastern Mediterranean (EMRO)	Egypt, Cairo	The Regional Director is Dr Ahmed Al-Mandhari from Oman. EMRO serves the countries of Africa that are not included in AFRO, as well as all the countries in the Middle East, except for Israel. Pakistan is also served by EMRO.

The countries that are members of the UN automatically become members of the WHO by accepting the WHO Constitution. Other countries can join by applying to the World Health Assembly where membership is determined by the vote taken at the annual meeting. The WHO comprises three bodies that are responsible for the operation of the organisation:

- **The World Health Assembly (WHA)**: This is the supreme decision-making body of the WHO. It determines the health policies of the WHO. The Assembly consists of delegates from the 194 member states (as in 2016). WHO is the world's highest health policy setting body and is composed of health ministers from member states. The members of the WHA generally meet every year in May in Geneva at the Palace of Nations, the location of the WHO headquarters. The main tasks of the WHA are to decide major policy questions, as well as to approve the WHO work programme and budget, and to elect and appoint its Director-General. The Health Assembly approves the WHO budget and the programme for the following year. It is also responsible for the appointment of the Director-General. This committee serves for a period of three years.

- **The Executive Council**: The council consists of 34 members, who must be technically qualified in the health field, and who serve for a period of three years. They are representatives of the different regions of the WHO. The council meets twice a year and, in addition to the functions mentioned above, it is responsible for preparing the agenda for the Health Assembly and for submitting advice and proposals for discussion at the assembly. Africa is currently represented by the following countries: Benin (2017–2020), Burkina Faso (2019–2022), Eswatini (2017–2020), Gabon (2018–2021) and Kenya (2019–2022).

- **The Secretariat**: The secretariat (or staff) of the WHO includes approximately 3 500 health professionals, other experts and support staff who work at the WHO headquarters in Geneva, in the six regional offices and in countries where the WHO assigns staff to offer technical assistance or assist in projects.

As of 2012, the WHO defined its role in public health as providing leadership on matters critical to health and engaging in partnerships where joint action is needed; shaping the research agenda and stimulating the generation, translation, and dissemination of valuable knowledge; setting norms and standards and promoting and monitoring their implementation; articulating ethical and evidence-based policy options; providing technical support, catalysing change, and building sustainable institutional capacity; and monitoring the health situation and assessing health trends.

The WHO makes use of various other groups and individuals to assist it in carrying out its functions. They include the following:

- **Consultants and advisers**: These are specialists in their particular fields who work for the WHO for varying periods on a temporary basis. These consultants may be used in specific countries and the regional offices, as well as in Geneva, to help with identified activities, projects and programmes.

- **Expert committees**: These are small international groups made up of experts from various countries. Expert committees usually consist of eight members selected by the Director-General from an advisory panel. Such committees are convened from time to time to advise on a particular technical subject, for example environmental pollution. At the close of their meetings such committees often publish their conclusions in a technical report.

- **The Advisory Committee on Medical Research**: This committee consists of 18 members and a chairperson. It advises the Director-General on matters of biomedical research and gives him or her guidance on the formulation of research policy. The members of this committee are usually appointed for a period of four years. A number of scientific groups consisting of about eight members draw up reports on highly specialised aspects of research programmes and assist the committee in its work.

- **Study groups**: A number of study groups also contribute to the work of the expert committees that offer technical advice to countries.

In 1948, the WHO defined health as 'a state of complete physical, mental and social well-being, and not merely the absence of disease or infirmity'. This definition is still appropriate today and is evident in the WHO's main objective, which is 'the attainment by all people of the highest level of health'. In order to achieve this objective, the WHO helps governments to fulfil their responsibilities for the health of their people. It is important to note that the WHO recognises the autonomy of member countries and will assist the government of a member state only if it is requested to do so. All planned activities of the WHO are founded on the following principles set out in the Constitution. These principles acknowledge that:

- the enjoyment of the highest attainable standard of health is one of the fundamental rights of every human being without distinction of race, religion, political belief, or economic or social conditions
- governments have a responsibility for the health of their people
- active cooperation on the part of the public is of the utmost importance in improving the health of the people.

The founders of the WHO and the UN clearly identified the relationship between security and justice and realised that neither of these two can survive without the other. A crucial part of this justice is to ensure that all people have equitable access to health services and a health-promoting environment. In other words, people must be given the means to attain and maintain optimal health for themselves, their families and their communities.

Important functions of the World Health Organization

In the 21st century, health is a shared responsibility, involving equitable access to essential care and collective defence against transnational threats. The core functions of the WHO in this era are the following:

- Providing leadership on matters critical to health and engaging in partnerships where joint action is needed
- Shaping the research agenda and stimulating the generation, translation and dissemination of valuable knowledge
- Setting norms and standards and promoting and monitoring their implementation
- Articulating ethical and evidence-based policy options
- Providing technical support, catalysing change and building sustainable institutional capacity
- Monitoring health situations and assessing health trends.

The Thirteenth General Programme of Work (GPW 13), which provides the framework for organisation-wide programming of the WHO work, budget, resources and results entitled 'Promote Health, Keep the World Safe, Serve the Vulnerable' covers the period 2019–2023. The WHO GPW 13 is structured around three key interconnected strategic priorities, namely (i) ensuring healthy lives and well-being for all at all ages, (ii) achieving universal health coverage, and (iii) addressing health emergencies and promoting healthier populations.

These priorities are linked to three bold targets as follows:

1. *Achieving universal health coverage* – one billion more people to benefit from universal health coverage to ensure achievement
2. *Addressing health emergencies* – one billion more people better protected from health emergencies
3. *Promoting healthier populations* – one billion more people enjoying better health and well-being.

WHO priorities are supported by three strategic shifts of stepping up leadership; driving public health impact in every country; and focusing global public goods on impact. The WHO is also committed to ensuring gender equality, equity and rights-based approaches to health that enhance participation, build resilience and empower communities.

The WHO operates in an increasingly complex and rapidly changing landscape. The boundaries of public health action have become blurred, extending into other sectors that influence health opportunities and outcomes. The WHO responds to these challenges using a six-point agenda that embraces the following:

1. Promoting development

Health development is directed by the *ethical principle of equity*. Access to life-saving or health-promoting interventions should not be denied for unfair reasons, including those with economic or social roots. Commitment to this principle ensures that the WHO activities aimed at health development give priority to health outcomes in poor, disadvantaged or vulnerable groups. Attainment of the health-related SDGs, preventing and treating chronic diseases and addressing neglected tropical diseases is the cornerstone of the health and development agenda of the WHO. (NB: Chapter 14 on sustainable development covers the SDGs and health priorities in South Africa in depth).

2. Fostering health security

One of the greatest threats to international health security arises from *outbreaks of emerging and epidemic-prone diseases*. Such outbreaks are occurring in increasing numbers, fuelled by factors such as rapid urbanisation, environmental mismanagement, the way food is produced and traded, and the way antibiotics are used and misused. The world's ability to defend itself collectively against outbreaks has been strengthened since June 2007, when the revised International Health Regulations came into force.

3. Strengthening health systems

For health improvement to operate as a *poverty-reduction* strategy, health services must reach poor and under-served populations. Health systems in many parts of the world are unable to do so, making the strengthening of health systems a high priority for the WHO. Areas being addressed include the provision of adequate numbers of appropriately trained staff, sufficient financing, suitable systems for collecting vital statistics, and access to appropriate technology, including essential drugs.

4. Harnessing research, information and evidence

Evidence provides the foundation for setting priorities, defining strategies and measuring results. The WHO generates authoritative health information, in consultation with leading experts, to set norms and standards, articulate evidence-based policy options and monitor the evolving global health situation.

5. Enhancing partnerships

The WHO carries out its work with the support and collaboration of many partners, including UN agencies and other international organisations, donors, civil society and the private sector. The WHO uses the strategic power of evidence to encourage partners implementing programmes within countries to align their activities with best technical guidelines and practices, as well as with the priorities established by countries.

6. Improving performance

The WHO participates in ongoing reforms aimed at improving its efficiency and effectiveness, both at the international level and within countries. The WHO aims to ensure that its strongest asset, its staff, works in an environment that is motivating and rewarding. The WHO plans its budget and activities through results-based management, with clear anticipated results to measure performance at regional, national and international levels.

The functions of the WHO are aimed at improving the underlying determinants of health. They include the following:

- Controlling and preventing specific infections, such as the communicable diseases and the parasitic infections. These remain the most serious health problems facing health workers in the developing countries.
- Conducting research into the epidemiology of cancer, cardiovascular diseases, genetic defects, mental disorders, and other non-communicable conditions.

- Helping governments to establish national health services. In connection with this, emphasis is laid on the importance of:
  - mobilising and utilising the available resources in the country
  - involving the members of the community in the healthcare system, especially at rural or at grass-roots level
  - adapting the structure of the health service to changing patterns of disease, as well as supplying and assisting with the training of the necessary specialised personnel
  - assisting governments in their efforts to reduce maternal and child mortality by giving advice on various matters and assisting in the provision of basic maternal and childcare services, as well as emphasising the importance of breastfeeding, adequate infant nutrition and family planning.

- Encouraging satisfactory environmental conditions as fundamental to the health of a community and stressing the importance of basic necessities such as sanitation, purification of water supplies, hygienic food handling and prevention of the pollution of land, air and water.

- Promoting occupational health in collaboration with the ILO, which is concerned with the economic and social well-being of workers; an important aspect of this part of the WHO's work is the detection and prevention of occupational hazards.

- Assisting governments of developing countries, where there is often a serious shortage of trained health workers, in the development of training programmes. The WHO also supplies teaching staff, books and other teaching material, if necessary. The WHO awards fellowships every year to health workers from various countries. These fellowships enable them to improve their knowledge and skills. On conclusion of the fellowships the recipients are required to serve in their own national health services.

- Collecting and publishing health statistics from various countries. These statistics are available on the WHO website. The WHO will help governments to improve their medical records, as medical records are not only necessary for the improvement of patient care but also an important source of information concerning the health of a country.

- Publishing a large number of technical and official manuscripts, including:
  - monographs
  - technical reports
  - public health papers
  - magazines (eg *World Health*). This is the WHO's own magazine, which is well-illustrated and contains a great deal of information about health matters around the world. It is a most readable publication and you should look for it in your library.

Conclusion

Achieving community, national and global quality health requires commitment at all these levels and cooperation among multinational agencies, national and regional authorities, communities and the private sector, as well as other stakeholders. It has been said that the world has become a village as travel is fast, easy and relatively cheap. Hundreds of thousands of people travel by road, sea and air every day, criss-crossing the world. Communicable diseases can be carried by these travellers without their knowledge, and across many countries, before the disease outbreak is even identified in the country of origin. This was seen with the occurrence of COVID-19 (coronavirus), which spread throughout the world in 2019/2020. These new global health risks require close collaboration and interdependence between nations. To assist in this process, the role of these multinational agencies becomes even more important in this millennium.

Self-assessment

1. What is the main function of the United Nations?

2. What do the following acronyms and abbreviations stand for?
   ILO; WHO; UNICEF; WFP; FAO

3. Discuss this statement: The functions of the WHO are aimed at improving the underlying determinants of health.

4. The World Health Organization played a crucial role during the COVID-19 (coronavirus) pandemic in 2019/2020. Critically analyse the role of the WHO in supporting African countries during the COVID-19 pandemic.

5. Outline what a UNICEF programme does for children in need.

Bibliography

Lee, L. & Ghanime, L. 2005. Environmental sustainability in 100 millennium development goal country reports. United Nations Development Programme. Energy and Environment Group. Bureau for Development Policy.

United Nations Development Programme (UNDP) South Africa. 2015. Sustainable developmental goals. Available: https://www.za.undp.org/content/south_africa/en/home/sustainable-development-goals.html (Accessed 11 September 2020).

United Nations Regional Information Centre (UNRIC). 2014. Available: http://www.unric.org/en/ (Accessed 11 September 2020).

United Nations (UN). 2015. Transforming our world: The 2030 agenda for sustainable development. Available: https://www.un.org/ga/search/view_doc.asp?symbol=A/RES/70/1&Lang=E (Accessed 11 September 2020).

World Health Organization (WHO). 1948. *Constitution of the World Health Organization.* Geneva: WHO.

World Health Organization (WHO). 2020a. Factsheets. Available: https://www.who.int/news-room/fact-sheets (Accessed 11 September 2020).

World Health Organization (WHO). 2020b. Thirteenth general programme of work (GPW). 2019–2023. Available: https://www.who.int/about/what-we-do/thirteenth-general-programme-of-work-2019---2023 (Accessed 11 September 2020).

Health policy and health systems in South Africa and the southern African region

Sindi Mthembu

Learning outcomes

After studying this chapter, you should be able to:

- Critically analyse the development of health policy and health systems in South Africa prior to the election of the first democratic government in 1994.
- Explain the purpose of the Constitution of South Africa and what influence it has on the health system.
- Describe the three spheres of the South African health system.
- List the legislation and the policy documents that have influenced the delivery of healthcare in South Africa since 1994.
- Discuss the Batho Pele principles and their objectives in the healthcare system.
- Compare patients' rights with patients' responsibilities.
- Explain the objectives of National Health Insurance (NHI) in the South African context.
- Discuss the implementation of the NHI in South Africa.
- Explain the purpose of the primary healthcare re-engineering in the South African health system.
- Describe the composition and functions of the primary healthcare and specialist support teams according to the primary healthcare re-engineering strategy.
- Outline the main functions of the school health nurse in meeting the requirements of the school health policy.
- Give a comprehensive definition of primary healthcare.
- Outline the principles that guide the NHI and link those to the primary healthcare principles.

- Discuss the role of the National Core Standards (NCS) in relation to the NHI.
- Outline what a comprehensive health system is and list the people who make up the health team.
- Explain the role of the Southern African Development Community in attaining health for the people in the region.

Key terms

Act: A written law of parliament or other legislative body that determines the legal practice in a specific activity.

Bill: A draft of a proposed law or Act.

Legislation: The process of making laws.

Legislature: The state body responsible for producing the laws or Acts.

Policy: A course of action, usually with determined goals proposed by the government, a business or an individual.

Promulgate: The process of accepting a bill and making it an Act in parliament or another legislative body.

Regulation: A document developed to guide the implementation of the law or Act.

Standard: A level of quality or measure serving as a basis or principle to which others should conform, or by which others are judged.

Introduction: The development of health policy and health systems in South Africa

In 1909, the South Africa Act (1909) united the four colonies, namely the Cape of Good Hope, Natal, the Orange Free State and the Transvaal, into a four-province union. The new country formed from this merger was known as the Union of South Africa. Through the South Africa Act, a three-tier government was established, with a central national government at the highest level, four provincial administrations at the second level and many local authorities at the third level.

The South Africa Act gave little attention to matters of health. The provincial administrations simply took over the functions of the previous colonial governments in this regard, although the central government accepted responsibility for the prevention of epidemics caused by communicable diseases.

Following a serious influenza epidemic (H1N1 virus commonly known as the Spanish Flu) in 1918, the Public Health Act 36 of 1919 was passed. This Act established a Department of Health (DOH) at central government level and assigned to it specific functions, while the other duties were allocated to either the provincial administrations or the local authorities.

The central government became responsible for the prevention of communicable diseases and other aspects of public health; the four provincial administrations were given the responsibility for all aspects of curative medicine; and the local authorities were responsible for environmental health issues. This allocation of duties and responsibilities to the different bodies led to a clear division between curative, preventative and promotive health services.

Following a referendum of registered white voters in 1961, the Republic of South Africa Act was passed. The Union of South Africa became known as the Republic of South Africa, and the head of state was no longer the governor-general but the state president. The three-tier system remained intact with separate services for white people and for people of colour.

In 1977, a new Health Act (Act 63 of 1977) was passed. This Act was designed to coordinate the health services of the Republic of South Africa, to determine suitable health policy and to ensure the full use of all available health services, thereby ensuring a comprehensive healthcare service. In order to achieve the objectives of a healthcare service, the three levels of government (national, provincial and local) were all involved in the delivery of healthcare. However, the ultimate responsibility for the health of the people of South Africa rested with the state at national level.

In 1994, South Africa held its first democratic election and in April of that year an African National Congress (ANC)-led government came into power and embarked on a programme of reconstruction and development. To enable this process, the Constitutional Assembly drew up the Constitution of the Republic of South Africa.

The Constitution of the Republic of South Africa, 1996

The Constitution determines the basic or fundamental rights of individual citizens and sets out the structure for a democratic process of government. The Constitution is the supreme law of the country, and aims to:

- heal the divisions of the past and establish a society based on democratic values, social justice and fundamental human rights
- improve the quality of life of all citizens and free the potential of each person
- lay the foundations for a democratic and open society in which government is based on the will of the people and where every citizen is equally protected by law
- build a united and democratic South Africa able to take its rightful place as a sovereign state in the family of nations.

Fundamental human rights

The fundamental rights of individuals are contained in Chapter 2 of the Constitution. As the cornerstone of the democracy, the Constitution enshrines the rights of all the people of South Africa and affirms the democratic values of human dignity, equality and freedom. The Constitution has specific health references in that it declares that everyone has the right to:

- a healthy environment
- access to healthcare services
- sufficient food and water
- social security.

Children in particular have the right to basic nutrition, shelter, basic healthcare services and social services. It also states that no one may be refused emergency medical treatment. The Constitutional Court guards these rights and determines whether actions taken by the state are in accordance with the constitutional provisions. In order to deepen the culture of democracy, parliament plans to adopt a charter of rights consistent with the provisions of the Constitution.

Government

According to the Constitution, parliament is the national legislative authority of the land and consists of two houses, the National Assembly and the National Council of Provinces.

- *The National Assembly* consists of between 350 and 400 members elected through a system of proportional representation. Members are elected for a term of five years.
- *The National Council of Provinces* consists of 54 permanent members and 36 special delegates (ie a total of 10 delegates from each province). The premier of a province usually heads the delegation from that province. The members serve to represent the interests of the provinces in the national sphere of government. For operational purposes, government is structured in three spheres, namely national, provincial and local. These spheres are distinctive, interdependent and interrelated. The word 'sphere' has replaced the old terminology of 'tiers' or 'levels'.

In Chapter 5 of the Constitution the leadership structure within the government is described. The president is the head of state and is elected by the National Assembly from among its members. The cabinet forms the national executive of government and consists of the president, the deputy president and the ministers. They are all appointed by the president and are responsible for the powers and functions of the executive assigned to them by the president. The president, together with the other members of the cabinet, exercises the executive authority by:

- implementing national legislation
- developing and implementing national policy
- coordinating the functions of state departments and administration
- preparing and initiating legislation
- performing any other executive function provided for in the Constitution or in the legislation.

According to the Constitution, each of the nine provinces has its own individual legislatures, which consist of between 30 and 80 members. The executive authority of each province is vested in the premier of that province. The executive council of a province consists of the premier, as head of the council, and members appointed from among members of the provincial legislature.

Local government

Local government is identified in the Constitution as the third sphere of government. This sphere of government is required to:
- provide a democratic and accountable government for local communities
- ensure the provision of services to communities in a sustainable manner
- promote social and economic development
- promote a safe and healthy environment
- encourage the involvement of communities and community organisations in the matters of local government.

The Constitution is the overlying Act and all other legislation must be written with this in mind. In other words, all other legislation must comply with the conditions imposed by the Constitution. Since 1994, several policy documents and pieces of legislation have been developed to support the principles of transformation and equity introduced by the first democratically elected government of South Africa. These are described briefly below.

The South African health policy

The White Paper on 'The Transformation of the Health System' was adopted in April 1997. It superseded the ANC's National Health Plan for South Africa and provided the policy framework for the transformation of the then new health system.

The health policy as outlined in the White Paper was based on the comprehensive primary healthcare (PHC) philosophy and approach as advocated at Alma Ata in Kazakhstan 1978. It is the approach that is adopted by the national government to provide accessible and appropriate healthcare to the majority of the people of this country. The implementation model for this approach to healthcare is the District Health System (DHS).

According to the White Paper, the establishment of the DHS is at the core of the entire health strategy, and its rapid implementation is therefore of the highest priority. The district health concept is based on the experiences of many countries that national and provincial levels of government are too far removed from the community to be responsive to local health needs. It is recognised internationally that many functions of government can be managed more effectively by decentralising them to small geographic and administrative units called districts.

The World Health Organization (WHO, 1986:9) defines a District Health System as follows:

> A DHS based on primary healthcare (PHC) is a more or less self-contained segment of the National Health System. It comprises first and foremost a well-defined population, living within a clearly delineated administrative and geographical area whether urban or rural. It includes all institutions and individuals providing healthcare at district, government, private or traditional level. A DHS therefore consists of a large variety of interrelated elements that contribute to health in homes, schools, workplaces and communities, through the health and other related sectors. It includes self-care and all healthcare workers and facilities up to and including at the first referral level and the appropriate laboratory, other diagnostic, and logistic support services.

According to the White Paper (1997) on the transformation of the health system, the structures that govern the provision of health services will have to respond to the structures of political governance in such a way that they can form an interface that is flexible as well as coordinating in nature. This governance structure is called the District Health Authority (DHA) and has a new separate statutory structure or a structure of local government. For the first 10 years of South Africa's new democracy, the policy set out within the White Paper has driven the new health system in the country and promoted equity and accessibility to comprehensive healthcare services.

Other legislation and policy documents that have influenced the delivery of healthcare during this period are the following:

- **Batho Pele**: 'People First' was conceived with the intention of transforming service delivery in the public sector. Good service delivery leads to happy customers and employee satisfaction for a job well done. This is a policy document that provides a policy framework to transform public service delivery and to improve client care through the process. It encourages health workers to be open and transparent, to treat all clients with respect and courtesy, and to inform people accurately about their right to appropriate care with the specific aim of meeting their individual needs. Batho Pele was founded on eight principles, but since the inception of the Good Governance Awards, two more principles have been added.

Table 3.1 Batho Pele principles

Principle	Description
1. Consultation	Communities will be consulted about the level and quality of public services they receive and where possible will be given a choice about the services offered.
2. Service standards	Citizens would know the level and quality of public service they are to receive and know what to expect.
3. Access	All citizens have equal access to the services to which they are entitled.
4. Courtesy	Citizens should be treated with courtesy and consideration.
5. Redress	If the promised standard of service is not delivered, citizens should be offered an apology, an explanation and an effective remedy; when complaints are made, citizens should receive a sympathetic positive response.
6. Value for money	Public services should be provided economically and efficiently in order to give citizens and communities the best possible value for money.
7. Information	Citizens should be given full, accurate information about the public service they are entitled to receive.
8. Openness and transparency	Citizens should be told how national and provincial departments are run, how much they cost and who is in charge.
9. Innovation and reward	Innovation can be new ways of providing better service, cutting costs, improving conditions, streamlining and generally making changes that tie in with the spirit of Batho Pele. It is also about rewarding the staff who 'go the extra mile' to make it all happen.
10. Customer impact	Impact means looking at the benefits that are provided to healthcare customers; it is how the nine principles link together to show how service delivery has improved overall.

- **The national drug policy**: This policy determined an acceptable structure to improve the supply of suitable drugs and ensure appropriate treatment regimens at acceptable cost. Essential drug lists have been developed that guide good practice at hospitals and at primary healthcare services.
- **HIV and AIDS policy and strategy**: The policy was introduced in 1999 and aimed at refocusing the country's response to the epidemic through an appropriate and effective programme. Through education the aim is to improve access to HIV testing and counselling, to improve treatment of sexually transmitted infections (STIs), and to improve the care and support of people living with HIV and AIDS (PLWA). It proposes to prevent new infections and maintain optimal health for those infected with the virus.

- **The Patients' Rights Charter**: This document sets the standard for quality patient care and informs both patients and health workers of their rights. It balances the rights and the obligations of the patient and sets the basic standards of good patient care for the health worker to attain.

Table 3.2 The Patients' Rights Charter and patient responsibilities

Patients' rights	Patients' responsibilities
Patients have the right to: • a healthy and safe environment • participate in decision-making, in health policy development and in issues that affect a person's own health • access to healthcare and to health workers who are courteous, empathetic and tolerant • knowledge of one's medical aid or insurance scheme • a choice of health service provider or health facility for treatment • confidentiality and privacy • informed consent • refusal of treatment • referral for a second opinion • continuity of care • complain about health services	Patients have the responsibility to: • advise healthcare providers of their wishes with regard to dying • comply with the prescribed treatment or rehabilitation procedures • enquire about the related costs of treatment and/or rehabilitation and arrange for payment • take care of health records in their possession • take care of their health • care for and protect the environment • respect the rights of other patients and health providers • utilise the healthcare system properly and not abuse it • know their local health services and what they offer • provide healthcare providers with the relevant and accurate information for diagnostic, treatment, rehabilitation or counselling purposes

Some examples of legislation that have had an impact on health and healthcare either directly or indirectly are given in Table 3.3.

Table 3.3 South African health and healthcare and related legislation

Title	Act number and year	Impact on health and healthcare
Foodstuffs, Cosmetics and Disinfectants Act	Act 54 of 1972	Ensures food safety and the protection of a country's consumers against food-borne diseases.
The Choice on Termination of Pregnancy Act	Act 92 of 1996	Allows women the right to reproductive choices.

Title	Act number and year	Impact on health and healthcare
The Employment Equity Act	Act 55 of 1998	Aims at promoting the constitutional right to fair employment practices.
Tobacco Products Control Act	Act 12 of 1999	Controls, prohibits or restricts smoking in public areas.
Pharmacy Act	Act 1 of 2000	Regulates and ensures the provision of quality pharmaceutical services.
Medicine and Related Substances Amendment Act	Act 59 of 2002	Provides for the statutory regulation of medication aimed at safeguarding patients against unsafe usage.
Mental Health Act	Act 17 of 2002	Ensures that both appropriate and adequate mental healthcare services are provided.
Traditional Health Practitioners Act	Act 22 of 2007	Controls the practice of traditional healers, registration of traditional practitioners and use of traditional medicine.
Medical Schemes Act	Act 131 of 1998	Regulates the functioning and control of certain activities of medical schemes to protect the interests of members of medical schemes.

The National Health Act 61 of 2003

The National Health Act (Act 61 of 2003) was signed by the president on 23 July 2004 and was an important step forward in the transformation of the South African health sector. Since 1994, health policy has been developed but implementation of the new policies has been handicapped because there has been no new health legislation to support the new health system, and because the old Act was entrenched in the policy of the previous government.

The Health Act is directly linked to the Constitution and sets out the framework within which the health system of the country must function. Regulations will now have to be developed to set out the broad legal and operational principles that are included in the Act. The contents of the Act are as follows:

- **Chapter 1** sets out the structure of the National Health System under the leadership of the Minister of Health.
- **Chapter 2** covers the rights of each citizen and is an extension of those listed in the Constitution. In healthcare, citizens have the right to:
  - emergency medical treatment
  - full knowledge of their condition
  - exercise informed consent
  - participate in decisions regarding their health

- be informed when they are participating in research
- confidentiality and access to health records
- lay complaints about the service as users.

They also have the responsibility to treat health workers with respect.

- **Chapter 3** outlines the structure of the National DOH.

- **Chapter 4** establishes the structure and functions of the nine provincial health services.

- **Chapter 5** describes the formation of district health services.

- **Chapter 6** deals with the registration and licensing of all health services, both public and private, with the National DOH.

- **Chapter 7** is dedicated to human resource planning that will ensure adequate numbers of well-trained health personnel who are distributed between all health services to meet the people's needs.

- **Chapter 8** outlines healthy practice in the use of human blood, blood products and human tissue and organs for transplant. It also addresses such issues as human cloning.

- **Chapter 9** ensures the rights of all citizens by providing for the establishment of a National Health Research Ethics Council and regional Health Research Ethics Committees to protect the public from unethical research.

- **Chapter 10** deals with maintaining the basic standards and norms that all health establishments are expected to attain.

- **Chapter 11** gives the power and the responsibility to the minister to develop the necessary regulations necessary to implement the Act.

- **Chapter 12** allows the appointment of the necessary people or committees to ensure that regulations are carried out.

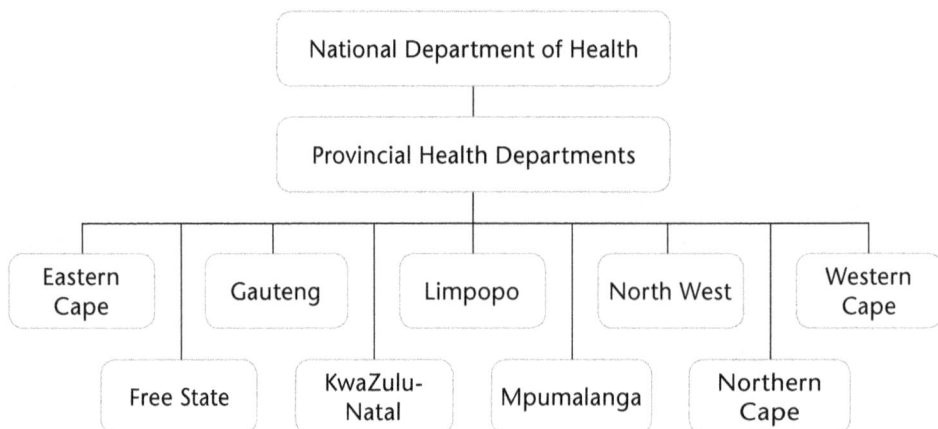

Figure 3.1 Organogram of the South African health departments

Provincial health departments

After the elections in 1994 the health authority was transferred from the former provinces and the so-called self-governing territories to the nine new provincial administrations that function as independent structures, each with its own budget. Each provincial structure has its own elected body, known as the legislature, that determines the law or legislation appropriate to the needs of that specific province.

District health services

The District Health System (DHS) is the vehicle by which all PHC is delivered. The legal and policy framework for the rendering of PHC services through a DHS at the level of local government is in place. The Local Government Municipal Structures Amendment Act 33 of 2000 and the Local Government Municipal Systems Amendment Act 1 of 2003 clearly articulate the role of local government in the rendering of the DHS and set out a proposed framework for the functioning of this level of governance. The DHS takes responsibility for developmental functions, providing cost-effective and accountable integration of intersectoral services that impact on health, such as water and sanitation, housing and environmental management. A National Health System based on this DHS approach is concerned with keeping people healthy, as it is with caring for them when they become unwell. The concepts of caring and wellness are promoted most effectively and efficiently by creating small management units of healthcare systems adapted to cater for local needs. The healthcare districts provide the framework for our health system, so that a single authority can take responsibility for the health of the population in its area.

The DHS has three main types of healthcare facilities:

1. District hospitals
2. Community health centres (CHCs)
3. PHC clinics.

Chapter 5 of the National Health Act 61 of 2003, which deals with the DHS, states that it should be fully implemented. This requires that the district and sub-district be well managed with respect to the principles of the DHS and well-funded by provinces. The DHS principles include:

- delivery of accessible, good-quality services in an equitable manner, ensuring that these services are comprehensive and not fragmented and that they are effectively and efficiently delivered
- local accountability, community participation, and a developmental and intersectoral approach accompanied by sustainability.

The DHS has to be adequately financed by the provinces to succeed. The challenge is to use the opportunity of restructuring at local government level to develop the DHS appropriately and to overcome the problems facing local governments, such as limited revenue, particularly in the rural areas. Another problem is the limited infrastructure, both capital and human, which is a problem most local governments have. Most important, however, are the structures in place that prevent the logical integration of PHC services run by the provinces and local governments. These include persistent differences in conditions of services and salaries of health workers employed by the different authorities and the lack of enabling legislation.

The South African healthcare system

The healthcare system in South Africa is a comprehensive system based on the principles of PHC as advocated by the World Health Organization (WHO).

A comprehensive healthcare system

A comprehensive healthcare system may be described as one that provides all people with maximum health benefits at a reasonable cost. It is an integrated and coordinated system of healthcare having promotive, preventative and curative components. It is a system that sees the individual as belonging to a family and a community, and operating in a specific social and physical environment from which he or she is inseparable and that has a profound influence on his or her health.

In such a system use is made of all community resources, and the participation of community members in the planning, organisation and evaluation of the services is encouraged. Promotive and preventative care operates at three levels:

1. Primary prevention
2. Secondary prevention
3. Tertiary prevention.

Primary prevention

At this point the person is not sick and does not present with the signs and symptoms of a disease. This level of disease prevention in the traditionally accepted meaning of the term consists of two stages, namely health promotion and specific protection.

1. **Health promotion**: Steps are taken to promote optimal health in individuals and communities by:
   - ensuring adequate nutrition
   - promoting high standards of environmental hygiene through the provision of suitable housing; satisfactory ventilation and the prevention of overcrowding; the efficient disposal of refuse and sewage; the provision of safe water supplies; and the control of rodents and insects, including flies

- encouraging satisfactory standards of personal hygiene and cleanliness
- ensuring suitable working conditions and the elimination of occupational hazards
- providing genetic counselling to people at risk
- promoting optimal psychological health through marriage guidance, vocational guidance and the use of good child-rearing practices
- the use of effective health education to achieve these aims and objectives
- ensuring that legislation and policy are appropriate to attain optimal health for all people.

2. **Specific protection**: This is achieved by:
   - immunisation
   - the use of protective clothing in industries, such as goggles and helmets
   - the wearing of seat belts in cars and crash helmets on motorcycles
   - the prophylactic use of drugs to prevent diseases such as malaria, and condoms in safe sexual practices
   - the elimination of vectors or the treatment of carriers of disease
   - the control of diseases in animals.

Secondary prevention

At this stage the person is already suffering from a disease and the measures that are taken are directed at rendering the patient non-infectious in as short a time as possible, preventing the spread of the disease, and stopping it from spreading. The success of this level of prevention is determined by the prompt and effective treatment of all sufferers. Secondary prevention is accomplished by:

- early diagnosis
- appropriate treatment, including isolation where necessary
- case-finding so that all persons suffering from the condition may be traced and treated
- notification of the disease to the appropriate authorities when legally required to do so and in the case of listed diseases such as tuberculosis and cholera
- treatment and control of the contacts who may be infected.

Tertiary prevention

Tertiary prevention is about the limitation of disability, and rehabilitation.

- **Limitation of disability**: At this level of prevention the concern is to stop the progress of the disease and to prevent complications. Prompt diagnosis, effective treatment and the early recognition of possible complications are important factors in the limitation of disability.

- **Rehabilitation**: At this level of prevention the aim is to return the person to his or her community, to ensure that his or her remaining capacities are fully utilised, and that further deterioration will be prevented. Where necessary, physiotherapy, vocational guidance, sheltered employment and social services such as disability grants should be made available.

Primary healthcare (PHC)

In 1978, the WHO introduced the concept of 'Health for all by 2000' at a conference held at Alma Ata in Kazakhstan. The Alma Ata Declaration highlighted major changes in the direction of healthcare. The concept of PHC was introduced, which is a comprehensive approach to healthcare that emphasises community-based rather than hospital-based healthcare. Health services are situated in the community close to the places where people live. It is a holistic approach to attaining health for all members in the community in that it promotes health by ensuring that the environment in which people live is healthy and has a positive impact on health. This means that health becomes the responsibility not only of health workers but of other sectors of the community whose work influences the environment and ensures safe water, adequate sanitation, food (agriculture), housing, roads and education.

Definition for primary healthcare

Primary healthcare is essential care based on practical, scientifically sound and socially acceptable methods and technology, made universally accessible to individuals and families in the community through their full participation and at a cost that the community and country can afford to maintain at every stage of their development in the spirit of self-reliance and self-determination.

(WHO, Alma Ata Conference, 1978)

PHC is an essential part of a comprehensive health service. PHC is an approach to healthcare that promotes the attainment by all people of a level of health that will permit them to live socially and economically productive lives. It is basically healthcare that is essential, practical, social and scientifically sound (evidence-based), ethical, accessible, equitable, affordable and accountable to the community.

This approach to healthcare places emphasis on the rights of an individual to participate as a member of the healthcare team. For such a programme to work, people need to be empowered by receiving information that is appropriate to the individual as well as the community, and to their specific needs. The information gained should enable them to make informed decisions that will contribute to their own good health.

PHC is not only a primary medical or curative care, nor is it a package of low-cost medical interventions for the poor and marginalised. On the contrary, it calls for the integration of health services into the process of community development, a process that requires political commitment, intersectoral collaboration and multidisciplinary involvement for success. The ultimate goal of PHC is better health for all. The core principles of PHC are:

- universal access to care and coverage on the basis of need (accessibility)
- commitment to health equity as part of development oriented to social justice (health promotion)
- community participation in defining and implementing health agendas (public participation)
- intersectoral approaches to health
- use of appropriate technology.

The WHO has identified five key elements to achieving that goal, which are:

- reducing exclusion and social disparities in health (universal coverage reforms)
- organising health services around people's needs and expectations (service delivery reforms)
- integrating health into all sectors (public policy reforms)
- pursuing collaborative models of policy dialogue (leadership reforms)
- increasing stakeholder participation.

The WHO has laid down certain basic principles for the organisation of PHC that can be summarised as follows:

- PHC should be shaped around the life patterns of the population and should meet all the daily health needs of the community.
- It should form an integral part of the national health system.
- PHC services should be integrated with other services concerned with community development, such as agricultural and educational services and communications.
- The local population should be actively involved in the healthcare activities.
- It should use an integrated approach that links promotive, preventative, curative and rehabilitative care to the services offered.
- Treatment should be as simple as possible and be carried out by health workers who have been suitably trained to perform such treatment according to their level of competency.
- There should be adequate facilities for prompt and efficient referral.

According to South Africa's health policy, the services offered in the healthcare system are based on the PHC philosophy and should include:

- environmental healthcare, including the supply of safe water and adequate safe sanitation

- maternal and child healthcare, including antenatal and delivery services, family planning services and well-baby clinics
- health promotion, including health education
- access to health data and health information
- prevention and control of communicable diseases, including access to immunisation services
- access to primary curative services for the treatment of minor ailments or common endemic conditions or diseases
- rehabilitative services
- services to persons in the community, including school health, workplace services and community development projects.

Re-engineering primary healthcare in South Africa

PHC is being re-engineered through four streams to improve timely access and to promote health and prevent disease. These streams are Municipal Ward-based Primary Healthcare Outreach Teams (WBPHCOTs); Integrated School Health Programme (ISHP); District Clinical Specialist Teams (DCSTs); and contracting of non-specialist health professionals.

PHC re-engineering (rPHC) was launched by South Africa's former Minister of Health, Dr Aaron Motsoaledi, in 2010. The aim is to improve performance of and access to healthcare services in South Africa. The main focus of PHC re-engineering is to:

- strengthen DHS effectiveness
- place greater emphasis on population-based health and outcomes, focusing on:
  - a new strategy for strengthening community-based services (including communities, households and schools)
  - a team approach to healthcare that includes all the PHC teams
  - more preventative strategies.

In an effort to increase life expectancy, decrease child and maternal mortality, lower the burden of disease from HIV and AIDS, tuberculosis and other chronic diseases and improve the effectiveness of the health system overall, the DOH has introduced three streams of healthcare services, focusing on:

- implementing ward-based PHC outreach (community-based care)
- strengthening school health services (a centralised system of ensuring child health)
- establishing district clinical specialist teams (DCSTs) with a focus on maternal and child health, as well as HIV and AIDS, tuberculosis and other chronic illnesses.

The new primary healthcare model within the DHS is shown in Figure 3.2.

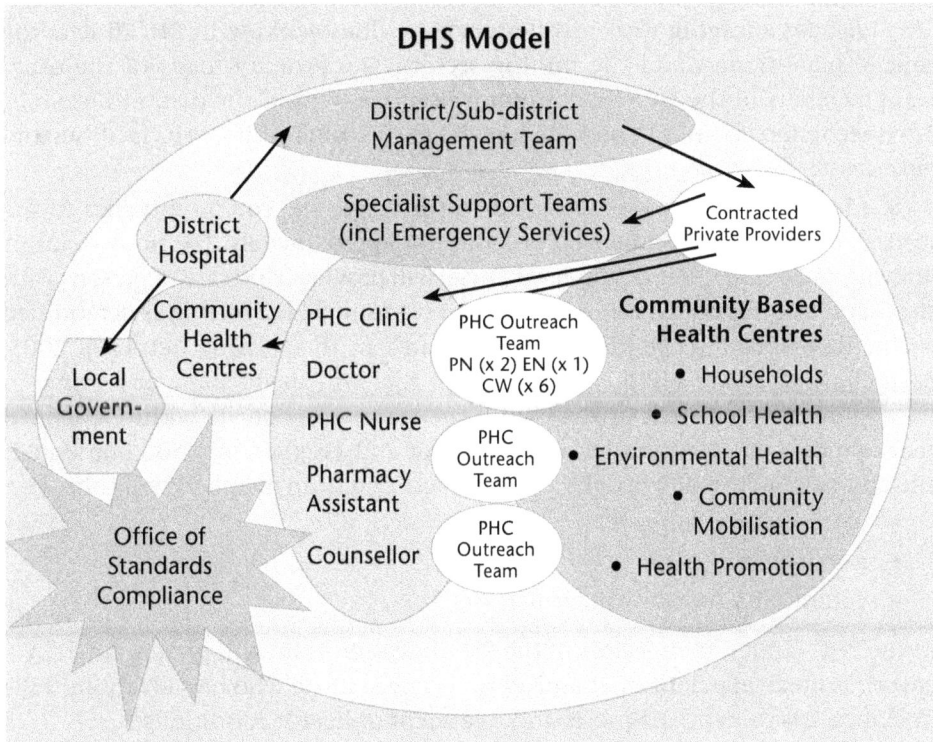

Figure 3.2 The new primary healthcare model within the District Health System
Source: PHASA (2011)

Every district is supported by a DCST consisting of:
- an obstetrician and a gynaecologist
- a paediatrician
- an anaesthetist
- a family physician
- an advanced midwife
- an advanced PHC nurse
- an advanced paediatric nurse.

The functions of the speciality teams are to:
- strengthen clinical governance (at PHC level and district hospitals)
- ensure that treatment guidelines and protocols are available and are used
- ensure that essential equipment is available and used correctly
- ensure that mortality-review meetings are held, are of good quality and that recommendations from these meetings are implemented
- support, supervise and mentor clinicians
- monitor health outcomes.

The family physician and advanced PHC nurse provide support at midwifery obstetrics units, PHC clinics, CHC clinics, PHC outreach teams and communities. This includes engaging with private-sector facilities working in PHC (including general practitioners and the mining sector). The primary focus of the other team members in the DCST is to improve services within the district hospitals. Their secondary focus is to provide support to the community, PHC facilities and outreach teams.

Staffing calculations estimate that, on average, six community healthcare workers (CHWs) can assume responsibility for approximately 250 households. A midwife and a staff nurse (a mid-level nurse) will provide basic care to persons with stable and uncomplicated general health problems in a PHC setting as determined by the new nurses' scope of practice stipulated in the Nursing Act 33 of 2005. Each clinic will have a PHC outreach team that will spend some of its time in the community and some at the clinic. The teams will operate within a defined geographical boundary and be responsible for and assigned to 1 500 households and approximately 6 000 people. The PHC outreach team members will consist of:

- a professional nurse (PN)
- a staff nurse (SN)
- community health workers (CHWs).

At the PHC clinics, the services of the PHC outreach team will be supported by a part-time medical practitioner and a PHC nurse (a nurse who has advanced skills in clinical assessment, diagnosis and treatment of health conditions).

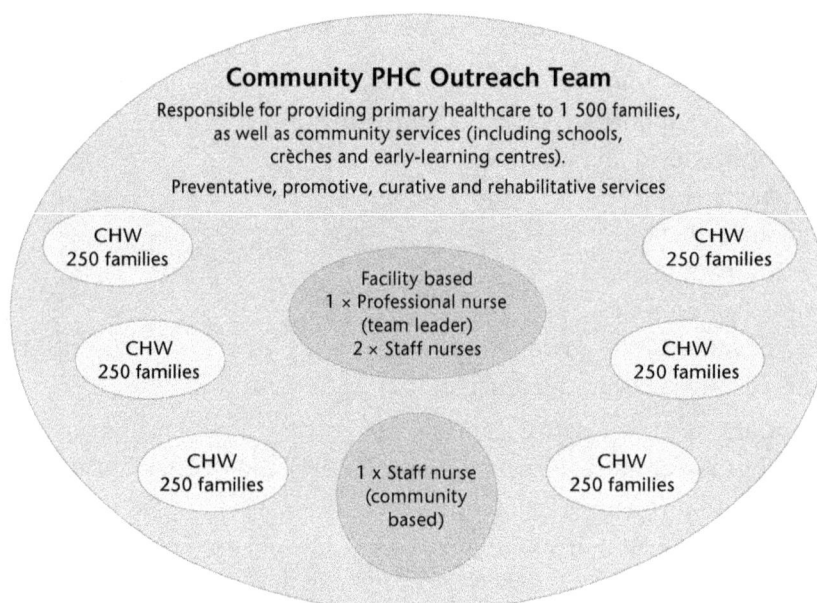

Figure 3.3 The primary healthcare outreach team
Source: Adapted from the National DOH PHC re-engineering document (2012)

The functions of PHC teams are to offer an integrated healthcare service at community, household and individual level. The core components of the integrated services are to:

- promote health (children, adolescents and women)
- prevent ill-health
- provide ante- and postnatal community-based support and intervention to reduce maternal mortality
- provide information and education to communities and households on a range of health and related matters
- offer psychosocial support
- screen for early detection and intervention of health problems and illnesses
- provide follow-up and support to persons with health problems (including lack of adherence to treatment)
- provide treatment for minor ailments, basic first aid and emergency interventions.

Table 3.4 The roles and functions of the primary healthcare outreach team

Total number and professional discipline	Role and functions of healthcare worker
1 × professional nurse (PN)	• Clinic-based services • Support/supervision of community-based services • Clinical support: early learning centres (ELCs), crèches, old-age homes, schools
2 × general nurses (GNs)	• Clinic-based services • Integrated management of childhood illness (IMCI), basic antenatal and postnatal care (normal pregnancies) • Immunisation • Repeats for stable, chronic patients • Treatment of minor ailments
1 × general nurse (GN)	• Support and supervise CHW services in the community • School health services • Community-based programmes (antenatal and postnatal care, immunisation campaigns) • Screening and support services to schools, ELCs, crèches and old-age homes
6 × community health workers (CHWs)	• Screening, assessment and referral, information and education, psychosocial support, basic home treatment, support of community campaigns, schools

➡

Total number and professional discipline	Role and functions of healthcare worker
Role of PHC clinic support staff (per PHC outreach team)	
Part-time doctor	Complex cases, clinical governance
Part-time PHC nurse	Complex cases, overall clinic management and supervision of support staff
Part-time (NA)	Observations, tests, support team members
Counsellor	Main focus: pre- and post-diagnosis counselling, HIV and AIDS, tuberculosis, chronic diseases, treatment adherence, support and counselling
Post-basic pharmacy assistant	Dispensing treatment, recording patient information

Source: Adapted from the National DOH PHC re-engineering document (2012)

The roles and functions of primary healthcare outreach teams

It is stipulated that three PHC teams are to be based in a facility with a catchment population of around 18 000 people. In each PHC clinic there will be a part-time medical practitioner, a PHC nurse practitioner, nursing auxiliaries, counsellors, post-basic pharmacist assistants and administrative support, in addition to cleaning and security services.

- **Medical practitioners**: The medical practitioner provides clinical support, supervision and clinical governance and manages patients who cannot be managed by the nurse practitioner.

- **PHC nurse practitioner**: The PHCN supports the PHC outreach team together with the part-time medical practitioner.

- **Pharmacy assistant**: The pharmacy assistants render all pharmaceutical services. The Pharmacy Council of South Africa (PCSA) registered the post-basic pharmacy assistant as a mid-level health worker to address the challenges facing the healthcare system with regard to the shortage of pharmacists.

- **Nursing auxiliaries**: The role of the nursing auxiliary is primarily to carry out the routine observations, weighing and measuring, basic diagnostic tests and basic support and care as and when required. The scope of practice and level of competence and skill of the nursing auxiliary is limited. Therefore, this category of nurse is unlikely to be able to play a more extended role in the PHC team.

- **Counsellors**: Currently there are a range of lay counsellors, adherence counsellors, directly observed treatment support (DOTS) workers, and pre- and post-HIV testing counsellors. Counsellors provide comprehensive and integrated treatment and psychosocial support.

- **Administrative support**: Support staff perform administrative duties, including information management.
- **CHWs**: Responsibilities include knowing the demography of the catchment population, knowing the epidemiology, health promotion and prevention (household and community), screening and referral, palliative care, social mobilisation, and linking resources to community needs in order to improve health.

School health nursing

A school health policy was adopted in South Africa in 2003; however, its implementation has been limited due to resource constraints. The adoption of the policy was a follow-up from the recommendations of the UN Convention on the Rights of Children. In 2012, the Ministers of Health and Basic Education presented an Integrated School Health Policy (ISHP), which outlines the role of the respective departments in addressing the healthcare needs of learners, with the aim of ensuring that a strong school health service operates according to clear standards across the country. This policy abides by the mandate of the DOH to have a health presence in every school. This entails the employment of more school health nurses and/or teams and deploying them at schools in each district.

The ISHP plays a crucial role in caring for and maintaining the health of the school-going child and lays the foundation for learners to be responsible for their own health. The WHO (1996) defines a school health programme as a combination of health services that focuses on learners' physical, mental and social well-being.

The school health team is led by a PN, who forms part of the multidisciplinary team (MDT), which may consist of a psychologist, CHWs, health promoters, an oral hygienist, social worker, speech therapist and occupational therapist. The school health nurse (SHN) uses an intersectoral approach by referring learners to other MDT members for further management and care if, needed.

In lower grades, nurses and other team members should screen learners for hearing, vision and dental problems. Learners in need of clinical intervention are referred to an appropriate facility. In high schools, the nurses will provide life-skills programmes for sexual and reproductive health, with a view to address HIV and AIDS prevention and the high number of teenage pregnancies. They will also deal with other social problems such as alcohol and drug use. The main roles of the healthcare teams at schools are therefore to:
- implement health education and promotion programmes in schools and crèches, based on assessed needs
- develop and disseminate health promotion messages
- identify appropriate and relevant health promotion material for use and distribution
- use a range of health promotion tools
- participate in health calendar days.

National health insurance in South Africa

The National Health Insurance (NHI) Fund is a health financing system that is designed to pool funds to provide access to quality affordable personal health services for all South Africans based on their health needs, irrespective of their socioeconomic status. The NHI will be a way of providing good healthcare for all by sharing the money available for healthcare among all South Africans. The NHI will be aimed at providing universal coverage. Universal coverage is defined by the World Health Organization (WHO) as the 'progressive development of a health system including its financing mechanisms into one that ensures that everyone has access to quality, needed health services and where everyone is accorded protection from financial hardships linked to accessing these health services'. The NHI will be for all South Africans in keeping with the fact that health is a basic right enshrined in the Constitution and hence cannot be for a selected few. Implementation of the NHI is based on the need to address structural imbalances in the health system and to reduce the burden of disease.

In South Africa, the NHI Fund will receive money from general tax revenue and from special contributions by individuals who earn above a specified level. The NHI will provide a mechanism for improving cross-subsidisation in the overall health system. Funding will be linked to an individual's ability to pay and benefits from health services will be in line with an individual's need for healthcare. The NHI White Paper in South Africa was gazetted on 30 June 2017. This White Paper lays the foundation for moving South Africa towards universal health coverage (UHC) through the implementation of the NHI and the establishment of a unified health system.

The objectives of the NHI are to:
- enable every person in South Africa to access good-quality healthcare irrespective of whether they are employed and thus to help South Africans become a healthier nation
- create fairness in the sharing of healthcare finance and other resources, including skilled health professionals
- provide funds to public and private healthcare providers on a fair basis so that equity and social solidarity will be achieved through the creation of a single fund. This will make it possible for everyone to get good-quality care, no matter what healthcare facility they go to
- procure or acquire services on behalf of the entire population and efficiently mobilise and control key financial resources
- strengthen the under-resourced and strained public sector to improve the performance of health systems.

The principles that guide the NHI in South Africa are the following:
- **The right to access**: Section 27 of the Bill of Rights of the Constitution states that everyone has the right of access to healthcare services, including reproductive healthcare, and that the state must take reasonable

legislative and other measures, within its available resources, to achieve the progressive realisation of these rights. The NHI will ensure reform of healthcare for the realisation of these rights.

- **Social solidarity**: This refers to the creation of financial risk protection for the entire population that ensures sufficient cross-subsidisation between the rich and the poor, and the healthy and sick.

- **Effectiveness**: This will be achieved through evidence-based interventions, strengthened management systems and better performance of the healthcare system that will contribute to positive health outcomes and overall improved life expectancy for the entire population.

- **Appropriateness**: This refers to the adoption of new and innovative health service delivery models that take account of the local context and acceptability and are tailored to respond to local needs. The health services delivery model will be based on a properly structured referral system rendered via a re-engineered PHC model.

- **Equity**: This refers to a health system that ensures that those with the greatest health needs are provided with timely access to health services. It should be free from any barriers, and any inequalities in the system should be minimised.

- **Affordability**: This means that services will be procured at reasonable costs that recognise health as not just an ordinary commodity of trade but as a public good.

- **Efficiency**: This will be ensured through creating administrative structures that eradicate duplication across the national, provincial and district spheres. The key will be to ensure that minimal resources are spent on the administrative structures of the NHI and that value for money is achieved in the translation of resources into actual health service delivery.

The roll-out of the NHI will be phased in over 14 years commencing in seriously under-served areas where people have difficulty accessing healthcare. The first phase of the NHI commenced in 2012 and was completed in 2017. This phase piloted various health system strengthening interventions focused at district and PHC level. The interventions implemented during this phase were mainly funded by a direct NHI Conditional Grant to provinces, although there were other funding mechanisms. The 10 NHI pilot districts were made up of one district in every province, except KwaZulu-Natal (KZN), which had two districts. Subsequently, KZN included a third district, which was solely funded through provincial funding. The NHI pilot districts were intended to become sites for innovation and testing throughout the implementation of the first phase of the NHI. The pilot districts were:

- OR Tambo (Eastern Cape)
- Thabo Mofutsanyana (Free State)
- Tshwane (Gauteng)

- UMgungundlovu and uMzinyathi (KZN)
- Vhembe (Limpopo)
- Gert Sibande (Mpumalanga)
- Pixley ka Seme (Northern Cape)
- Dr Kenneth Kaunda (North West)
- Eden (Western Cape)
- Amajuba (the additional district included by KZN).

The interventions for the pilot sites were as follows:

- *Ward-based primary healthcare outreach teams (WBPHCOTS)*: responsible for the provision of promotive and preventative healthcare to households.

- *The integrated school health programme (ISHP)*: aimed at providing a range of health promotion and preventative services to school-going children at their place of learning.

- *General practitioner (GP) contracting*: aimed at increasing the number of GPs at PHC facilities to improve the quality and acceptability of care.

- *Ideal clinic realisation and maintenance model (ICRM)*: aimed at increasing quality of services through the establishment of minimum standards.

- *District clinical specialist teams (DCST)*: responsible for supporting clinical governance, undertaking clinical work, research and training.

- *Centralised chronic medicine dispensing and distribution (CCMDD)*: aimed at improving distribution of medicines to patients through the provision of chronic medication at designated pick-up points closer to communities.

- *Health patient registration system (HPRS)*: with the ultimate goal of a fully electronic patient recordkeeping system but has started with data capturing of patients and generation of electronic files.

- *Stock visibility system (SVS)*: aimed at improving oversight of stock through an electronic stock monitoring system, and thereby reducing stock-outs by allowing for appropriate and timely ordering.

- *Infrastructure projects*: to improve health infrastructure and ensure increased access and quality of the NHI pilot districts.

- *Workload indicator for staffing needs (WISN)*: a WHO planning tool conducted to help facility managers make more efficient staffing decisions.

The implementation of the NHI is a government priority and forms part of the 10 Point Plan implemented by the Department of Health to improve the health system in South Africa. The 10 Point Plan focuses on the following priorities:

1. Provision of strategic leadership and creation of a social compact for better health outcomes
2. Implementation of the NHI

3. Improving the quality of health services
4. Overhauling the healthcare system by:
   - refocusing on PHC
   - improving the functionality and management of the health system
5. Improving human resources, planning, development and management
6. Revitalisation of infrastructure, with a focus on:
   - accelerating the delivery of health infrastructure through public–private partnerships (PPPs)
   - revitalising primary-level facilities
   - accelerating the delivery of health technology and information communication technology (ICT) infrastructure
7. Accelerated implementation of the HIV and AIDS and sexually transmitted infections (STIs) national strategic plan and reduction of mortality due to tuberculosis and associated diseases
8. Mass mobilisation for better health for the population
9. Review of the drug policy
10. Strengthening research and development.

The implementation of the NHI is gradually being introduced in the country, with full implementation in 2026. The timeline is as follows:

- **Phase 1**: from 2012 to 2017, focused on piloting health system strengthening (HSS) initiatives; the establishment of the NHI Fund and key institutions; and the moving of central hospitals to the national sphere.

- **Phase 2**: from 2017 to 2022, will be focused on ensuring the NHI Fund is fully functional and has the required management and governance structures so that the purchase of services and population registration can begin. This involves passing the NHI Bill, which was introduced in 2019, and making amendments to several pieces of legislation.

- **Phase 3**: from 2022 to 2026, will signal the introduction of mandatory prepayment and the contracting of accredited private hospital and specialist services as well as the finalisation of the Medical Schemes Amendment Act.

When the NHI is fully implemented, there will be only one health system in the country. South Africans will be able to access health services from any doctor or clinic, public or private, that is certified and accredited by the NHI. The system will provide a comprehensive PHC package of healthcare services, and all healthcare will be provided at the primary healthcare level, whilst hospitals and specialists will only be for referral. It is proposed that the basic NHI package will cover the following services: HIV and tuberculosis, reproductive healthcare, optometry and mental health.

The National Core Standards

The National Core Standards (NCS) are the national drive and instruments used by the DOH to improve, together with the NHI, the quality of healthcare. The legal context of the NCS for the health sector is the National Health Act (61 of 2003), which promotes good-quality healthcare services and healthcare standards. The NCS are seen as a basis for quality. Quality of care is about getting the best results possible, within the available resources. Quality of care is defined by the WHO as 'the level of attainment of health systems' intrinsic goals for health improvement and responsiveness to the legitimate expectations of the population'. Patients' experiences of healthcare are important in gauging and shaping a health system's approach to quality.

The purpose of the NCS, therefore, is to set a benchmark for quality of care, and to provide a framework for the national accreditation of health establishments. In this regard, the DOH identified six focus areas which have been introduced to aid the implementation of the NHI:

Patient rights:

1. Improving the values and attitudes of staff, managers and patients.
2. Reducing waiting time.
3. Ensuring cleanliness of hospitals and clinics.

Patient safety, clinical governance and care:

4. Keeping patients safe and providing reliable care.
5. Infection prevention and control.

Clinical support services:

6. Ensuring availability of medicines, supplies and equipment.

The NCS are structured in seven cross-cutting domains. The first three domains, namely patient rights; safety, clinical governance and care; and clinical support services, represent the core business of delivering quality healthcare to users and patients. The remaining domains, namely public health; leadership and corporate governance; operational management; and facilities and infrastructure, are the support systems for healthcare delivery. Internal clients and staff are important stakeholders in achieving these standards.

Table 3.6 The seven domains of the National Core Standards and six focus areas

National Core Standards and six priorities

National Core Standards	Six Priorities	
1. Patient rights	2. Safety, clinical risk	**Patient Rights:** 1. Values and attitudes 2. Waiting times 3. Cleanliness
	3. Clinical support services	
4. Public health 5. Leadership & corporate governance 6. Operational management 7. Facilities & infrastucture	**Clinical Support Services:** 6. Availability of medicines and supplies	

In the six priorities column, top right: **Patient Safety, Clinical Governance & Care:** 4. Patienty safety 5. Infection prevention and control

Source: Adapted from RSA (2011)

The Office of Health Standards Compliance

The Office of Health Standards Compliance (OHSC) is an independent body established in terms of the National Health Amendment Act 12 of 2013 to ensure that both public and private health establishments in South Africa comply with the required health standards. The OHSC has been established to assure quality of health services and it will be key in the certification of health establishments throughout the country. The Inspectorate will ensure compliance with norms and standards, and the Ombudsperson will enforce accountability and impose corrective measures, where necessary.

The objectives of the OHSC are to protect and promote the health and safety of users of health services by doing the following:

- Monitoring and enforcing compliance by health establishments with norms and standards prescribed by the Minister of Health in relation to the national health system.

- Ensuring consideration, investigation and disposal of complaints relating to non-compliance with prescribed norms and standards for health establishments in a procedurally fair, economical and expeditious manner.

The functions of the OHSC are set out in Section 29 of the Health Act, and include the following:

- Advise the Minister of Health on determining norms and standards that are to be prescribed for the national health system and on the review of such norms and standards.

- Inspect and certify health establishments as compliant or non-compliant with prescribed norms and standards or, where appropriate, withdraw such certification.

- Investigate complaints relating to breaches of prescribed norms and standards.

- Monitor indicators of risk to develop an early warning system related to serious breaches of norms and standards and report breaches to the Minister without delay.

- Make recommendations for intervention by national, provincial or municipal health departments or by individual health establishments to ensure compliance with prescribed norms and standards.

- Publish information relating to prescribed norms and standards through the media and, where appropriate, to specific communities.

- Recommend to the Minister quality assurance and management systems for the national health system.

The multidisciplinary healthcare team

Delivery of care is the responsibility of a multidisciplinary team (MDT) of health practitioners, health workers, the community and the patient. In PHC the patient is a trusted member of the team and is required to take responsibility for his or her own health. Community members are required to be involved in the process of fostering an environment that helps the people within that community attain optimal health for themselves.

The role of most of the MDT in PHC settings has been deliberated in the section on PHC re-engineering above. The MDT consists of the following:

- **Professional nurses**: PNs work at all levels of care, both as generalists and as specialists, with an additional qualification registered with the South African Nursing Council (SANC). Below is a brief description of a few such specialists who work in community healthcare settings and implement PHC:
  - *PHC nurses*: These nurses are general nurses with a Diploma in Clinical Nursing, Health Assessment, Treatment and Care, and they must also be qualified for Midwifery. They usually work in a PHC clinic or CHC, or in special clinics at district hospitals. These nurses deal mainly with the curative aspects of PHC. The duties performed by these nurses require that they have additional training in diagnostic skills and techniques, in clinical assessment and in appropriate pharmacology and treatment skills.

- *Occupational health nurses*: This category of nurse is concerned with providing a healthy and safe working environment for employees. Occupational health nurses hold an additional qualification in Occupational Health and are employed by industrial or commercial organisations to provide a comprehensive healthcare service that includes the promotion of health, the prevention of injury and ill health and the early detection of disease.
  - *Other categories of nurses*: Both enrolled or staff nurses and auxiliary nurses assist the professional nurses to implement healthcare. They are valuable members of the team and perform valuable care, especially in rural communities where there is a shortage of professional nurses.

- **Pharmacists**: Pharmacists have become more integrated into the national healthcare system and offer more extensive services as part of the PHC services in both the preventative, promotive and curative health services.

- **Medical doctors**: There are about 216 191 registered medical doctors in South Africa (Health Professions Council of South Africa, 2014), the majority of whom live in urban areas, work in the private sector and concentrate mainly on curative medicine. Nevertheless, they play an essential role in the delivery of PHC.

- **Traditional healers**: In South Africa, there were an estimated 190 000 traditional healers in 2007 (Nxumalo et al, 2011). The traditional healers have close ties with their communities and exert considerable influence. The Traditional Healers Act 22 of 2007 has been promulgated and allows traditional healers who fulfil certain criteria to register. The registered practitioners are now recognised as members of the health practitioners' team and their patients will be able to claim from their medical aid for services rendered by them.

- **Other members of the health team**: These include social workers, physiotherapists, speech therapists, occupational therapists, dieticians, nutritionists, lay counsellors and others.

- **Community healthcare workers**: In 2003 the DOH recognised the need to formalise training for CWHs in order to ensure the safety of the workers and also to acknowledge their contribution to healthcare in the community. With the increasing number of people living with HIV and AIDS, the role of CWHs in the healthcare team has become increasingly important.

There are shortages of staff in all the categories of professional health practitioners in South Africa. This situation is worse in rural areas than in urban areas. The SANC website has reliable information on the geographical distribution of the population of South Africa versus nursing personnel; visit www.sanc.co.za for this information.

Health policy in the Southern African Development Community

The Southern African Development Community (SADC) was established in Windhoek in 1992, to encourage closer cooperation among the people and governments of the region. The treaty is legally binding and requires partner countries to coordinate and rationalise their policies and strategies for sustainable development. The SADC consists of 14 member countries in the southern part of Africa, whose governments together address the needs of about 365 million people living in the region.

The following countries are involved in this agreement: Angola, Botswana, the Democratic Republic of Congo, Lesotho, Malawi, Mauritius, Mozambique, Namibia, Seychelles, South Africa, eSwatini (formerly Swaziland), Tanzania, Zambia and Zimbabwe.

The heads of state meet once a year at a regional summit, but operational aspects of the organisation are the responsibility of various sectoral committees that meet at least twice a year. In August 1997, a Health Sector Committee was established to improve cooperation in addressing common health problems affecting the member states.

The goal of the Health Sector Committee was to identify strategies to attain 'an acceptable level of health for all citizens by promoting, coordinating and supporting the individual and collective efforts of the member states' (SADC, 2010). The committee adopted the WHO global targets for 2002, as the basis of the joint regional initiative. To pursue this goal the member states accepted a protocol based on five principles:

1. Mutual respect and equality of member states through striving for health policies that are consistent throughout the region
2. Coordination, sharing and support through:
   - determining data that will be collected and that will identify regional trends and priorities
   - conducting research that will determine ways to improve the health of the people in the region
   - promoting health through healthy public policy, health education and producing appropriate educational material
   - determining ways of using the limited resources, including human resources, available in the region optimally to meet the needs of the people
3. Commitment to the PHC approach in order to attain optimal health for all, with special attention being given to strategies to control tuberculosis, malaria and HIV and AIDS, and to improve child health
4. Efforts made to improve access to healthcare at all levels and to improve referral systems
5. Equity promoted to achieve better health through development strategies, including economic strategies.

The aim of the SADC is to create a community providing for regional peace and security, and an integrated regional economy. As a regional institution it has laid the basis on which regional planning and development in southern Africa could be pursued. It also provides the desired instrument with which member states should move along the path towards eventual economic integration. Furthermore, the SADC forms one of the building blocks of the African Economic Community.

As a member of the SADC, South Africa's focus is on regional cooperation for the socioeconomic development of the southern African region. South Africa's membership of the SADC provides an opportunity to tackle, in a coordinated fashion, together with other member states, issues such as sustainable regional economic growth, HIV and AIDS, illegal immigration and refugees, and narcotics and arms smuggling into the region.

The SADC Health Policy plans to raise the regional standard of health for all citizens to an acceptable level by promoting, coordinating and supporting efforts of member states to improve access to high-impact health interventions. This framework was developed by the SADC Health Ministers and approved by the SADC Council of Ministers in September 2000. It proposes policies, strategies and priorities in the following areas:

- health research and surveillance
- health information systems
- health promotion and education
- HIV and AIDS, and sexually transmitted diseases
- communicable and non-communicable control
- disabilities
- reproductive health
- human resources development
- nutrition and food safety
- violence and substance abuse.

Conclusion

As shown in this chapter, the South African health system is constantly under review so that it is able to provide quality care for all its citizens. The current and most challenging change is the implementation of the NHI; it will be interesting to watch the progress of this initiative.

Self-assessment

1. Explain how the Constitution of South Africa ensures that the health rights of people in South Africa are protected.
2. List three laws that have influenced the delivery of healthcare in South Africa since 1994.
3. Compare patients' rights with patients' responsibilities.
4. Discuss the progress and achievements to date with the implementation of the National Health Insurance.
5. Define primary healthcare (PHC).
6. Describe the roles and responsibilities of the PHC outreach teams.
7. What is the contextual background of PHC re-engineering in South Africa?
8. Explain the role of the Office of the Health Compliance Standard and how its objectives are achieved.
9. What is the role of the Southern African Development Community (SADC) in strengthening health-related policies in southern Africa.

Bibliography

African National Congress (ANC). 1994. A national health plan for South Africa. Available: http:// www.anc.org.za/ancdocs/policy/health.htm (Accessed 21 September 2020).

Declaration of Alma-Ata. 1979. International Conference on Primary Health Care, Alma-Ata, USSR, 6-12. Available: http://www.who.int/publications/almaata_declaration_en.pdf (Accessed 21 September 2020).

Dennill, K., King, I. & Swanepoel, T. 1999. *Aspects of Primary Health Care.* Cape Town: Oxford University Press.

Department of Health (DOH). 2011. *National Core Standards for Health Establishments in South Africa.* Pretoria: Department of Health.

Department of Health (DOH). 2012. Integrated school health policy. Available: www. education.gov.za (Accessed 21 September 2020).

Department of Health (DOH). 2013. *Integrated School Health Policy.* Pretoria: National Department of Health, National Department of Education.

Department of Health (DOH). 2017a. *National Health Insurance.* Government Gazette, Pretoria.

Department of Health (DOH). 2017b. *National Health Insurance Policy: Towards Universal Health Coverage.* Pretoria: National Department of Health.

Department of Health (DOH). 2017c. NHI White Paper. Pretoria: National Department of Health.

Department of Health (DOH). 2017d. National Health Act, 2003: National Health Insurance Policy: Towards Universal Health Coverage. Pretoria: Department of Health.

Department of Health (DOH). nd. Evaluation of Phase 1 implementation of interventions in the National Health Insurance (NHI) pilot districts in South Africa, Evaluation Report, Final. NDOH10/2017-2018.

Department of Health (DOH). nd. Patients' rights charter. Available: https://www.justice.gov.za/VC/docs/policy/Patient%20Rights%20Charter.pdf (Accessed 11 September 2020).

Health Professions Council of South Africa (HPCSA). nd. Summary of registered persons. Available: www.hpcsa.co.za (Accessed 21 September 2020).

Nxumalo, N., Alaba, O., Harris, B., Chersich, M. & Goudge, J. 2011. Utilization of traditional healers in South Africa and costs to patients: Findings from a national household survey. *Journal of Public Health Policy,* 32(1): 124–136.

PHASA. 2011. The implementation of PHC re-engineering in South Africa. Available: https://phasa.org.za/2011/11/15/the-implementation-of-phc-re-engineering-in-south-africa/ (Accessed 21 September 2020).

Republic of South Africa (RSA). 1996. Constitution, Act 108 of 1996. *Government Gazette.* Pretoria: Government Printer. Available: http://www.gov.za/constitution (Accessed 21 September 2020).

Republic of South Africa (RSA). 1997. Batho Pele principles. Available: www.info.gov.za/whitepapers/1997/118340.pdf (Accessed 21 September 2020).

Republic of South Africa (RSA). 2003. National Health Act No. 61 of 2003. *Government Gazette.* Pretoria: Government Printer.

Southern African Development Community (SADC). 2010. Health sector policy framework. Available: www.sadc.int/themes/health (Accessed 21 September 2020).

World Health Organization (WHO). 1978a. Alma Ata Declaration on primary health care. Available: http://www.who.int/publications/almaata_declaration_en.pdf (Accessed 21 September 2020).

World Health Organization (WHO). 1978b. Primary health care. Report of the international conference on primary health care. Geneva: WHO.

World Health Organization (WHO). 2003. The core principles of primary care. Available: www.who./whr/2003/chapter 7/en/index1.html (Accessed 21 September 2020).

World Health Organization (WHO). nd. Health financing for universal coverage: What is universal coverage? Available: www.who.int/health_financing/universal_coverage_definition/en/ (Accessed 21 September 2020).

4 Promoting health through health education

Shanti Ramkilowan

Learning outcomes

After studying this chapter, you should be able to:

- Define health promotion and health education.
- Explain how health education forms part of the three levels of disease prevention.
- Describe the different teaching methods that can be used in health education.
- Discuss the principles of successful health education programmes.

Key terms

Preventative medicine: A medicine or other treatment designed to stop disease or ill health from occurring.

Self-determination: The process by which a country or person controls its/his/ her own statehood or life.

Therapeutic: Relating to the healing of disease; administered or applied for reasons of health.

Introduction

The first international conference on health promotion held in Ottawa in 1986 was a response to growing expectations for a new public health movement around the world. A series of actions was then launched to achieve the goal of 'Health for All' by the year 2000 and beyond. Since then, the World Health Organization (WHO) health promotion conferences have established and developed the global strategies for health promotion.

The three basic strategies for health promotion identified in the Ottawa Charter were to advocate for health (ie to boost the factors which encourage health), enable all people to achieve health equity, and mediate through collaboration across all sectors.

The fundamental requirements for improvement in health are peace, shelter, education, food, income, a stable eco-system, sustainable resources, social justice and equity.

Definition of health promotion

The Ottawa Charter defines health promotion as the process of enabling people to increase control over, and to improve, their health. To reach a state of complete physical, mental and social well-being, an individual or group must be able to identify and realise aspirations, to satisfy needs and to change or cope with the environment.

(WHO, 1986)

The Ottawa Charter recognises that both the individual and the community have to be involved in the process of promoting health. Giving people the information they need through health-education programmes enables them to become more skilled in making healthy choices. This remains an important role for the health practitioner. However, health promotion cannot happen in isolation. A good health promotion programme must include activities that aim to make conditions favourable, through advocacy for health, by:

- assisting in the development of good public health policy that promotes health
- encouraging a supportive, healthy environment through political, social, cultural and economic development
- strengthening community involvement in health issues and care
- changing health services from curative-centred to more comprehensive, holistic healthcare.

Health promotion embraces a broad range of activities, including health education to empower individuals and/or communities to achieve optimum health status. In this way health promotion is about building capability. Health promotion programmes must include the whole spectrum of human growth and development from birth to old age. Some examples of health promotion activities include healthy lifestyle programmes, health surveillance, substance abuse programmes, stress management and research to promote good health.

Health education

Health education is an important component of health promotion and of preventative medicine. It is an active process directed at changing people's attitudes and influencing their behaviour in health-related matters. Health education is one of the measures of health promotion. Although health education is a process that is part of health promotion, it is not a term to be used interchangeably with health promotion. There is a vast difference between health education and health promotion. Health education involves providing individuals with information in relation to health-related topics, whereas health promotion is a broader concept. Health education enables people to take an increased interest in and responsibility for their own health. Health education programmes assist in fulfilling specific needs of a person or group of individuals, using specialised knowledge and skills. Health education helps build knowledge, skills and positive attitudes about health. It motivates individuals and communities to improve and maintain their health, prevent disease and reduce risky behaviours.

Definition of health education

The WHO defines health education as 'any combination of learning experiences designed to help individuals and communities improve their health, by increasing their knowledge or influencing their attitudes'.
(WHO, 2020)

All the members of the healthcare team are involved in providing health education – the doctors, nurses (and especially community nurses), social workers, physiotherapists, environmental officers, agricultural extension officers, pharmacists and community-based healthcare workers. Teachers in particular have an important role to play as it is much easier to modify behaviour and instil healthy habits in children than it is in adults. Health education includes personal education and development, mass media information and education.

Health education forms part of comprehensive healthcare at all three levels of prevention:

- **Primary prevention** focuses on information and campaigns to give people what they need to prevent them from becoming infected or ill. These include immunisation campaigns and campaigns that promote condom use to prevent the spread of sexually transmitted infections (STIs), including HIV and AIDS.
- **Secondary prevention** refers to educational and other strategies that minimise the risks of ill health by encouraging early diagnosis and treatment that will limit the course of the disease and prevent recurrence.
- **Tertiary prevention** is the education given to someone who has a disease or condition that results in an illness. It aims to ensure that treatment is taken properly and that complications do not occur.

Outcomes of health education

The process of a good health-education programme is to communicate with people and give them the information they need to attain good health. Health education should aim to achieve the following goals:

- Encourage people to value their health and to regard it as something that is worth striving for. Health education will not be effective unless the people who are involved in the process are value-positive about health and believe that it is worth making an effort to achieve a state of well-being.

- Help people to understand the principles of healthy living. This should include the principles of mental, social and physical health.

- Empower people to deal with their own health problems, where possible, and to know when to seek help. Empowerment includes giving people the necessary information concerning health services and encouraging them to make full use of the services that are available.

- Provide people with the necessary knowledge about diseases and conditions that are common in their community so they can take appropriate preventative steps, or if diseases do occur, they can seek early medical assistance.

Teaching methods

Everyone learns in a different way. It has been proven that learning is more effective if people participate in the learning process and when the learning can be applied to real-life situations. There are different methods of teaching, including the following:

- **Formal lesson or lecture**: This is the most common method of teaching and is best suited to convey information to a large group of people. It is cost-effective, but is often also the least effective method as the learner listens to the lesson but does not participate in the learning process in any other way.

- **Demonstration**: This method works well in smaller groups and for one-on-one learning situations. It takes more time but is a good learning experience as the learner listens, sees and does. It is ideal for teaching patients the skills they need to improve self-care. An example is teaching patients with diabetes mellitus how to give themselves insulin injections.

- **Group discussion**: This method can be used very successfully in health education. A group is regarded as two or more people who interact with each other. In health education they must have a common interest or goal and the 'teacher' should help them to work together, to share information and to solve common problems they experience regarding health issues.

- **Role play**: This is a method of teaching where the participants act out real-life situations and problems; these are then discussed and possible solutions are determined. Role play offers a safe environment where people can discuss problems and determine different ways of dealing with them.
- **Games**: They have limited application but can be used successfully as they bring an element of fun into learning.
- **Case study**: This learning process is based on a real-life situation or challenge. It looks at what has happened and how the situation could have been different. This method can be used to help learners to develop problem-solving and decision-making skills.

Teaching aids and media

People remember more if they hear, see and do activities in the process of learning. Therefore, audio-visual aids such as pictures, diagrams, PowerPoint presentations, videos, CDs and DVDs are useful. However, these teaching aids must be suitable and appropriate for the situation, for example, if a chart is used it must be big enough for the group to see and simple enough to get the message across.

Mass-media education and information is popular; it raises public awareness and offers advice on health risks. It can take the form of advertising, marketing and news information, through daily newspapers, television, radio and the internet.

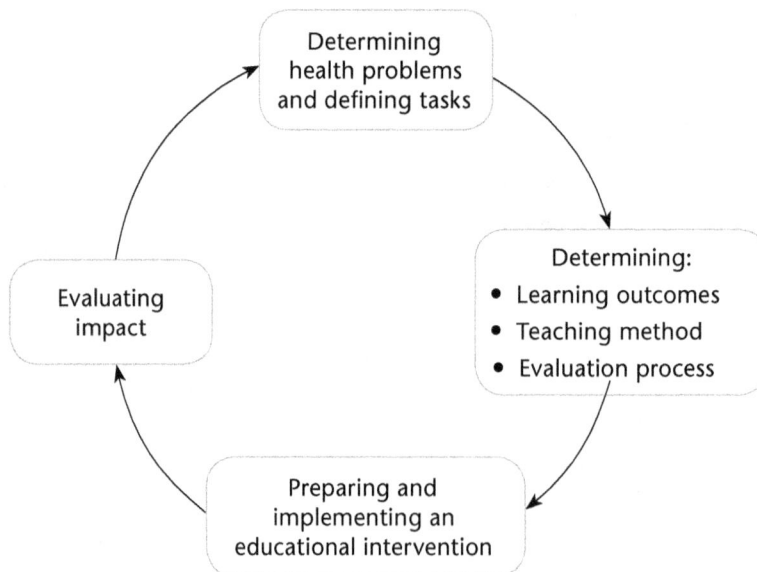

Figure 4.1 Process of developing a health education intervention

Planning a health education session

It is important that careful thought goes into planning a health education session. Several factors must be considered in addition to determining the venue, time available, duration of the session, and seeking permission from relevant authorities. The following is a useful guide for a health educator planning an education session:

- **Title of the topic**: Select a topic that has been identified as a need in the community, for example learning about the advantages of breastfeeding.

- **Set the objectives**: The objectives determine the content of the topic and set the boundaries or limits. The objectives should be well defined and limited in number.

- **Target group**: Know the audience well, determine their level of knowledge, the language they speak, the age group, their cultural orientation and how they feel and what they know about the topic.

- **Teaching method**: Determine the method you will use to deliver the education session, for example a group discussion or a combination of methods. It is important to relate information to people's everyday experiences for better understanding.

- **Teaching aids:** Decide on the teaching aids that you will use to keep their interest and facilitate understanding of the discussion. Choose teaching aids that are suited to the target group, topic and venue, such as colourful posters or a PowerPoint presentation.

- **Content**: Make sure that you have a good knowledge of the topic under discussion. Determine what the audience already knows about the topic and adapt the content accordingly. The content should have an introduction, a body, conclusion, summary and method of evaluation. Use key words and phrases rather than detailed sentences.

- **Summary**: A summary is a good way of ensuring that all the main points of the topic have been covered.

- **Evaluation**: The evaluation will indicate if the objectives or goals of the teaching session have been met. The method of evaluation should be included in the plan, for example decide whether you will be using verbal questioning or practical tasks to assess their knowledge.

Organisations promoting health through education

The following are examples of organisations involved in promoting health through education:

- **Government departments**: The Department of Health produces vast quantities of material that is available for distribution at national, provincial and district level.

- **Professional organisations**: The South African Medical Association, the Pharmaceutical Society of South Africa, the South African Nursing Council and professional nursing associations encourage their members to get involved in health education and to offer information through their publications.
- **Non-governmental organisations**: The Red Cross Society, the South African National Tuberculosis Association, the Health Systems Trust, the Cancer Association of South Africa and many others are actively involved in health-education programmes that aim to inform the public about the early signs and symptoms of certain conditions. These organisations also encourage the public to seek medical advice and make use of the available services, such as education programmes for HIV and AIDS prevention and management.

Important principles for success in health education

For teaching to be effective, the health educator must know and understand the following principles that promote success in health education:

- Health education is more than simply providing the public with information about some aspect of health. If people's attitudes and health-related behavioural patterns are to be changed, it is essential that they be motivated to change.
- Health educators should know the community in which they work. They should understand the attitudes, values and beliefs that influence behaviour.
- Health education is most effective when the educator is a member of the community in which she or he serves.
- Educators should use basic communication skills and teach in the language of the target group to facilitate understanding of what is being taught.
- Topics must be relevant and important to the community and not what the educator deems to be important. Therefore, education should follow general discussions with the community.
- Health educators should gain the support of the leaders who best represent the opinions of the community in order to ensure success.
- The modification of behaviour that is being sought should bring as little change as possible to the way of life of the target group.
- The community should be actively involved in the programme.
- The health educator should be enthusiastic about the topic and create a good, stimulating teaching and learning environment.
- The application of the principles of teaching and learning will enhance the success of the health-education programme.
- The health educators should know their limitations and be able to evaluate their own teaching. Evaluation is an important aspect of health education. Changes in behaviour towards health may not be observed immediately.

However, progressive changes can be seen over a period of time, for example improved compliance with treatment programmes such as weight loss in obese persons, or better nutrition management within families. Questionnaires and follow-up visits are useful to obtain feedback.

Conclusion

Health education is the basis of preventative medicine and an important component of public healthcare and promotive health. There are many conditions that seriously threaten the health of certain groups and that cannot be prevented or controlled without change occurring in the way the people in those groups live their lives. Health education is an important part of that process, but on its own it has limited value in promoting the health status of a community or group. Health education has to be seen as a part of the broader range of health-promoting activities if it is to be a successful tool to help people attain optimal health for themselves and their communities.

Self-assessment

1. Define health promotion and health education.
2. Identify one disease or condition that you are familiar with and plan a health-education session using the following headings:
    * Title
    * Target group
    * Teaching method and teaching aids
    * Content to be covered
    * Evaluation.
3. Identify what the outcomes will be of the teaching programme that you decided on in question 2. (What must people know and what skills must they have learnt?)
4. Explain the principles that make up a good health-education programme.

Bibliography

Boyd, M.D., Graham, B.A., Gleit, C.J. & Whitman, N.I. 1998. *Health Teaching in Nursing Practice: A Professional Model.* Stamford, CT: Appleton & Lange.

Coulson, N. & Goldstein, S. 1998. *Promoting Health in South Africa: An Action Manual.* Sandton: Heinemann.

Denehy, J. 2001. Health education: An important role for school nurses. *The Journal of School Nursing,* 17(5), 233–238.

Ehlers, V.J. 2002. *Teaching Aspects of Health Care*. 2nd edition. Cape Town: Juta.

Guilbert, J.J. 1998. *Educational Handbook for Health Personnel*. 6th edition. Geneva: WHO.

Hattingh, S. & Acutt, J. 2011. *Occupational Health – Management & Practice for Health Practitioners*. 4th revised edition. Cape Town: Juta.

Nutbeam, D. 2019. Health education and health promotion revisited. *Health Education Journal*, 78(6):705–709.

World Health Organization (WHO). 1986. Ottawa Charter for health promotion: An international conference on health promotion. Geneva: WHO. Available: https://www.who.int/healthpromotion/conferences/previous/ottawa/en/ (Accessed 12 March 2020).

World Health Organization (WHO). 2020: What is health promotion? Available: https://www.who.int/westernpacific/news/q-a-detail/what-is-health-promotion- (Accessed 15 September 2020).

Epidemiology and health information

Shanti Ramkilowan

5 CHAPTER

Learning outcomes

After studying this chapter, you should be able to:

- Define the following terms: epidemiology, statistics, data and information.
- Describe the uses of epidemiological studies.
- Define what is meant by demographic data and health data.
- Define what is meant by International Classification of Diseases (ICD).
- Define what is meant by health information management systems.
- Describe common basic epidemiological measurements or rates.
- Explain how health statistics may be used to improve practice.
- Briefly describe different epidemiological methods.

Key terms

Data: Known facts and collected statistics.

Epidemic: An epidemic occurs when there is a larger than expected increase in the number of cases of a disease in a community or geographic area.

Epidemiology: The study of the distribution and determinants of health-related conditions and events in populations and the application of this study to the control of health problems.

Information: Facts and data gathered about an issue of importance to researchers.

Rate: A measurement of the change in a quantity in a stated period of time.

Statistics: The systematic collection, organisation, analysis and interpretation of numerical data pertaining to any subject.

Introduction

Epidemiology is a science that studies disease in order to determine the causes of that disease. This science grew out of the study of the epidemics of communicable diseases, such as cholera, plague and smallpox, which occurred during the 19th century. The main areas of concern of the early epidemiologists were the communicable diseases, but many of these diseases are now controlled, or in the case of smallpox, eradicated from the world. Epidemiologists have now turned their attention to the 'new' epidemics such as coronary artery disease, road accidents and malignant disease, all of which play an important part in the health of populations today. However, the emergence of new communicable diseases such as HIV and AIDS, and the increase in the number of people presenting with tuberculosis, has brought the attention of epidemiologists back to communicable diseases.

Using epidemiology in healthcare practice

The health practitioner uses epidemiology as the basis for providing good and appropriate healthcare. The basic process of conducting an epidemiological study is to determine questions that will generate data or information that can be used for planning, managing and evaluating activities required to promote health and to prevent and control disease. It is a form of problem solving using questions, or basic epidemiological tools, to find answers.

The following questions are used by health professionals to solve health problems and determine best practices:

- **What?** What is the nature of the health problem, disease or condition, and what are its manifestations and characteristics?

- **Who?** Who is affected? Reference should be made to age, sex, race, religious group, occupation, socioeconomic status, personal habits and whether the condition that occurs is hereditary. Other issues, such as nutritional and immune status, would also be identified here.

- **Where?** Where does the problem occur? Is it related to where the person lives or the place where he or she works? Issues related to whether the area is urban or rural, the altitude above sea level, desert or farmable land, environmental status and access to health services will all be identified.

- **When?** When does it happen in relation to the day, seasons, months or years? Or does it happen as a result of a certain activity? When are the health problems at their most severe or when in the year does the incidence of certain conditions, such as diarrhoea, or diseases such as measles, increase?

➡

- **How?** How does the health problem, the disease or the condition occur? Is there a microorganism, a chemical substance or an environmental factor that causes the disease? Are certain groups susceptible or are there other contributing factors that influence the health problem, disease or condition?
- **Why?** Why does the problem occur? Are there reasons for its occurrence or for its persistence?

Based on the data and information gained from the answers to these questions, an intervention or way of solving the problem can be identified and implemented.

So, what next? Has the problem been resolved completely or partially? Has the intervention been successful? This is the evaluation part of the process and can be done using the same questions again to see if the answers have changed. The problem can be reassessed if the intervention was not successful to come up with new ideas to solve the problem.

Epidemiological studies are used in a number of different situations to ensure and improve healthcare. Studies can be used to:

- determine the extent of a problem, or how, what and when a problem occurs in a community
- study the distribution of the disease or find out where it occurs
- construct theories concerning the causation of the disease or determine why it occurs
- develop programmes and interventions that are designed to prevent the condition or reduce the incidence
- evaluate such programmes to determine whether or not the problem has been resolved.

Epidemiology is a quantitative science. This means that it deals in quantities of something that is measurable. However, it is very difficult, if not impossible, to measure health directly. The epidemiologist therefore measures the amount of ill health that is present in a population and then infers or deduces the state of health of the people from the data obtained. To do this, statistics are identified and used as tools in epidemiology. The following types of data are collected as the basis of epidemiological studies:

- Demographic data, which include population and vital statistics
- Health data, which include morbidity and mortality statistics.

Demographic data

The collection of population data is based on the formation of categories or divisions. All persons presumed to have certain characteristics in common are placed in a particular division or category. These categories include age, sex, race or ethnic group, marital status, income level and occupation. Other categories can be included, such as religion, socioeconomic status and place of residence. The data that are obtained supply information concerning the composition of the population, as well as its distribution. The most important source of such data is the national census, which is carried out every 5 to 10 years. A census is designed to count all the people in the population.

In the years between censuses the figures are kept up to date by adding births and immigrants to the census figures and subtracting deaths and emigrants. The most common basic epidemiological measurements (rates) are:

- Crude birth rate (CBR):

$$\frac{\text{Number of live births in a calendar year}}{\text{Total population}} \times 1\ 000$$

- Crude death rate (CDR):

$$\frac{\text{Number of deaths in a calendar year}}{\text{Total population}} \times 1\ 000$$

These are known as crude rates because the age and sex composition of the population is not taken into account.

More refined mortality (death) rates may also be used, such as:

- Perinatal death rate:

$$\frac{\text{Number of deaths of infants in the first week of life in a calendar year}}{\text{Number of live births in that year}} \times 1\ 000$$

- Neonatal death rate:

$$\frac{\text{Number of deaths of infants during the first four weeks of life in a calendar year}}{\text{Number of live births in that year}} \times 1\ 000$$

- Infant mortality rate (IMR):

$$\frac{\text{Number of deaths of infants during the first year of life in a calendar year}}{\text{Number of live births in that year}} \times 1\ 000$$

- Maternal mortality rate (MMR):

$$\frac{\text{Number of deaths due to pregnancy or childbirth in a calendar year}}{\text{Number of live births in that year}} \times 1\ 000$$

Other specific death rates may be used, such as cause-specific death rates. For example, the number of deaths as a result of drowning in a calendar year, or the number of suicides. It is possible to compute cause-specific death rates because it is compulsory to enter the cause of death on a death certificate. Rates of natural population increase are calculated as follows:

$$\frac{(\text{Births} - \text{deaths}) + (\text{immigration} - \text{emigration})}{\text{Total population}} \times 100$$

For example:

$$\frac{\text{CBR (eg 17.2)} - \text{CDR (eg 8.2)}}{17.2 - 8.2 = 9.0 \text{ per 1 000}}$$

Therefore, the rate of natural increase is 9.0 per 1 000 or 0.9 per 100. The rate of natural increase is usually expressed as a percentage; in this case it is 0.9 per cent.

The rate of natural increase indicates how fast a population is growing. Some parts of the world are now seeing smaller increments of growth, and some, such as Japan, Germany and Spain, are actually experiencing population decreases.

In the past year, the population of the African continent grew by 30 million. The Continent of Africa is home to 1.2 billion people (2016), up from just over 477 in 1980. Population in South Africa as per statistics South Africa was 59,62 million (July 2020). By the year 2050, annual increases will exceed 42 million people per year and the total population will have doubled to 2.4 billion, according to the United Nations.

This has important implications for world health as it is doubtful that food production can be increased sufficiently to feed all these people in a relatively short time, or if sufficient educational and employment opportunities and sufficient housing can be provided. It will also impact on the healthcare services that will be required to meet growing needs.

The Births, Marriages and Deaths Registration Act 81 of 1963 makes it compulsory to register all births and deaths and these registration records form another important source of data. The numerical data that are collected through the registration of these 'vital' events in the lives of people, such as birth, marriage and death, are referred to as *vital statistics*.

Health data

Health data are factual numerical data concerning the health of a group of people or the population as a whole. This includes data or statistics concerning disease (morbidity) and death (mortality). Health data are commonly obtained from the following sources:

- Hospital records are a useful source of morbidity data.
- Notification records of specified diseases. In all countries, it is mandatory to report certain diseases to the local health authorities. In South Africa, regulations promulgated under the new National Health Act 61 of 2003 list the conditions that have to be notified.
- Clinic records.
- Records from schools and school health services.
- Records from private health practitioners.
- Records of medical examinations from large organisations, such as the mines or the defence force.
- Epidemiological survey reports.

The epidemiologist uses the data to calculate the frequency of a condition in a particular population. This is referred to as a rate. Rates are expressed as the number of people or cases per 100, 1 000, 10 000, or 100 000 people, which makes it possible to compare the frequency of a disease, condition or cause of death among different groups. The rates most commonly used for this purpose are prevalence and incidence rates.

Prevalence and incidence rates

Prevalence and incidence rates provide information concerning the levels of disease in a population, the rate of disease development and the risk of disease. The prevalence rate is a measure of existing disease in a population at a particular time, whereas the incidence rate reflects the number of new cases developing in a population at risk during a specific time period.

$$\text{Prevalence rate} = \frac{\text{Total number of people suffering from the disease at a given time}}{\text{Total number of people in the population at the same time}} \times 100$$

One can calculate the presence of a specific disease; eg in a survey of the prevalence of tuberculosis in a population of 2 000 nursing students attending a particular nursing training college, 50 students were reported to have the disease already. The prevalence rate of tuberculosis in this population would be:

$$\frac{50 \times 100}{2\,000} = 2.5\%$$

This means that 2.5 per cent of students already have the disease in this particular population group.

$$\text{The incidence rate} = \frac{\text{Number of new cases of a disease during a specific time}}{\text{Number of people in the population who are at risk from the disease at the given time}} \times 100$$

Using the example above, one could follow the remaining students (ie 1 950 students) in this group over a period of time, eg one year, and note the number of new cases of tuberculosis among these students. If there were 10 new cases, the incidence rate of tuberculosis would be:

$$\frac{10 \times 100}{1\ 950} = 0.5\%$$

This means that the incidence of new cases is 0.5 per cent over a period of one year.

Incidence rates are more applicable to acute conditions such as infectious or communicable diseases like tuberculosis or HIV and AIDS, while prevalence rates are more useful when dealing with chronic conditions such as malnutrition or ischaemic heart disease.

International Classification of Diseases

The International Classification of Diseases (ICD) was endorsed by the 43rd World Health Assembly in 1990 and came into use from 1994. The ICD is the international standard classification of all diseases and conditions, achieved by giving them certain codes that are internationally recognised. Important functions of the ICD are listed below:

- It is used to classify diseases on health records such as a patient's health file and vital records such as death certificates.
- It enables the storage and retrieval of diagnostic information for epidemiological purposes and is used as a basis for the compilation of national mortality and morbidity statistics.
- It is also used to analyse the general health situation of population groups and to monitor the incidence and prevalence of diseases and other health problems, eg HIV and AIDS, tuberculosis, diabetes and various types of cancer.

Using health statistics

Statistics consist of data that are usually expressed as numbers. These numbers mean very little on their own and at this stage are often referred to as *raw data* (eg the outbreak of the coronavirus (COVID-19) at the end of 2019). Once the data are applied to the actual situation and the variables or conditions in which they occur, an analysis is done. This determines whether the situation or practice is good or identifies areas that are problematic and need improving, or whether a change in practice is required. In other words, data provide meaning to a given situation. Data now become information that can be used by the health practitioner to solve problems or prove that the health interventions or practices are successful. This research process is the basis of good healthcare as health practitioners can generate information to improve the care they give their clients. This is referred to as *determining best practice*.

Statistics ———————→ Data ———————→ Information

Information generated through this process will enable healthcare authorities to plan the type, the size and the location of such services on the basis of factual information. This information can also be used to determine:

- which conditions need to be prioritised
- areas of high or increasing incidence of disease, thus drawing attention to problem situations, eg the global coronavirus outbreak (COVID-19) and multiple-drug-resistant tuberculosis
- the extent of ill health occurring in a certain area at a given time or over a period of time
- a picture of the distribution of a disease, potentially giving important clues to the factors associated with the disease and that may contribute to its occurrence
- the information necessary for epidemiological and medical research
- the authorities responsible for allocating scarce resources based on the area with the greatest need
- the basis on which preventative health programmes are planned
- the evaluation of the effectiveness of such preventative health programmes.

Health information systems

A health information system captures and processes information about the health of individuals and the activities of a healthcare system.

(WHO, 2008)

Health information management systems

Health information is the data related to a person's medical history, including symptoms, diagnoses, procedures and outcomes. A health information management system is a system that is designed to manage a person's health data. The system collects, stores and manages a patient's medical records electronically. This electronic system protects digital and traditional medical information vital to providing quality patient care.

Health information systems benefit the health industry by improving cost control, speeding up the retrieval time of information compared to manual retrieval, improving accuracy of patient care, increasing service capacity, and reducing personnel costs.

Epidemiological research methods

Observational methods refer to studies that make use of observational methods. These can be further divided into the following categories:

- **Descriptive studies**: These studies describe patterns of disease in human populations and are concerned with the frequency and the distribution of disease (how, when and where).

- **Analytic studies**: These studies are designed to answer the question why and examine the relationship between the factors operating in the situation and try to explain the reasons for the disease pattern. Analytic studies often involve a comparison of disease frequencies in different groups.

- **Experimental methods**: These methods are used to test the efficiency of some preventative measures, eg immunisation. Let us presume that a new 'cold' vaccine has been developed. In order to test its efficacy, two groups of people are selected, the experimental group and the control group. The vaccine is administered to the experimental group and not to the control group. When anyone in either group develops a cold, it is recorded. If, at the end of the experiment, significantly fewer people in the experimental group developed colds, we may accept that the vaccine is an effective measure in the prevention of colds.

Epidemiology and demography are the foundations on which community health is planned and their importance to all health workers cannot be overemphasised.

Conclusion

The collection of accurate data allows the epidemiologist to plan for and provide appropriate healthcare. Without this data, it is not possible to understand what the population's health problems are, or where and how they occur.

Self-assessment

1. List five sources from which health data may be obtained.
2. Describe the types of question that health professionals use to collect data.
3. Describe the value or uses of epidemiological studies in order to improve healthcare.
4. Briefly explain three epidemiological research methods used by epidemiologists to generate data.

Bibliography

Erlich, R. & Joubert, G. 2014. *Epidemiology: A Research Manual for South Africa*. Cape Town: Oxford University Press Southern Africa.

Stanhope, M. & Lancaster, J. 2015. *Public Health Nursing: Population-Centered Health Care in the Community*. Washington, NC: Mosby.

The Guardian. 2016. Population growth in Africa – grasping the scale of the challenge. Available: https://www.populationmedia.org/2016/01/11/population-growth-in-africa/ (Accessed 13 September 2020).

Vaughn, J.P. & Morrow, R.H. 1989. *Manual of Epidemiology for District Health Management*. Geneva: WHO.

World Health Organization (WHO). 2008. Framework and standards for country health information systems (Health Metrics Network). Available: https://www.who.int/healthinfo/country_monitoring_evaluation/who-hmn-framework-standards-chi.pdf (Accessed 14 September 2020).

Non-communicable diseases

Shanti Ramkilowan

Learning outcomes

After studying this chapter, you should be able to:

- Explain what a non-communicable disease is.
- Differentiate between acute and chronic diseases.
- Explain what is meant by primary, secondary and tertiary prevention.
- Discuss the priority chronic diseases in South Africa using the following headings: aetiology, preventative measures and care.
- Discuss the care for patients with chronic non-communicable diseases.

Key terms

Acute disease: Refers to a disease or condition that produces signs and symptoms suddenly or soon after exposure to the cause.

Aetiology: The cause of disease or reason why it occurs.

Chronic disease: This disease or condition is usually the result of an acute illness from which the person does not recover fully. A chronic disease produces signs and symptoms over a varying period of time and results in only partial recovery.

Hospice: A nursing home or haven where very ill or terminally ill patients are cared for, made as comfortable as possible and allowed to die with dignity.

Keratosis: The formation of a horny growth of skin tissue found in the elderly.

Leukoplakia: Precancerous white patches on mucous membranes.

Malaise: Feeling uneasy or unwell.

> **Non-communicable diseases (NCDs)**: A broad term that refers to all conditions not caused by a microorganism and that are therefore not transferable from one person to another.
>
> **Remission**: The abatement of an illness that may be temporary or permanent.
>
> **Trauma**: Injury or death caused by an unanticipated or unexpected event.

Introduction

According to the Global Action Plan for the Prevention and Control of NCDs 2013–2020, non-communicable diseases – mainly cardiovascular diseases, cancers, chronic respiratory diseases and diabetes – are the biggest cause of death worldwide (WHO, 2013). More than 36 million people die annually from NCDs (63 per cent of global deaths), including 14 million people who die prematurely before the age of 70. More than 90 per cent of these premature deaths from NCDs occur in low- and middle-income countries and could have largely been prevented. Most premature deaths are linked to common risk factors, namely tobacco use, unhealthy diet, physical inactivity and harmful use of alcohol.

These risk factors are the result of lifestyle choices and therefore the incidence of the diseases can be reduced drastically if people simply change to healthier lifestyles. Intervention at the family and community level is essential in the prevention and control of NCDs.

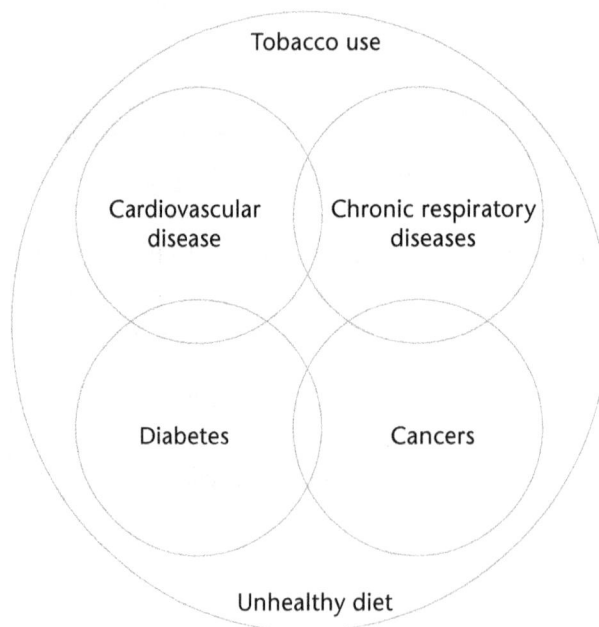

Figure 6.1 The world's biggest killer diseases and the shared risk factors
Source: Adapted from WHO (2013)

The global action plan (2013–2020) passed by the World Health Organization (WHO) encourages the establishment of programmes for the prevention and control of NCDs to help millions of people affected by these lifelong diseases. The strategy has a particular focus on low- and middle-income countries and vulnerable populations. According to the global action plan, up to 80 per cent of heart disease, stroke and type 2 diabetes, and over a third of cancers, can be prevented by eliminating the shared risk factors.

Key facts

- Non-communicable diseases (NCDs) kill 41 million people each year globally.
- Over 85 per cent of these 'premature' deaths occur in low- and middle-income countries.
- Cardiovascular diseases account for most NCD deaths, or 17.9 million people annually, followed by cancers (9.0 million), respiratory diseases (3.9 million), and diabetes (1.6 million).
- These four groups of diseases account for over 80 per cent of all premature NCD deaths.
- Tobacco use, physical inactivity, the harmful use of alcohol and unhealthy diets all increase the risk of dying from an NCD.
- Detection, screening and treatment of NCDs, as well as palliative care, are key components of the response to NCDs.

Source: WHO (2018b)

Non-communicable diseases

The prevention and control of non-communicable diseases

The WHO has identified the following six objectives for the prevention and control of NCDs:

- Reduce the level of exposure of individuals and populations to the main common and shared risk factors, namely tobacco use, unhealthy diet, physical inactivity and the harmful use of alcohol.
- Strengthen healthcare for people by providing cost-effective interventions, with priority given to cardiovascular diseases, diabetes, chronic respiratory diseases, cancer, oral health and sickle cell disease.
- Raise the priority accorded to NCDs at national level; integrate prevention and control of NCDs into policies and plans across all government departments.
- Establish and strengthen national policies and plans in line with the primary healthcare approach.

- Promote research for the control and prevention of NCDs.
- Promote partnerships for the control and prevention of NCDs.

Non-communicable diseases can be acute or chronic. They often result in long-term health problems that require the patient to seek help that is not only medical in nature. Therefore, the management of these diseases requires action not only by the nurse and doctor but also by other members of the multidisciplinary team, such as a physiotherapist, speech therapist, occupational therapist, psychologist and social worker.

In South Africa, the incidence of chronic diseases has increased, resulting in higher morbidity and mortality rates. According to the WHO country profiles (WHO, 2018b), in the year 2016 the South African population totalled 56 015 000, with total deaths for that year at 526 000. NCDs were estimated to account for 51 per cent of all deaths. It is clear from these statistics that there is an increased need for healthcare.

Table 6.1 Main health risk factors in the South African population

Main health risk factors in South Africa
Harmful use of alcohol
Physical inactivity
Salt/sodium intake
Tobacco use
Raised blood pressure
Diabetes
Obesity

Source: WHO (2018b)

Management of these chronic diseases should occur at primary, secondary and tertiary level.

1. Primary prevention

Primary prevention includes strategies to prevent chronic diseases from occurring. This can be done through health promotion and health education. The aim is to reduce or modify risk factors by living a healthy lifestyle and thereby reducing the risk of getting a chronic condition, for example by paying attention to patterns of food consumption, alcohol and tobacco use and physical activity levels. If people change their dietary habits and participate in regular physical activity, they can reduce the incidence of NCDs substantially.

Eating for health requires a diet that includes fresh fruit and vegetables, nuts and whole-grain foods and adequate fluid intake. Fatty, salty and sugar-rich foods should be reduced and, if necessary, a low-calorie diet should be introduced to help people reach and maintain normal body weight.

Daily exercise of at least 10 minutes, or three times a week for 30 minutes, is advocated, such as cycling or brisk walking.

Health promotion also includes having the appropriate health policies and services available to support people in attaining and maintaining optimal health.

2. Secondary prevention

This level is aimed at early diagnosis, adequate treatment and ongoing care that will ensure that the effect of the chronic condition on the health and functioning of the individual is kept to a minimum. Treatment can include a number of therapeutic interventions such as medication, chemotherapy, surgery, radiation, physiotherapy and occupational therapy. The main objective of this treatment is to contain the impact of the disease and to allow the person to attain and maintain optimal health for as long as possible. During this time, the chronic disease can go into remission and the person will then be free of all symptoms for a period of time, which may be months or years.

3. Tertiary prevention

The third management stage recognises that the person with a chronic disease has some form of disability or function loss due to the condition. The objective at this level of care is to ensure that there is no further loss of function in the affected organs or limbs and that the disease is contained to prevent further disability. This requires good patient management, support and monitoring.

Caring for patients with chronic NCD

Care should be evaluated in relation to the needs of the individual patient. It must be appropriate and holistic, and include the following three components:

1. **Medical/nursing needs**: Appropriate medicine and equipment must be made available and be easily accessible to the patient.
2. **Psychosocial needs**: Patients must be informed about the disease and the options they may follow in the management of the disease. Once patients are empowered with this knowledge, they are able to make the necessary decisions regarding the disease and how they will live with the disease. Some form of support system is necessary for patients and their family or friends to ensure that patients adhere to the treatment and care plan determined for them. This strategy will enable patients to attain optimal health within the constraints that the disease may place on their lives.

3. **Quality of life**: The individual patient and the status of the chronic condition and the patient's adjustment to having the chronic condition are assessed and reassessed from time to time. If interventions have been successful, the disease will be under control or the condition of the patient will improve. There will be less disruption of the individual's daily life, allowing them to enjoy an improved quality of life.

Adherence to or compliance with the treatment regimen is an important part of the successful treatment of chronic diseases and the prevention of complications. In diseases like hypertension, diabetes and epilepsy, medication must be taken as prescribed every day for the remainder of the patient's life. Failure to keep to the determined regimen will usually result in the disease becoming acute, with the patient requiring special care by a doctor or, in the absence of a doctor, a nurse.

For patients to adhere to the treatment plan determined for them, they have to be well informed about their condition and their treatment and they must accept the whole care plan determined for them by the multidisciplinary team. For this to happen, patients must become team members in their own care and must have a support system where they can find help in their day-to-day living. This support can be given by family members or by community support groups. The nurse's role in the successful patient care plan is to facilitate the holistic care plan and educate the patient to ensure that he or she understands and accepts the care. If the patient does not accept his or her care plan, they are unlikely to adhere to the treatment determined for them.

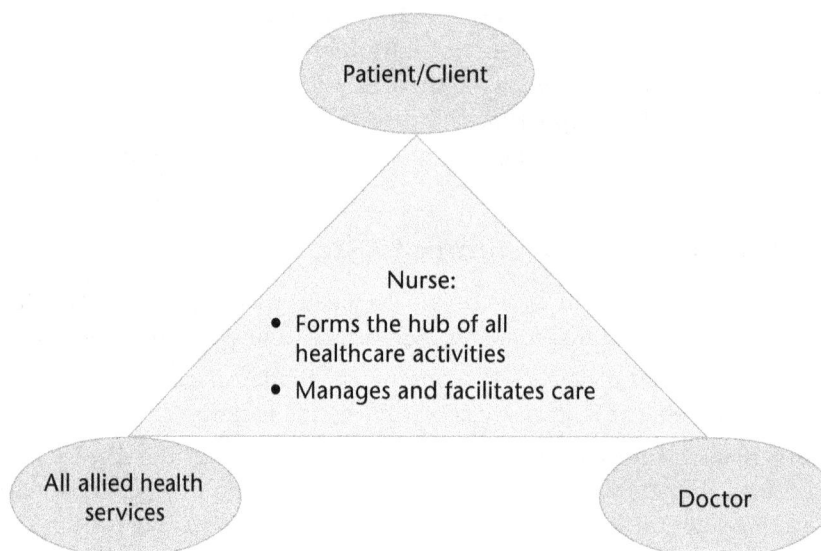

Figure 6.2 The role of the nurse in facilitating care

The most common forms of chronic diseases experienced in South Africa are cardiovascular diseases (these are a group of disorders of the heart and blood vessels and include hypertension, ischaemic heart disease/coronary artery disease, cerebrovascular disease, rheumatic heart disease/rheumatic fever, peripheral arterial disease, deep vein thrombosis and pulmonary embolism), arthritis, diabetes mellitus, cancers, chronic respiratory diseases such as asthma, and obesity and depression.

Burden of disease

A country's burden of disease refers to the assessment of mortality, morbidity, injuries, disabilities and other risk factors specific to that country. Quantifying the disease burden in a way that is internationally comparable is not an easy task. The Global Burden of Disease (GBD), a comprehensive global research study, introduced a new metric for measuring the burden of disease in an area, called the disability-adjusted life years (DALYs). The DALYs is an incidence-based measure quantifying the health gap between the actual health status of a population and a specified norm.

South Africa has a quadruple burden of disease: HIV and Aids, other communicable diseases, NCDs and injuries. This means that the country has substantially higher numbers of sick people who are sicker than those in other countries. On average, South Africa's burden of disease is four times higher than that of developed countries, and in most instances almost double that of developing countries.

Arthritis

Arthritis means joint inflammation, but the term is used to describe around 200 conditions that affect joints, the tissues that surround the joint, and other connective tissue. It is a rheumatic condition.

Aetiology

Rheumatoid arthritis is perhaps the most common chronic disease in this group and affects more women than men. The disease can affect other organs, but the main feature is the sudden inflammation of joints that occurs during the productive years of life. The causes of the disease are unknown but there are contributing factors such as abnormal immune mechanisms, infection and other metabolic factors. The patient presents with fatigue, general malaise, a fever and general aches especially in the limbs, hands and feet. Later the pain may be in one particular joint and after the acute phase the joint may be less painful but stiffness and physical changes occur, eventually resulting in limitations in movement and functioning of the affected joints.

Preventative measures

During the acute phases, patients should be put on bed rest to reduce the permanent impact of the inflammation of the joint. The doctor will usually order anti-inflammatory drugs and something for pain. A healthy balanced diet will assist in the healing process. About 5 to 10 per cent of patients will eventually become disabled despite treatment.

Nursing care

Nursing problems will be determined from the nursing assessment of the patient and from the records. Care will be determined according to the identified problems or needs of the patient and can include the following:

- Informing patients about the disease and how the effect on the joints can be reduced. This also includes important information about the treatment prescribed by the doctor, about adherence and about the aids available to assist patients to maintain their independence for as long as possible
- Ensuring that medications are available for patients and that they are aware of side-effects and any other related matters
- Helping patients with bathing, hygiene, dressing and other daily activities they are unable to do for themselves due to disability and, if necessary, using home-based care services to offer this service
- Promoting mobility and preventing further injury by positioning joints in a way that will avoid contractures, or referring patients to a physiotherapist to learn exercises to maintain optimal use of the joints
- Reconstructive surgery, if necessary.

Cancer

The types and the rates of cancer experienced in this country are increasing. Cancer is a major killer throughout the world and is a worrying trend in the South African statistics.

According to the Cancer Association of South Africa (CANSA) the main cancers affecting men in South Africa are prostate cancer, which is the most common, followed by colorectal cancer, lung cancer, cancer of unknown primary (CUP), Kaposi sarcoma, bladder cancer, Non-Hodgkin's lymphoma, malignant melanoma, oesophageal cancer and cancer of the stomach. Table 6.2 shows the top 10 most common cancers affecting men in South Africa.

Table 6.2 Top 10 most common cancers affecting men (2018)

Type of cancer for all men	Actual no of cases	Estimated lifetime risk	Percentage of all cancers
Prostate cancer	7 057	1:19	19.18%
Colorectal cancer	1 943	1:79	5.28%
Lung cancer	1 791	1:80	4.87%
Cancer of unknown primary (CUP)*	1 740	1:91	4.73%
Kaposi sarcoma	978	1:320	2.66%
Cancer of the bladder	942	1:152	2.56%
Non-Hodgkin's lymphoma	932	1:221	2.53%
Malignant melanoma	869	1:187	2.36%
Oesophageal cancer	848	1:178	2.31%
Cancer of the stomach	767	1:204	2.08%

*   Although doctors are able to identify areas affected by cancer, they are not always able to pinpoint the source, or starting point, of the cancer. This type of cancer is called a cancer of unknown primary (CUP) or occult primary tumour.

Source: Adapted from CANSA (2018)

The main cancers affecting women in South Africa are breast cancer, cervical cancer, cancer of unknown primary (CUP), colorectal cancer, uterine cancer, lung cancer, Non-Hodgkin's lymphoma, malignant melanoma, Kaposi sarcoma and cancer of the oesophagus. Both breast and cervical cancer have been identified as a national priority. Table 6.3 shows the top ten most common cancers affecting women in South Africa.

Table 6.3 Top 10 most common cancers affecting women (2018)

Type of cancer for all women	Actual no of cases	Estimated lifetime risk	Percentage of all cancers
Breast cancer	8 230	1:27	21.78%
Cervical cancer	5 735	1:42	15.17%
Cancer of unknown primary (CUP)*	1 691	1:124	4.47%
Colorectal cancer	1 620	1:134	4.29%
Cancer of the uterus	1 256	1:145	3.32%
Lung cancer	936	1:195	2.48%
Non-Hodgkin's lymphoma	870	1:296	2.30%

➡

Type of cancer for all women	Actual no of cases	Estimated lifetime risk	Percentage of all cancers
Malignant melanoma	755	1:311	2.00%
Kaposi sarcoma	669	1:555	1.77%
Oesophageal cancer	650	1:326	1.72%

* Although doctors are able to identify areas affected by cancer, they are not always able to pinpoint the source, or starting point, of the cancer. This type of cancer is called a cancer of unknown primary (CUP) or occult primary tumour.

Source: Adapted from CANSA (2018)

Millions of people die from cancer each year, accounting for 9.6 million deaths worldwide (WHO, 2018a). Research for a universal cure continues and the treatment of cancers keeps improving based on the research outcomes, and as a result the cure rate continues to rise.

Age Standardised Cancer Incidence Rates
ALL MALES: 2009

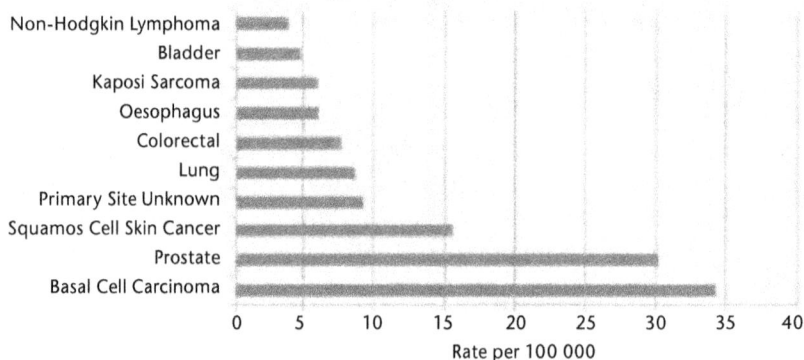

Age Standardised Cancer Incidence Rates
ALL FEMALES: 2009

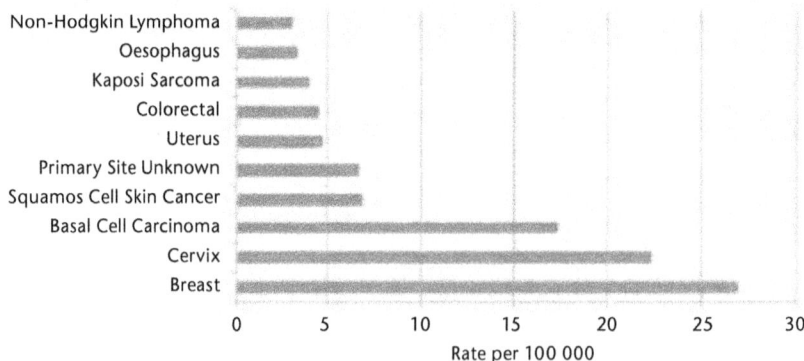

Figure 6.3 Age standardised cancer incidence rates for men and women (2009)
Source: NICD (National Cancer Registry) (2009)

Although the distribution of cancer is worldwide, there are variations in incidence and type:

- Some cancers are found more often than others; cancers of the lung, breast, cervix, stomach and colon are common, while those of the tonsil and pharynx are rare.
- The incidence and type of cancer vary from country to country and even from region to region within a country. Variations also occur between sex, population and age groups.
- Lung cancer is a growing health problem in South Africa in both sexes although males far exceed females. Tobacco use is the most important risk factor for cancer.
- Infection with high-risk human papillomavirus (HPV) is known to be a cause of cervical cancer. Other risk factors associated with cervical cancer are sexual behaviour, low socio-cultural level and smoking.
- Around one-third of deaths from cancer are due to behavioural and dietary risks: high body mass index, low fruit and vegetable intake, lack of physical activity, tobacco and alcohol use.

Aetiology

There is no single cause of cancer. It occurs as the result of an unfavourable interaction between biological, socio-cultural and environmental factors. Some of the contributing factors are discussed below.

Biological factors

The biological factors include genetic endowment, age, gender and ethnicity and race.

- **Genetic endowment**: The genes that you have received from your parents and grandparents may either protect you from cancer or predispose you to it. Certain carcinomas show a familial incidence, for instance, it has also been shown that the daughters of mothers who have breast cancer are more likely to develop this form of cancer than the general female population.
- **Age**: Although cancer occurs in all age groups, the incidence increases rapidly with increasing age. The death rate in females rises from less than 10 per 100 000 for girls under the age of 10 years to 100 per 100 000 by the age of 40 years and 1 000 per 100 000 by the age of 85.
- **Gender**: There are also variations in the incidence of the different types of cancers associated with the sexes, eg the incidence of lung cancer is higher in males than in females.

- **Ethnicity or race**: Certain types of cancer occur more frequently in some ethnic groups than in others. Examples of such variations are:
  - cancer of the nasopharynx is rare in all ethnic groups except in the Chinese, where it is common.
  - cancer of the stomach is very common in the Japanese population.
  - carcinoma of the cervix is extremely rare in Jewish women.

Socio-cultural factors

- **Economic**: Cancer mortality rates are highest in the lower economic classes. There is also a difference in the type of cancer that is most common in a particular economic group. Carcinomas of the colon and the testes, as well as leukaemia, are cancers of the wealthy, while cancers of the mouth and the cervix are more frequent among the poor.
- **Cultural**: Many cancers have their origins in habits and customs that are culturally transmitted and socially approved. Examples are cancer of the skin due to sunbathing, cancer of the liver due to food-storage methods, cancer of the colon due to the 'Western-type diet', cancer of the stomach due to the national diet of the Japanese and cancer of the mouth in the Philippines due to the chewing of betel nut and slaked lime.

Environmental factors

- **Occupational**: There are many occupations in which workers are exposed to known carcinogens daily. Consequently, they run a high risk of developing a certain kind of malignancy. The first occupational cancer to be identified was carcinoma of the scrotum, which was described by Percivall Pott in 1775. He had observed a high incidence of this condition among children who were chimney-sweeps and therefore he attributed this to be due to the presence of soot that collected on the skin of the scrotum and which, because of the poor standards of hygiene at that time, was seldom washed off. Since then a long list of such occupationally induced cancers has been compiled. The following are but a few examples of particular malignancies that have been linked to a particular occupation: cancer of the lung in miners, mesothelioma in those who work with asbestos and cancer of the bladder in aniline dye workers.
- **Chemical**: Many hundreds of substances with which people come into contact daily have been shown to have carcinogenic properties. Examples of these are asbestos, vinyl chloride, creosote, tar and benzine.
- **Tobacco**: Smoking has been linked to cancer of the lung and tongue.
- **Sunlight**: The ultraviolet rays of the sun are carcinogenic and the incidence of cancer of the skin is highest among fair-skinned people, especially those who live in countries that have many hours of sunlight each day. People who work out of doors, such as farmers, fishermen, sailors and gardeners,

as well as those who spend many hours sunbathing, are particularly prone to cancer of the skin. The condition is common in people with albinism.

- **Viruses**: Certain viruses are associated with cancer. The herpes virus is associated with cancer of the cervix and hepatitis B with liver cancer.
- **Aflatoxins**: These toxins are produced by certain strains of fungus that contaminate foods such as beans, groundnuts and cereals that have been incorrectly stored. Aflatoxins are linked to cancer of the liver.

Preventative measures

Because environmental factors play a major role in the aetiology of cancer, many cancers are preventable, and the WHO estimates that about one-third of all cancers can be prevented if timely and appropriate steps are taken.

Primary prevention: It is of the greatest importance and involves vigorous and effective health education aimed at promoting positive health; healthy living habits must be instilled during childhood and the danger of behaviours such as smoking must be stressed.

The promotion of a safe environment in which chemical pollution is strictly controlled and standards of environmental hygiene are high is an essential part of a preventative health programme.

A healthy diet containing natural foods should be encouraged. The diet should consist of relatively high amounts of carbohydrate, particularly unrefined cereals such as maize, whole wheat, unpolished rice, and fruit and vegetables. Such a diet would also be high in fibre. Intake of meat and saturated fats should be reduced, and processed foods avoided. Harmful methods of preparing and storing foods should be modified. Specific prevention involves the treatment of precancerous conditions such as cervical erosions and polyps, as well as the avoidance of known carcinogens such as tobacco, ultraviolet rays and X-rays. Vaccination against human papillomavirus (HPV) and hepatitis B virus is recommended.

Secondary prevention: The early diagnosis of cancer is required. Members of the public should be taught to recognise early warning signs and precancerous lesions and be encouraged to get medical advice immediately should they occur. Early warning signs or precancerous lesions commonly present as:
- changes in bowel or bladder habits
- a sore that does not heal
- unusual bleeding or discharge
- a thickening or lump in the breast or anywhere else in the body
- indigestion or difficulty in swallowing
- pigmented moles or obvious changes in a wart or a mole
- coughing or hoarseness
- leukoplakia of the mucous membrane of the mouth
- senile keratoses
- cervical erosions.

The prognosis is far better if the cancer is discovered in its early stages. This makes case finding particularly important in secondary prevention. Many carcinomas can be diagnosed using relatively simple techniques. For example, carcinoma of the rectum can be detected on rectal examination and the presence of occult blood in the stools, and carcinoma of the breast by self-examination of the breast. In areas where cancer of the mouth is common, health workers can be trained to carry out the necessary examinations.

Nursing care

Once the condition has been diagnosed, prompt treatment is essential. The treatment of cancer may involve the use of one or more of the following: surgical excision of the neoplasm, radiation therapy and/or chemotherapy. It is beyond the scope of this book to deal with the treatment in greater detail.

Patients who have been treated for carcinoma with surgical interventions, chemotherapy or radiation usually require support and rehabilitation. The Cancer Association of South Africa (CANSA) plays an important role in this process by assisting people who are suffering from cancer or recovering from having had cancer. Support and assistance are also given to the patient's family.

Those cancer patients who are not cured require appropriate care, pain management and other medical or nursing interventions that will allow them to maintain their independence and an optimal quality of life for as long as possible. Then they must be cared for to allow them to die in peace with dignity, free from pain and suffering minimal discomfort. Care must be holistic and requires the participation of a multidisciplinary team. The Hospice Association of South Africa is the umbrella body for hospices or organisations that offer a programme of palliative care for dying patients and their family.

Ischaemic heart disease

Hypertension has been identified as one of the five priority conditions that need to be managed to prevent associated disease such as strokes and heart attacks from occurring. The WHO defines hypertension as a consistent blood pressure above 160/95 mmHg; to reduce the risk of associated diseases occurring, a blood pressure below 140/90 mmHg must be maintained. In 1998 it was found that 16 per cent of adult men and 13 per cent of adult women were hypertensive, and only about a quarter of these were on treatment and controlled. Adherence to the treatment regimen was therefore identified as being poor.

As a result, the incidence of coronary artery disease is a major health problem affecting all South Africans. Historically, white South Africans have a much higher incidence of heart disease than black South Africans, but the number of other groups, especially Indians, presenting with ischaemic heart disease is increasing at an alarming rate. This increase is attributed to changes in diet and lifestyle.

Aetiology

There is no single cause of coronary artery disease; rather it is the result of an interaction between many factors. These risk factors include a high serum cholesterol, high blood pressure and cigarette smoking. Risk factors of lesser importance are diabetes mellitus, obesity, lack of regular exercise, psychological stress and certain personality characteristics. These risk factors have a cumulative effect and if one risk factor is present in an individual, his or her chances of developing ischaemic heart disease double; if two or more of these risk factors are present then the chances increase four to five times.

Coronary heart disease commences early in life and even in boys, certain pathological features may be present. The first step in the disease process is a thickening of the inner lining of the blood vessels of the heart and elsewhere in the body due to the deposition of fatty material, mainly cholesterol. This leads to a narrowing of the coronary arteries and may be followed many years later by the formation of a blood clot in the diseased arteries, which obstructs the flow of blood to the heart muscle and leads to the typical heart attack.

Other important factors that are associated with diseases of the heart and vessels are the following:

- **Genetic factors**: Heart diseases tend to be more prevalent in some families than in others and also in certain sections of the population. A group of Afrikaans families have an inherited condition transmitted by a dominant gene that causes hyperlipidaemia, and unless the condition is diagnosed early and treated, those affected will die of heart-related conditions in early adulthood. There is, however, a close association between serum cholesterol levels and diet. Diets high in saturated fats and foods rich in cholesterol, such as meat, eggs, milk, cream and butter, and low in grains and carbohydrates, have been referred to as the 'fatty way to heaven'.

- **Personality type**: People who have a Type-A personality are considered to be more at risk for coronary heart disease, as they tend to be more competitive, aggressive, hardworking and impatient than people with other personality types. They are always rushing to meet a deadline and trying to do as many things as possible at the same time. The stress they generate can become unhealthy if combined with general risk factors of lifestyle such as obesity, lack of exercise, high serum cholesterol levels and smoking.

- **Age**: Death rates from coronary artery disease increase progressively with age, and although heart attacks among younger men are on the increase, it is the older age groups that have the highest incidence.

- **Sex**: Men are more likely to suffer from ischaemic heart disease than women and about four times as many men as women will die from this group of diseases before they reach the age of 65 years. The incidence in women, however, increases after menopause.

- **Smoking**: There is a connection between smoking and the risk of ischaemic heart disease, and the risk increases with the number of cigarettes smoked. A person who smokes 30 cigarettes a day has a greater chance of developing ischaemic heart disease than one who smokes 10. Smoking is implicated in ischaemic heart disease because it aggravates the atherosclerotic changes in the blood vessels.
- **Diabetes mellitus**: Diabetics are more likely to suffer from atherosclerosis than non-diabetics and they are therefore more likely to suffer from these heart diseases.
- **Lack of exercise**: Exercise decreases the risk of coronary artery disease because it lowers blood cholesterol levels, reduces the clotting tendency of the blood and increases the efficiency of the heart.

Preventative measures

Primary prevention: As improved medical care and high-technology intensive coronary care units have done little to reduce mortality rates, and nothing to reduce the incidence of the condition, it is essential that health workers should turn their attention to primary prevention and particularly to health promotion. Health education aimed at promoting a less harmful way of life should start in childhood. This way of life should include healthy dietary habits, and education about nutrition should be started at the antenatal clinic. Throughout life the aim should be to reduce the amount of animal fat in the diet, to increase the amount of vegetables, fruit and whole grains and to attain a moderate kilojoule intake. Prevention of obesity in infancy and childhood is important: chubby babies tend to become obese adults. Breastfeeding should be encouraged as there is evidence that infants who have been breastfed are less likely to develop coronary artery disease in later life than those who have been artificially fed.

It is important that regular physical exercise be continued after leaving school as research has shown that participation in sport declines rapidly after leaving school.

Secondary prevention: Case finding is the first step in secondary prevention, and the screening of high-risk groups is necessary if the incidence of heart attacks is to be reduced. This includes regular:

- blood pressure checks and treatment of hypertension
- blood tests for high serum cholesterol levels
- urine and blood glucose tests for late-onset diabetes mellitus.

In no other condition is prompt treatment more vital than in the case of a myocardial infarction or heart attack. Statistics reveal that most deaths occur before the patient reaches a hospital, and appropriate early intervention reduces mortality rates significantly. Pre-hospital care that provides for airway maintenance, cardiac compression and defibrillation is important for the survival and full recovery of the patient.

Nursing care

- The importance of immediate intervention requires community participation. Education of people in cardiopulmonary resuscitation (CPR) is therefore an important part of the successful management of a heart attack.

- Mobile intensive care ambulances or helicopters with highly trained personnel can ensure that the patient receives the correct treatment needed to survive and to reduce complications.

- Where possible, patients are admitted to intensive care units where specialist care continues. Limitation of disability can be facilitated by early diagnosis, prompt and efficient treatment and the prevention of complications.

- Rehabilitation should always be commenced on admission and should certainly include emotional support and reassurance. Rehabilitation is aimed at returning the patient to a full, useful and productive life, and this is possible in about 90 per cent of cases. However, although most people will be able to return to work, they must be made to realise that some change in their way of life will be inevitable. Their diet may have to be modified, smoking stopped and a more relaxed attitude to life adopted. A programme of graded exercises must be started as soon as possible, as exercise reduces serum cholesterol levels, opens up collateral circulation to the heart muscle and increases the efficiency of the heart.

Rheumatic heart disease

Chronic rheumatic heart disease is the most common cardiac condition found in children and young adults, particularly those from lower-level socio-economic groups. The incidence of streptococcal infections, and therefore of rheumatic fever, is associated with poor housing, overcrowding and inadequate ventilation.

Aetiology

There is a positive correlation between the incidence of an acute streptococcal infection of the upper respiratory tract and the prevalence of chronic rheumatic heart disease in a community. About 3 per cent of children who have had a streptococcal infection will develop acute rheumatic fever about two weeks later. This is thought to be due to an immunological response to the toxins of the streptococcus. The incidence of both acute streptococcal infections and acute rheumatic fever reaches a peak in the 6- to 15-year age group. Rheumatic fever tends to recur and a child who has had one attack is likely to have subsequent attacks. Acute rheumatic fever presents with fever, painful and swollen joints with tender nodules under the skin and, in a number of cases, cardiac involvement. Pericarditis, myocarditis and endocarditis may all occur. Some children recover completely from rheumatic fever, but a number are later found to be suffering from chronic rheumatic heart disease.

In chronic rheumatic heart disease there is permanent damage to one or more of the valves of the heart. These become deformed and narrowed, and the heart is consequently unable to function efficiently. Any of the valves may be affected but the mitral valve is the one most commonly involved. This leads to either mitral stenosis or mitral regurgitation. Subacute bacterial endocarditis, thromboembolic disease and cardiac failure are frequent complications of chronic valvular disease of the heart.

Treatment of chronic valvular disease may be medical or surgical. Surgical treatment requires major cardiac surgery and, in some cases, replacement of the damaged valves. There appears to be a familial susceptibility to rheumatic fever, but it is not clear whether this is due to genetic or environmental influences.

Preventative measures and nursing care

Primary prevention: The prevention of chronic rheumatic heart disease is through the prevention of the acute streptococcal infection. Prevention includes all measures designed to promote health, such as improving the socio-economic status of the community, the provision of adequate housing and ventilation, the prevention of overcrowding and the promotion of adequate nutrition.

Effective health education programmes should provide information on the signs and symptoms of acute streptococcal infections, the importance of receiving prompt and effective treatment, and the possibility of rheumatic fever occurring a few weeks later. Unfortunately, this does not solve the problem as more than one-third of cases presenting with acute rheumatic fever have no history of a previous acute streptococcal infection.

Secondary prevention: Early diagnosis and case finding is important. If an outbreak is identified at a school, throat swabs should be taken from all members of the high-risk group. Prompt treatment of streptococcal infections requires adequate doses of the appropriate antibiotic, and if rheumatic fever is diagnosed, prolonged, complete bed rest is necessary. Children who have had rheumatic fever must be followed up, prophylactic antibiotics supplied as required and heart function monitored. If necessary, patients should be referred to specialist cardiac clinics for assessment and surgical interventions if necessary.

Cerebrovascular disease

A cerebrovascular accident (CVA) is commonly called a stroke. It is a condition that affects all age groups but mainly older adults.

Aetiology

A CVA is caused by a cerebral haemorrhage, a thrombosis or an embolism. Strokes occurring in younger people are usually the result of cerebral emboli that are associated with atrial fibrillation, rheumatic heart disease, subacute bacterial endocarditis and myocardial infarction or, less commonly, a ruptured cerebral

early and well managed, patients can live a normal life and have a good quality of life. It is a disease that results from a deficit in production or utilisation of the hormone known as insulin that causes hypo- and hyperglycaemia to occur.

Aetiology

Diabetes mellitus is a result of insulin deficiency, which hampers the metabolism of carbohydrates, proteins and fats. Causes of the disease are both genetic and environmental. The genetic relationship is not well understood but a family history of the disease is regarded as a risk factor for developing the disease. Obesity is also a risk factor for the disease, especially in adults. Over time diabetes can damage the heart, blood vessels, eyes, kidneys and nervous system. Diabetes is divided into two distinct types:

- **Type 1:** This type affects children and young adults. It is the more severe of the two types; it tends to run in families and is more common in some racial groups, for example Asians, than in other groups. This type is usually insulin-dependent, and patients will be required to have daily injections of insulin for the rest of their lives. If the disease is not managed well, vascular and neurological complications will occur.
- **Type 2:** This type of diabetes is the less severe form of the disease and occurs mainly in the older adult and accounts for about 80 per cent of all diabetes cases. It is often associated with unhealthy lifestyles that result in obesity, hypertension and arteriosclerosis.

Preventative measures

To prevent diabetes, preventative measures similar to those for cardiovascular disease must be introduced. Healthy lifestyle and a healthy diet with reduced sugar and saturated fat are necessary to avoid obesity or to reduce weight if obesity is already present. Regular exercise is important and smoking should be avoided.

Early diagnosis and good management of the condition is crucial, as Type 2 diabetes often goes undiagnosed until a patient presents with an associated disease such as hypertension, a stroke or cardiovascular disease. If possible, special screening programmes should be introduced to check people who may be at risk. Pregnant women with diabetes must be referred for special care.

Nursing care

The earlier the disease is diagnosed and treated, the lesser its impact of the disease or disability. Self-monitoring and the promotion of self-care through good patient education and empowerment are important. Patients must know how to test their urine/blood and administer insulin, recognise symptoms of hypo- and hyperglycaemia, and know how to treat the symptoms and when to seek help. Regular clinic attendance and compliance with the treatment regimen is vital.

Appropriate care for diabetes mellitus must be available at all health services to:
- relieve symptoms
- prevent acute metabolic and long-term complications
- screen for retinopathy, kidney-related disease and cholesterol levels
- ensure the permanent availability of oral diabetic medication, insulin, syringes and other drugs used in the treatment of diabetes and its associated conditions.

Through good management of the disease, the patient can look forward to a productive and good quality life. Good management will also reduce the economic burden on the individual, the family and the community.

Trauma and disability

Trauma is an increasingly significant health problem throughout the world. The WHO states that trauma is responsible for 16 per cent of the world's burden of disease. The incidence of trauma is set to increase, especially in the developing world, over the next decade.

Trauma can be the result of an accident or a violent deed inflicted wilfully by one person on another. An accident is an unanticipated or unexpected event that results in death or injury to a person or persons and/or damage to property. South Africa has among the world's highest trauma rates for accidents and violence.

According to the WHO, nearly half of all accidents occur in the home. Far from being the havens of safety that we imagine homes to be, they are nearly as dangerous as the roads. The kitchen is the most dangerous room in the house and more accidents take place there than anywhere else. It is difficult to estimate the extent of the problem. Although it is quite easy to establish how many people die or are admitted to hospital as a result of domestic accidents, it is not easy to find out how many people are less seriously injured in accidents at home each year.

Preventative measures

Preventative programmes have been initiated in South Africa to prevent trauma. The 'Arrive Alive' campaign is well known and aims to reduce dangerous behaviour on the roads. It focuses on the four main reasons for traffic accidents and the associated injuries:
- drinking and driving
- speeding
- not using safety belts
- vehicles that are not roadworthy.

Campaigns to reduce abuse, especially to reduce the abuse of women and children, have been instituted annually over the past few years with little visible success. Rape of both women and children is alarmingly high in South Africa and the forensic aspects of handling these victims bring a new dimension to healthcare. Nurses must know how to handle these cases and what to do in the absence of a doctor. The process of handling the patient and the associated injuries may determine whether the perpetrator is successfully convicted and whether the person attains full recovery.

Nursing care

Trauma requires more than the treatment of the physical injuries. Counselling and psychological support are also needed to heal and bring people to a state of full recovery or at least to reduce the impact of the incident on their lives.

Effective trauma management is an important factor in determining the outcome of the trauma. Poor outcomes can often be attributed to poor management during the first hour after the incident has occurred. In trauma this hour is often referred to as the 'golden hour'. Trauma management should start at the site of the incident with pre-hospital care. The care continuum then continues in the casualty or trauma unit through to rehabilitation.

Conclusion

Many NCDs end up as chronic conditions. Prevention is therefore better than cure, because 'care' is often not possible. Therefore, programmes instituted for the management of chronic diseases must include prevention strategies. This forms the beginning of the continuum of healthcare in the management of NCDs. Health information is the next important step as a patient armed with appropriate information has the best ally to prevent or successfully manage these diseases, which are so often linked to lifestyle. Early diagnosis and appropriate treatment are next in the disease management process and must be followed by adherence to the treatment regimen if successful outcomes are to be reached. The key to success in the management of NCDs lies with the affected person and his or her active participation in the care continuum.

Self-assessment

1. Most chronic diseases can be prevented or managed by good preventative measures. Discuss the healthy lifestyle you would promote to prevent the development of these chronic diseases.
2. List the warning signs of cancer.
3. Identify the top ten cancers in men and women in South Africa.
4. List six main health risk factors that lead to the development of non-communicable diseases.
5. Explain what is meant by primary, secondary and tertiary disease prevention.
6. Discuss the care of patients with chronic non-communicable diseases.

Bibliography

Cancer Association of South Africa (CANSA). 2018. Fact sheet on the top ten cancers per population group. Available: https://www.cansa.org.za/files/2018/07/Fact-Sheet-Top-Ten-Cancers-per-Population-Group-NCR-2014-web-July-2018.pdf (Accessed 1 March 2020).

Clark, M.J.D. 2015. *Population and Community Health Nursing*. 6th edition. Hoboken, New Jersey: Pearson Education.

Department of Health. 1998. Guidelines, manuals and instructions. Available: https://www.westerncape.gov.za/your_gov/55/documents/guides/N- (Accessed 10 March 2020).

Department of Health. 2006. *A Strategic Vision for Non-communicable Diseases*. Directorate: chronic diseases, disabilities and geriatrics. Pretoria: Government Printer.

Department of Health (Western Cape Government). 2013. Chronic care. Available: http://www.westerncape.gov.za/service/chronic-care (Accessed 24 September 2020).

Diabetes South Africa. 2015. Managing diabetes. Available: https://www.diabetessa.org.za/managing-diabetes/- (Accessed 25 February 2020).

Health Systems Trust. 2000. *South African Health Review*. Durban: The Press Gang.

Hospice Palliative Care Association of South Africa. 2015. Available: https://hpca.co.za/palliative-care/ (Accessed 25 February 2020).

Long, B.C., Phipps, W.J. & Cassmeyer, V.L. 1995. *Adult Nursing: A Nursing Process Approach*. London: Mosby.

National Institute for Communicable Diseases (NICD). 2004. National Cancer Registry: Incidence of histologically diagnosed cancer in South Africa. https://www.nicd.ac.za/wp-content/uploads/2019/12/2004-Cancer_Registry_2004.pdf (Accessed 25 February 2020).

National Institute for Communicable Diseases (NICD). 2009. National Cancer Registry: 2009 report. Available: https://www.nicd.ac.za/centres/national-cancer-registry/ (Accessed 18 September 2020).

Novartis Foundation. 2015. Available: https://www.novartisfoundation.org (Accessed 8 March 2020).

World Health Organization (WHO). 2013. Global NCD action plan for the prevention and control of communicable diseases 2013–2020 Available: https://www.who.int/nmh/publications/ncd-action-plan/en/ (Accessed 25 February 2020).

World Health Organization (WHO). 2018a. Cancer key facts. Available: https://www.who.int/en/news-room/fact-sheets/detail/cancer (Accessed 25 February 2020).

World Health Organization (WHO). 2018b. Non-communicable diseases (NCD) country profiles, 2018. Available: https://www.who.int/nmh/publications/ncd-profiles-2018/en/ (Accessed 25 February 2020).

World Health Organization (WHO). 2018c. Non-communicable disease fact sheet, June 2018. Available: https://www.who.int/news-room/fact-sheets/detail/noncommunicable-diseases (Accessed 25 February 2020).

Microbiology and the transmission of infection

Joy Cleghorn

Learning outcomes

After studying this chapter, you should be able to:

- Describe a typical cell and its contents.
- Discuss how microbes can be destroyed.
- Classify pathogenic microorganisms associated with the transmission of infection and disease.
- Discuss how common microbes cause infections and diseases.
- Discuss reservoir of infections in relation to the host and carriers.
- Describe the importance of immunisation for children and diseases included in the South African schedule.

Key terms

Commensal: A microbe that coexists with the human host to its benefit but that leaves the host unaffected.

Fomites: Inanimate objects or material on which disease-producing agents may be conveyed.

Immunity: Refers to the body's resistance to infection; immunity may be general or specific.

Infection: The invasion of a host by pathogenic microorganisms that can cause the infected person to present with a disease.

Microorganisms (or microbes): A microscopic organism or single-celled plant or animal.

Non-pathogenic microorganisms: The vast majority of microorganisms fall into this group, are part of the ecology and exist for the benefit of humans and their health.

Pathogenic microorganisms: A small number of microorganisms fall into this group and are harmful to humans and animals. They are microbes that cause diseases.

Saprophyte: Organisms such as mould, fungus or bacteria that absorb their nutrition directly through the cell membrane from the host.

Vector: An animal host that carries microorganisms from one human host to another.

Zoonosis: A disease affecting animals, which can be transferred to humans.

Introduction

Microbiology is the scientific study of microorganisms. These microorganisms, or microbes, consist of single cells or cell clusters, except for viruses, which are microscopic but not cellular. These microbial cells differ from those in humans, animals and plants in that they are able to live alone. People are the most common reservoir of these microbes and are responsible for transmitting them from one person to another. The vast majority of microorganisms are non-pathogenic and support other functions that contribute to the normal activities of our daily lives. A relatively small number are associated with infection and disease, and it is these that will be discussed in this chapter.

If the microbe is pathogenic, and the human recipient of that microorganism does not have the necessary resistance to prevent reproduction of that organism or to resist the biochemical processes of the cells, the person will become ill and show the signs and symptoms of disease. However, if the host is healthy, has a high natural state of immunity and lives in a healthy environment, he or she can usually resist the infection. This immunity to disease can be artificially stimulated through immunisation, which enables people to develop immunity to specific diseases.

Developing countries have high rates of poverty and associated poor environments and malnutrition. As a result, the natural resistance of the population, and especially of children, is low. This results in infection rates and the incidence of disease being higher in such communities. Conditions such as HIV and AIDS reduce the resistance of those infected with the virus, leaving them with little or no resistance to other infections. It is these secondary infections that often prove fatal to those living with HIV and AIDS, and not the primary disease. Malnutrition causes a decreased immune function, leaving the person vulnerable to infection; infection leads to a decreased ability to absorb nutrients, thereby leaving the person vulnerable to a secondary infection. This cycle is illustrated in Figure 7.1.

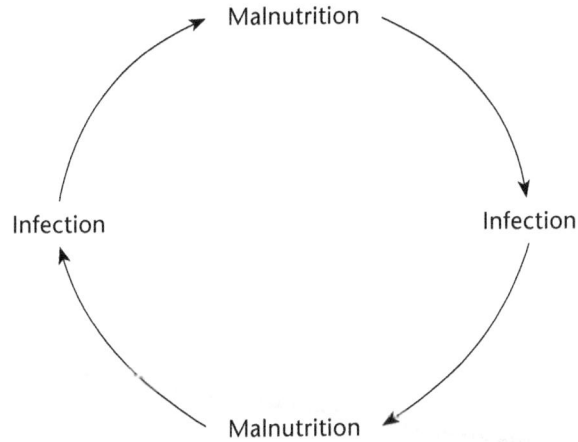

Figure 7.1 Cycle of malnutrition and infection

The single-cell microorganism

The majority of microorganisms consist of a single cell. Microorganisms have many of the characteristics of a typical cell as described below. The cell is visible only under a microscope and consists of a small speck of protoplasm containing a nucleus, and this is surrounded by a cell membrane. It is made up of the components described below and shown in Figure 7.2.

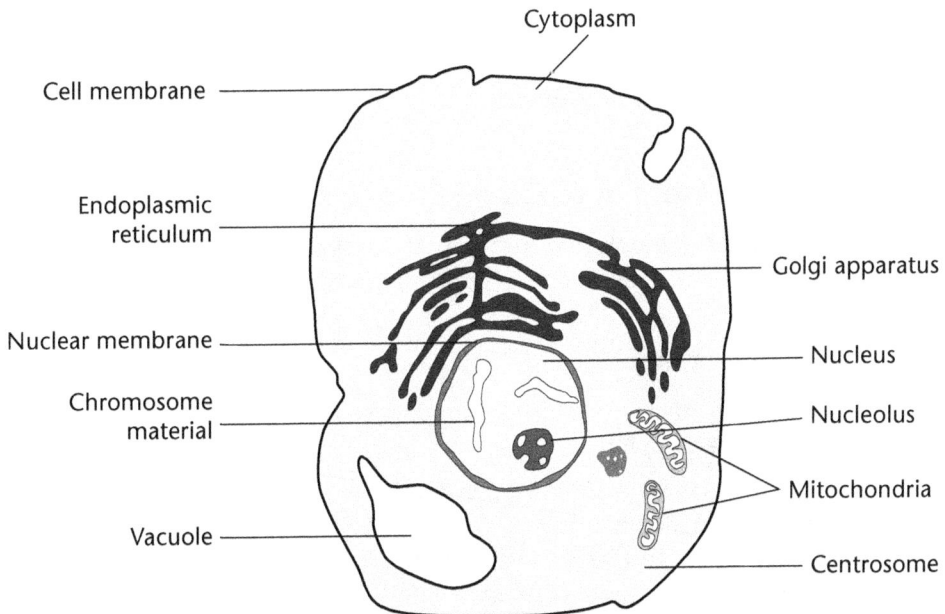

Figure 7.2 A typical cell

Protoplasm

Protoplasm is a transparent jelly-like substance containing mineral salts, gasses and organic substances such as proteins, carbohydrates, fats and enzymes.

The nucleus

The nucleus is a transparent, colourless structure, spherical or ovoid in shape, which is in turn surrounded by a nuclear membrane. The nucleus may contain one or more rounded structures known as nucleoli. The nucleus is vital and without it the cell dies. It controls all the activities of the cell and is essential for cell division, as well as for the transmission of hereditary characteristics to the next generation. The nucleus stains readily because it contains a substance known as chromatin. Chromatin contains DNA (deoxyribonucleic acid) and carries the genes, which are responsible for heredity or the transfer of characteristics from one generation to another.

Other structures present in a typical cell are:

- the **centrosome**, which is a small area near the nucleus that contains two **centrioles**, structures that are active during cell division
- the **mitochondria**, which are rod-shaped structures enclosed in a membrane and that take part in the processes necessary for the release of energy from food within the cell. They have been called the 'power plants of the cell'
- the **Golgi apparatus**, which is a fairly large structure and quite easy to see when a stained cell is viewed under a microscope. The Golgi apparatus is thought to have a secretory function
- the **ribosomes**, which are minute structures concerned with protein synthesis.

Living characteristics of microbes

In this section we examine the environmental needs of microorganisms as living structures, as well as their replication, movement and the production of toxins.

Supportive environment

As living structures, microbes require a supportive environment to grow and to reproduce. They need the following:

- **Energy**: This is necessary for growth, reproduction, movement and many other processes. Some microbes obtain this energy from the sun, but most derive it from a process known as the oxidation of organic or inorganic substances, which releases energy.
- **Oxygen**: Some microbes make use of free or atmospheric oxygen and this group is known as aerobic organisms. Others obtain oxygen by breaking

down inorganic substances such as nitrates and cannot grow in the presence of free oxygen. These are anaerobes. A third group, the facultative anaerobes, will grow in any environment whether free oxygen is present or not.

- **An optimal temperature**: This is essential for growth and multiplication. Temperatures that are too high or too low will either stop growth or kill the microorganism. Most human pathogens grow best at a body temperature or 37 °C, but there are exceptions. Generally, there is a range of optimal temperatures and growth will usually continue between 20 °C and 40 °C.

- **An optimal pH or hydrogen ion concentration**: Very few microbes will grow in a medium that is too acidic or too alkaline, and pathogens that affect humans grow best at a pH of 7.3, which is similar to the pH of the body fluids and slightly alkaline. Exceptions do exist, however, and the vibrio, which causes cholera, prefers a more alkaline medium of about 8.3.

- **Moisture**: Most microbes are destroyed by drying and require moisture for growth and reproduction. However, there are those such as *Mycobacterium tuberculosis* that will remain alive for some time in the air and in dust, and the spores of other bacteria such as *Bacillus anthracis* that can remain alive indefinitely without moisture.

- **Darkness**: Darkness promotes the growth of microbes, as sunlight with ultraviolet rays will destroy many microbes. Light also inhibits their growth and reproduction.

Reproduction

Different groups of microbes replicate in different ways.

- *Bacteria* multiply by simple fission. The cell grows until it reaches the maximum size for the species and then divides into two identical daughter cells. Under favourable conditions bacteria will divide as often as once every 30 minutes.

- *Viruses* replicate themselves within the cells of the host, and in the process affect the cell and may even destroy it.

- *Pathogenic protozoa*, such as the plasmodia that causes malaria, have complicated life cycles.

Toxin production

Poisonous substances known as toxins are the important end products of some pathogenic bacterial metabolism.

An *exotoxin* is a toxin that diffuses out and away from the bacterial cell. *Clostridium tetani*, the causative organism of tetanus, produces a powerful exotoxin, and although the organism is present only at the site of entry, its toxins will be found circulating throughout the body, causing the disease signs and symptoms.

Endotoxins, on the other hand, remain within the bacterial cell and are set free only when the cell disintegrates. Generally, exotoxins are more powerful than endotoxins. It is the *virulence* of a microorganism that determines its ability to cause disease and this is directly related to the type of toxin the microorganism produces.

Spore formation

A spore is formed when the round or oval area within the microorganism becomes surrounded by a thick wall that enables it to survive even the most unfavourable conditions such as exposure to high temperatures, drying and chemical disinfectants. When conditions become favourable for growth of the microorganism, the spore once more becomes a functional cell. This is not a reproductive process because only one bacterial cell results from a spore. Spores are extremely difficult to destroy. Boiling and the use of disinfectants are not effective; the only way to ensure their destruction is to use steam under pressure. Exposure to a temperature of 121 °C for 15 minutes will kill some spores.

Flagella

Certain microbes are motile or capable of movement. They propel themselves along with long, thin, whip-like processes, known as flagella.

Capsules

Some bacterial cells, such as the pneumococcus and *Yersinia pestis*, are surrounded by a jelly-like capsule consisting of polysaccharides. The capsule protects the organism against unfavourable conditions.

Laboratory examination of microorganisms

When microorganisms are examined in the laboratory, three methods are used: the Gram stain, the development of an artificial culture and the cultivation of colonies of bacteria.

Gram stain

Bacteria are far easier to examine under a microscope if they are stained. A number of stains may be used, but the Gram stain is probably the one most frequently used. On the basis of this stain, bacteria may be divided into two classes: Gram-positive bacteria that stain blue, and Gram-negative organisms that stain red.

Artificial culture media

Microbes such as bacteria can be grown in the laboratory if the conditions of their natural environment are duplicated. The incubation of these bacteria requires the correct temperature, pH, oxygen state and nutrients. They are grown on a *nutrient agar* or a jelly-like broth containing all the necessary nutrients and to which an extract derived from seaweed, known as agar, is added. Further additives such as blood and serum may be used. The medium is poured into a flat, round glass container called a Petri dish and the bacteria or other microorganism is added from a swab or other source obtained from the infected patient. This is not the only method used to culture microorganisms as technological advancements occur all the time.

Colonies

The bacteria cultivated in a Petri dish in an incubator at 37 °C, will reproduce so rapidly that after only 24 hours clusters of small oval or round dots may be seen on the surface of the medium with the naked eye. These are called colonies and each colony consists of more than a million bacteria.

Destroying pathogenic microorganisms

Pathogenic microorganisms can be destroyed by physical methods, chemical methods, chemotherapeutic agents and antibiotics. These will all be explained in this section.

Physical methods

The physical methods used are heat, pressurised steam, drying, ultra-violet light, filtration and cold.

Heat

There are two common methods – dry heat and moist heat:

- **Dry heat**: Incineration is the most effective way of dealing with healthcare risk waste such as soiled dressings and potentially infectious material resulting from patient care. At the correct temperature, it totally destroys all microorganisms.
- **Moist heat**: Pasteurisation is a method used to destroy pathogens in milk, wine, fruit juices and other liquids. Boiling is the most common method of pasteurisation. Water boils at 100 °C and will destroy most bacteria, but not spores or certain viruses. However, if the article being pasteurised is not covered completely by the boiling water, or if the container is not kept boiling for the required time, the article may not be pasteurised. It is an easy and convenient way of destroying most pathogens, and a wide variety of articles, such as baby bottles, can be boiled.

Pressurised steam

Steam under pressure is used in an autoclave. By increasing the pressure of the steam in the autoclave to above atmospheric pressure the temperature will be raised. The time required for sterilisation depends upon the temperature of the steam. The higher the temperature, the shorter the time necessary to render the article sterile; for example, at 120 °C, 30 minutes is required, while at 132 °C, depending on the autoclave, only 3 minutes is required.

Drying

Most microbes require moisture for their growth and multiplication. Depriving them of moisture will inhibit their growth and destroy many of them. However, certain bacteria, such as *Mycobacterium tuberculosis*, can remain alive for some time in dust, while spores are extremely resistant to a dry environment and will stay alive for years without moisture.

Ultraviolet light

Exposure to the direct rays of the sun for a sufficiently long time will destroy most microorganisms. The number of pathogens that are found on contaminated articles such as pillows, linen and clothing can be greatly reduced by placing the items in the sun for about eight hours. It is important to remember that the ultraviolet rays cannot penetrate through an article so the articles must be turned in order to expose all the surfaces to the ultraviolet rays. It is also important to note that a contaminated article must first be washed and be free of organic matter before the rays will have an effect on the pathogens.

Ultraviolet germicidal irradiation (UVGI) is a technology that uses a short wavelength of ultraviolet light to disinfect surfaces, air and water.

Filtration

This is a process whereby a liquid is passed through a porous medium in order to remove microorganisms from the solution. It is used for the sterilisation of substances such as vaccines and drugs that may be damaged by heat.

Cold

Exposure to very low temperatures will inhibit the growth of microbes but will not necessarily destroy them. In fact, temperatures of minus 70 °C are used to preserve cultures containing viruses or bacteria. These will begin multiplying again when the culture is warmed.

Chemical methods

There are a large number of chemicals that destroy or prevent the growth and multiplication of bacteria. A chemical that can destroy bacteria is called a bactericidal and a chemical that stops multiplication of bacteria is called a bacteriostatic. This method of high-level disinfection/sterilisation should not be used unless there is no other method available. A good disinfectant and sterilant should ideally:

- be inexpensive, non-toxic and non-corrosive
- act effectively in the presence of organic matter
- not deteriorate during storage
- be effective against a wide variety of microorganisms.

To ensure that a disinfectant is effective, use one that is appropriate for the material to be disinfected. It must be the correct concentration and the material to be disinfected must be in contact with the fluid for the correct length of time. A disinfectant will not penetrate organic matter and must always be followed by thorough cleaning with a detergent in order to remove organic matter.

Disinfectants are used on inanimate objects and antiseptics are used on human tissue. Common disinfectants are the following:

- **Alcohol:** a 70 per cent solution is regarded as the most effective disinfectant and will destroy a large number of microbes but not spores. Seventy per cent alcohol can be used as both a disinfectant and an antiseptic.
- **Halogens:** chlorine is an example of a halogen and is widely used for the treatment of water (0.1 to 0.2 ml of sodium hypochlorite (bleach) can be added to 1 litre of water and left to stand for 20 minutes) and also for disinfecting babies' feeding bottles, crockery and similar articles. Iodine is most commonly used as a tincture of iodine for application to the skin. Chlorine as a hypochlorite solution is commonly used as a surface disinfectant in hospitals.
- **Oxidising agents:** these include *disinfectants* such as hydrogen peroxide, commonly used for sterilising heat-labile instruments such as endoscopes. Hydrogen peroxide is also used to disinfect surfaces and air by means of aerosolising the chemical.

Chemotherapeutic agents

These are specific chemical substances that will inhibit the growth and multiplication of microorganisms in the body and, in some cases, destroy them, without harming the patient. One of the earliest chemotherapeutic agents used was quinine, which was used in the treatment of malaria. The sulphonamides can also be used as chemotherapeutic substances.

Antibiotics

These are substances derived from living organisms such as fungi, which will inhibit the growth and multiplication of microorganisms in the body or destroy them. Penicillin was the first antibiotic to be used in the treatment of disease. Although it was discovered by Sir Alexander Fleming in 1929, it was not used until 1940. For any antibiotic to be effective it is necessary that the appropriate antibiotic be used in adequate doses. Today, large numbers of antibiotics are available but due to misuse and abuse over the years many existing and emerging resistant strains of bacteria can no longer be treated using common antibiotics. Some bacteria have become resistant to all existing antibiotics.

Portals of entry

Pathogens may enter the body of a new host via a number of routes, as illustrated in Figure 7.3.

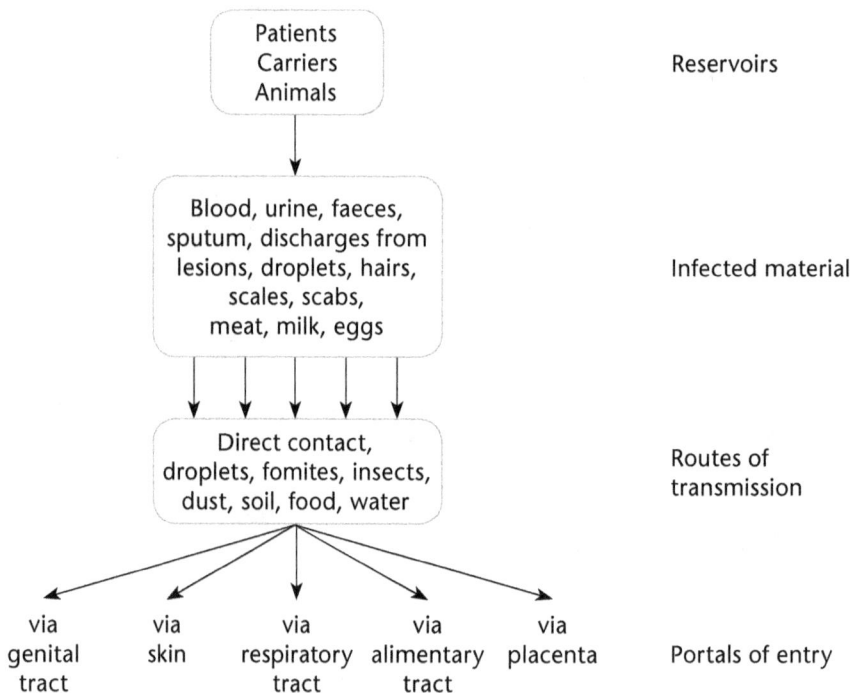

Figure 7.3 Summary of the routes of transmission of pathogens

Pathogens enter the body of the host through the skin or mucous membranes through:

- the nose, mouth or conjunctiva, for example seasonal influenza, SARS-CoV-2 (COVID-19)
- a break in the skin, such as a cut or scratch, causing tetanus and gas gangrene

- unbroken skin, for example the larvae of the *Schistosoma haematobium*, or the hookworm
- the gastrointestinal tract by the ingestion of infected food or water, for example typhoid fever, dysentery and food poisoning
- the inhalation of infected droplets or dust, as in pulmonary tuberculosis
- any tube inserted into a patient, such as a urinary catheter, intravenous therapy, etc, as it becomes an additional portal of entry through which organisms can enter the body
- the genital tract, as in gonorrhoea
- the placenta to the foetus, for example in the case of syphilis.

Classification of microorganisms

Most microorganisms can be classified into the following broad groups:
- bacteria
- viruses
- fungi
- parasites (protozoa – helminths).

Bacteria

Bacteria may be classified according to their morphology or shape, as illustrated in Figure 7.4.

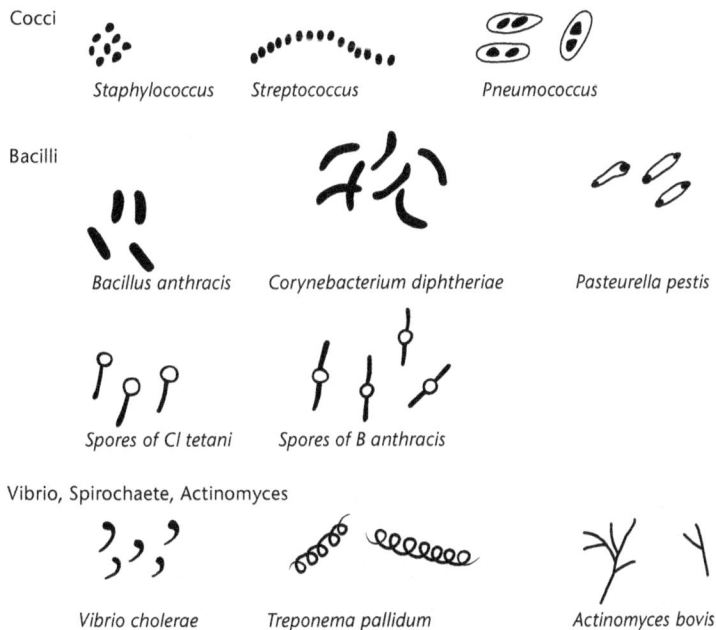

Figure 7.4 Morphological classification of bacteria

Gram-positive cocci

- *Streptococci* usually occur in a chain formation and are important human pathogens that are responsible for a number of serious diseases.
- *Streptococcus pyogenes* is the causative organism of scarlet fever, tonsillitis, cellulitis, mastoiditis, impetigo and septicaemia.
- *Enterococcus faecalis* is found in wound infections, urinary tract infections and endocarditis.
- *Staphylococcus aureus* occurs in clusters resembling a bunch of grapes and is an important cause of food poisoning, wound infection, boils, carbuncles and septicaemia. It often causes outbreaks of secondary infections in hospitals and is resistant to many antibiotics.
- *Staphylococcus epidermis* is usually non-pathogenic and occurs normally on the skin, but it may cause bacterial endocarditis if it enters the bloodstream.

Gram-negative cocci

- *Neisseria gonorrhoeae* causes urethritis in males, cervicitis in females and ophthalmia neonatorum (neonatal conjunctivitis).
- *Neisseria meningitidis* causes meningococcaemia and meningitis.

Gram-positive bacilli

- *Bacillus anthracis* is a spore-forming Gram-positive organism that causes anthrax. The disease is spread to people through the eating of contaminated meat, through the handling of infected material such as wool or animal hides, or through the ingestion of spores. The spores can exist in adverse conditions for a long period of time. In 2003, in an act of bioterrorism, *Bacillus anthracis* spores were sent to ordinary American citizens through the United States postal system, causing some outbreaks of anthrax across the country.
- *Clostridium tetani* is the causative organism of tetanus (lockjaw). It has a 'drumstick' appearance when viewed under a microscope, because of a round terminal spore. It enters the body through a penetrating wound in the skin, frequently one that is contaminated with soil or animal excreta. In South Africa, tetanus used to occur commonly in newborn babies who had their umbilical cord dressed with mud or cow dung. It also occurs in drug users sharing needles.
- *Clostridium botulism* is a bacterium that produces several toxins of which the best known is its neurotoxin that causes flaccid muscular paralysis seen in botulism. It occurs in the soil where it is a saprophyte, and may contaminate food such as canned fish, meat and vegetables. Ingestion of infected food leads to a severe type of food poisoning.

- *Clostridium perfringens* is an anaerobic, sporing bacillus that occurs in the intestine of humans and animals, as well as in the soil. It is the organism most frequently responsible for gas gangrene. Wounds that are fairly extensive and associated with muscle damage and that are contaminated with soil are the ones most likely to be infected. Gas gangrene commonly occurs in war situations.

- *Clostridium difficile* causes colitis associated with antibiotic usage and pseudomembranous colitis.

- *Corynebacterium diphtheriae* causes infections of the throat, pharynx, tonsils and nose, known as diphtheria.

- *Bacillus cereus* causes food poisoning.

Gram-negative bacilli

- *Escherichia coli* is an opportunistic pathogen and may cause urinary tract infections, wound sepsis and abscesses.

- *Salmonellae.* The most important pathogens in this class are *Salmonella typhi* and *S. paratyphi*, which are the causative organisms for typhoid and paratyphoid fever respectively. They are present in the urine and faeces of carriers and sufferers of the diseases.

- *Shigellae.* These are *Shigella shigae, S. sonnei* and *S. flexneri*, the causative organisms of a group of gastrointestinal diseases known as the bacillary dysenteries.

- *Bordetella pertussis* is a short, capsulated bacillus, which is the causative organism of whooping cough, an acute infection of the lower respiratory tract occurring in infants and young children.

- *Brucella* are primarily pathogens in animals such as cattle and goats. They cause an infection in these animals known as brucellosis that can be transmitted to humans through the ingestion of unpasteurised milk and cheese. *Brucella abortus* infects cattle, *B. suis* infects pigs and *B. ovis* infects sheep.

- *Yersinia pestis* is the causative organism of bubonic plague, which is transmitted through rodents. It is transmitted to humans via the bite of infected rats or fleas. Buboes refer to painfully swollen lymph nodes.

- *Legionella pneumophila* grows in stagnant water, for example unused water pipes in buildings, and causes Legionnaires' disease and Pontiac fever.

- *Vibrio cholerae* causes cholera, is found in contaminated faeces and water supplies and can be carried by flies.

Acid-fast bacilli

- *Mycobacterium tuberculosis* is the causative organism of tuberculosis. The *bovine strain* is transmitted from an infected cow to humans via milk. The *human strain* is transmitted via airborne droplets of sputum from an infected person. This organism can survive in the atmosphere for some time.

- *Mycobacterium leprae* and *M. lepromatosis* are the causative organisms of leprosy, also known as Hansen's disease, a disease that has virtually disappeared from the developed countries of the world. However, it is still common in the less-developed countries of Africa.

Spirochaete

These are slender, spiral, motile microorganisms. *Treponema pallida* is the causative organism of syphilis, a disease transmitted almost exclusively by sexual intercourse. Spirochaete will not multiply in artificial media.

Rickettsiae

These microorganisms are transmitted to humans via the bite of bloodsucking insects such as fleas, mites, ticks and lice. The organisms gain entry to the body by inoculation. Rickettsiae are similar to bacteria in many ways. They are sensitive to at least some of the antibiotics and they multiply by simple fission; however, like viruses, they will grow and multiply only in living tissues. In size they are more similar to viruses than bacteria. Rickettsiae are responsible for diseases such as epidemic typhus and tick-bite fever, which occur in South Africa, and Rocky Mountain Spotted Fever, Trench Fever and Q Fever, found in other parts of the world.

Viruses

Most viruses, but not all, are ultra-microscopic and can be seen only if an electron microscope is used. Viruses do not reproduce by simple fission as bacteria do but replicate themselves by producing an exact copy of themselves within the cells of living tissues.

Viruses are cultivated in chick embryos or tissue cells that are kept alive in a suitable fluid, as they will not live in artificial media. The structure of a virus is very different from that of a typical cell. Viruses are important pathogens and the causative organisms of many communicable diseases such as measles, poliomyelitis, mumps and influenza SARS-CoV-2, commonly known as coronavirus disease 2019 (COVID-19).

Coronavirus (COVID-19)

Coronavirus disease is a new viral disease caused by the Severe Acute Respiratory Syndrome Coronavirus (SARS-CoV-2). COVID-19 generally causes mild to moderate illness, although patients with co-morbidities become more ill and may require oxygen therapy and/or ventilation, and despite the treatment may die.

COVID-19 was first discovered in the Chinese city of Wuhan in late 2019 and in 2020 swiftly spread across the globe causing an international pandemic. In South Africa alone, as of the 21 January 2021, there were 1 369 426 positive cases and 38 854 deaths.

To avoid the spread of the disease, there are basic principles that must be strictly adhered to are the following:

- Maintain social distancing (1.5–2 metres).
- Wear a mask (universal masking).
- Practise cough etiquette.
- Do not touch your face unless your hands are clean (ie sanitised or washed).
- Use 70 per cent alcohol-based hand sanitiser and wash hands with soap and water.
- Clean and disinfect surfaces on a regular basis.

Medical staff involved with direct care for patients who have tested positive for COVID-19 are required to wear personal protective equipment (PPE), which includes gowns, visors and face shields.

Staff involved with aerosol-generating procedures (AGP), for example intubation, suctioning, taking of throat and naso-pharyngeal swabs, are required to wear an N95 respirator (filtration up to 95 per cent particles) instead of a surgical mask for additional protection.

Figure 7.5 is a diagrammatic representation of the SARS-CoV-2 organism.

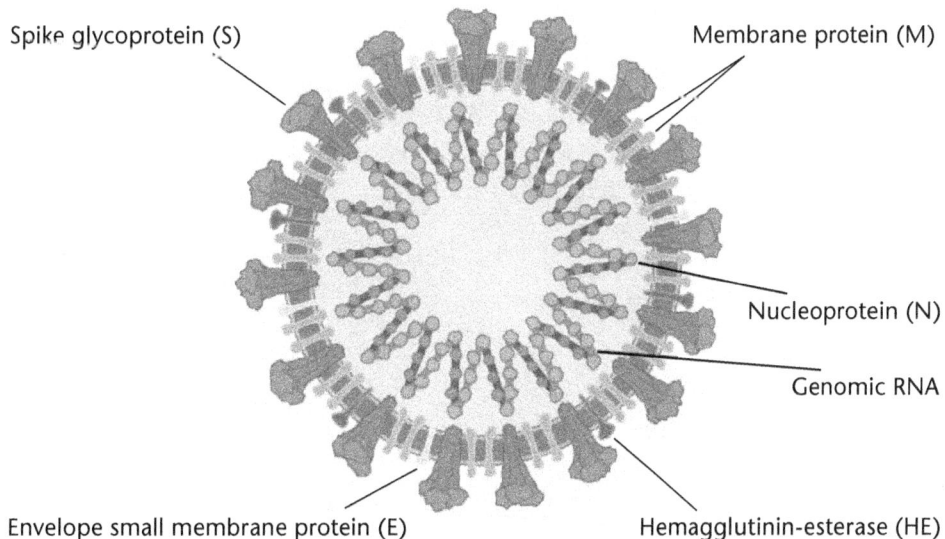

Figure 7. 5 Diagram of the SARS-CoV-2 organism
Source: Encyclopaedia Britannica, Inc.

Although viruses are frequently transmitted via droplets, there are other routes of transmission:

- *Arboviruses* are transmitted via arthropod vectors such as mosquitoes and are the causative organisms of diseases such as yellow fever and Dengue fever.
- *Enteroviruses* are transmitted via infected faeces. The poliomyelitis virus and the coxsackie viruses are examples of enteroviruses.
- *Rhinovirus* and *Coronaviridae* are responsible for the common cold; there are a large number of viruses in these groups.

Some viruses may be inoculated into the body. The rabies virus and the virus that is responsible for infective hepatitis may enter the body in this way.

Fungi

There are many different kinds of fungi, but most of those pathogenic to humans form long, branching, interlacing filaments, or hyphae. These are known as mycelia. Diseases caused by fungi are called *mycoses*, and those which affect the skin, such as ringworm and athlete's foot, are known as the *dermatomycoses*. An important infection that affects mainly small children, women and debilitated patients is thrush. It is caused by a yeast-like fungus, *Candida albicans*. *Candida auris* is another relatively new fungus causing healthcare-associated infections.

Protozoa

These single-celled microorganisms vary greatly in shape, size and structure, and are motile in some stages of their development. They are generally much larger than bacteria. Most protozoa are non-pathogenic, but some do cause diseases such as malaria, bilharzia and amoebic dysentery.

Entamoeba histolytica – this organism occurs in two forms, a vegetative form and a cystic form, as illustrated in Figure 7.6.

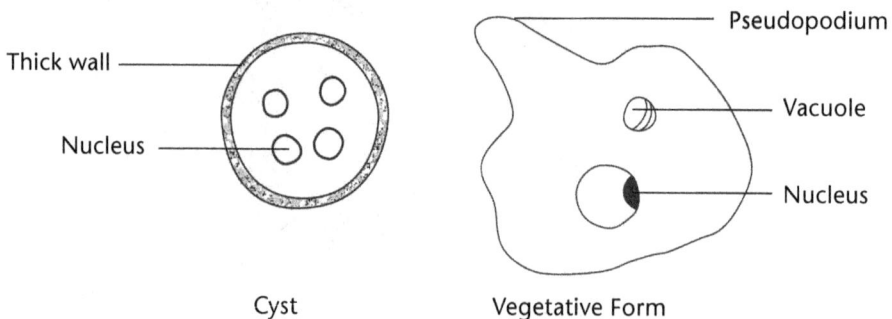

Figure 7.6 Cystic and vegetative forms of *Entamoeba histolytica*

In the vegetative form the shape is continually changing as the organism thrusts out and draws back finger-like protrusions known as pseudopodia. The cystic form consists of round, multinucleated, thick-walled cysts that can withstand the most unfavourable conditions for considerable periods of time. These cysts are excreted in the faeces of carriers and sufferers and may contaminate water, food, raw vegetables and hands. The cysts can also be spread by flies. After ingestion by a human being, the cysts hatch out and live and multiply in the large intestine. After an incubation period of a few weeks the patient presents with pyrexia, abdominal pain and diarrhoea with blood and mucus in the stools. The condition is known as amoebic dysentery.

Plasmodium falciparum, P. vivax, P. ovale and *P. malariae* – these protozoa are the causative organisms of malaria. They undergo one stage of development in the female *Anopheles* mosquito and one in humans.

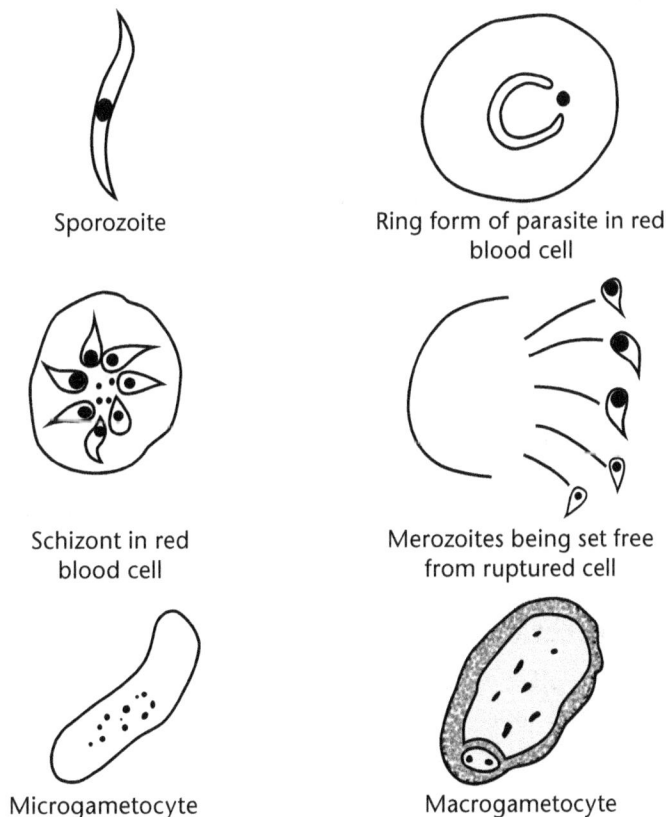

Sporozoite	Ring form of parasite in red blood cell
Schizont in red blood cell	Merozoites being set free from ruptured cell
Microgametocyte	Macrogametocyte

Figure 7.7 Stages of development of *Plasmodium falciparum*, one of the causative organisms of malaria

Most of the merozoites will enter other red blood cells, but some will develop into male and female gametocytes that will be sucked up by the mosquito and undergo developmental changes in the mosquito.

Humans are the reservoir and the disease is transmitted to a susceptible host via the bite of an infected female *Anopheles* mosquito. The mosquito injects sporozoites, which are in her saliva, into the new host.

Trypanosoma – a slender, elongated protozoon, with a single flagellum. It is the causative organism of trypanosomiasis, or sleeping sickness, which is transmitted via the bite of an infected tsetse fly. There are two types of trypanosomes:

1. *American trypanosomiasis*, causing Chagas disease.
2. *African trypanosomiasis*, caused by *Trypanosoma rhodesiense* or *T. gambiense*.

T. rhodesiense can also be transmitted from an animal vector to a person.

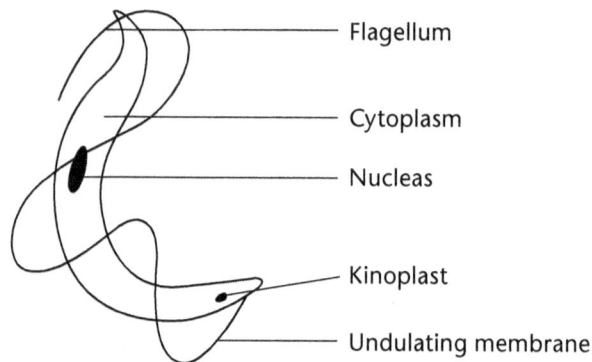

Figure 7.8 Trypanosoma

Toxoplasma gondi – this protozoon causes toxoplasmosis. This disease is frequently undiagnosed in human beings as the affected person has no symptoms. It can be passed to the foetus from an infected mother and causes congenital defects such as blindness and hydrocephalus. Toxoplasmosis is a disease of cats, which excrete the oocyst in their faeces. Human beings may acquire the infection through close contact with the animal.

Reservoirs of infection

A reservoir is a safe place where the organism can survive and multiply and is usually a warm and moist place with nutrients, which is ideally away from sunlight/UV light.

Sometimes the reservoir can be one and the same as a host; for example, a patient with psoriasis (reservoir) is spreading skin squames and is infected at the same time (the host).

Infection is spread by droplet contact or is airborne and this can take place via hands, bedding, equipment, food, dust, soil, etc, or via a vector such as a mosquito.

The microbes will be spread by secretions and excretions, such as droplets from the respiratory tract, sputum, pus from a wound, faeces or urine.

Carriers are people who harbour and transmit the causative organism of a disease without showing any of the signs and symptoms. They are often unaware that they are carrying the microbe in their body. The condition of the carrier may be *temporary or permanent*. During the convalescent period the person may appear well but may still transmit the microorganisms for a variable time. Some of these people may, however, go on to become permanent carriers who will excrete the microorganisms for many years. Such carriers are sometimes difficult to detect because they excrete the pathogens only intermittently. Carriers play an important part in the transmission of certain infections:

- *Diphtheria*: The carrier usually harbours the microbe in the nose and throat, and it is transmitted via droplets and fomites.
- *Dysentery*: In bacillary and amoebic dysentery the carrier excretes the microorganisms in watery stools, and milk and food may become contaminated through poor hygienic standards.
- *Meningococcal meningitis*: This meningococcus is found in discharge from the carrier's nose and throat and is distributed via droplets and fomites.
- *Poliomyelitis* is excreted in the faeces of sufferers and in that of convalescent and healthy carriers.
- *Infected animals*: Diseases of animals that can be transmitted to humans are known as *zoonoses*. Rabies, plague, anthrax, tapeworm and toxoplasmosis are a few examples of the zoonoses. Humans become infected either by direct contact with the animal, by eating the flesh or drinking the milk of the animal, or by indirect contact with soil, dust, wool or hides that harbour the pathogen.

Immunity

The immune system of the body is a complex combination of cell and chemical activities that assists the body to resist infection and certain diseases such as malignant growths. Immunity can be general (non-specific) or specific.

General (or non-specific) immunity

This is dependent on the state of general health of the individual, as well as the normal defences of the body, such as an intact healthy skin and mucous membrane, the action of the white blood cells, the lymph, and the body's secretions. Generally, someone who is in an adequate state of nutrition and who is not fatigued or suffering from psychological stress or disease has a high resistance to infection.

Specific immunity

This is due to the presence of certain specific antibodies in the blood; it may be either innate or acquired. Another form of immunity is herd (or community) immunity.

- *Innate immunity* applies to certain ethnic groups or species that have a higher resistance to some infections than others.
- *Acquired immunity* is illustrated in Table 7.1.
- *Herd (or community) immunity* is when a large enough proportion of the population has been vaccinated and therefore has immunity, making the spread of the disease from person to person unlikely. Herd immunity gives protection against an outbreak when one person becomes ill.

Table 7.1 Acquired immunity

Active	Passive
The body produces its own antibodies against specific microorganisms. It takes some time for this type of immunity to develop, usually a few weeks. This type of immunity lasts for many years, often for a lifetime.	The person receives ready-made antibodies as prophylaxis to prevent him or her from getting a known disease to which they may be exposed. It is of short duration and lasts only a few weeks or months.
Naturally acquired	**Naturally acquired**
The person suffers from an infection such as measles and produces antibodies against the measles virus.	The newborn infant receives antibodies from its mother via the placenta.
Artificially acquired	**Artificially acquired**
A vaccine or toxoid is administered either by injection or orally. This stimulates the body to form antibodies.	A serum containing ready-made antibodies is administered to someone who has been in contact with an infection or who is suffering from one, such as diphtheria.

Immunisation

Immunisation is a method of inducing an active artificial immunity in a susceptible person by the administration of a vaccine or a toxoid.

A vaccine is a suspension containing the dead or weakened organisms of a disease, while a toxoid is a saline suspension containing the toxins of the microorganisms. Effective immunisation of all children is probably the most important step in the prevention of many of the communicable diseases.

The Department of Health adopted the Expanded Programme of Immunisation (EPI (SA)) as advocated by the World Health Organization (WHO) in 1995.

Since then, the WHO has continued its work to prevent millions of deaths by promoting access to vaccinations; the most recent WHO initiative is the Global Vaccine Action Plan, released on 9 December 2019. Progress has been made in many areas, including the following:

- Two of the three poliovirus types have been eradicated.
- Rubella has been eliminated in 81 countries.
- Maternal and neonatal tetanus have been eliminated in all countries, except 12.
- Most low- and middle-income countries have introduced at least one new vaccine.
- Global child mortality has dropped by one-quarter.

Table 7.2 Expanded programme on immunisation – EPI (SA)

Age	Vaccine	Also known as	Protects against
Birth	OPV (0)	Oral polio vaccine (trivalent)	Polio
Birth	BCG	Bacille Calmette-Guerin vaccine	Tuberculosis
6 weeks	OPV (1)	Oral polio vaccine (trivalent)	Polio
6 weeks	RV (1)*	Rotavirus vaccine	Rotavirus
6 weeks	PCV (1)	Pneumococcal conjugate vaccine	Pneumococcal diseases
6 weeks	DTaP-IPV-HiB (1)	Pentavalent vaccine (5 in 1)	Diphtheria, tenanus, acellular pertussis (whooping cough), inactivated polio vaccine, haemophilus influenza type B
10 weeks	DTaP-IPV-HiB (2)	Pentavalent vaccine (5 in 1)	Diphtheria, tenanus, acellular pertussis (whooping cough), inactivated polio vaccine, haemophilus influenza type B
14 weeks	RV (2)*	Rotavirus vaccine	Rotavirus
14 weeks	PCV (2)	Pneumococcal conjugate vaccine	Pneumococcal diseases
14 weeks	DTaP-IPV-HiB (3)	Pentavalent vaccine (5 in 1)	Diphtheria, tenanus, acellular pertussis (whooping cough), inactivated polio vaccine, haemophilus influenza type B

➡

Age	Vaccine	Also known as	Protects against
6 months	Measles vaccine (1)	Measles vaccine	Measles
9 months	PCV (3)	Pneumococcal conjugate vaccine	Pneumococcal diseases
12 months	Measles vaccine (2)	Measles vaccine	Measles
18 months	DTaP-IPV-HiB (4)	Pentavalent vaccine (5 in 1)	Diphtheria, tenanus, acellular pertussis (whooping cough), inactivated polio vaccine, haemophilus influenza type B
6 years	Td vaccine	Tetanus and reduced strength diphtheria vaccine	Tetanus, diphtheria
12 years	Td vaccine	Tetanus and reduced strength diphtheria vaccine	Tetanus, diphtheria

* Note: Do not administer any dose of rotavirus vaccine to a child who is more than 24 weeks old.

Immunisation against some of the following diseases may be advisable for people who are exposed to them, for example:

- doctors and nurses against hepatitis B, pertussis (whooping cough)
- travellers who are going into areas where certain infections are endemic, eg yellow fever, typhoid, hepatitis A (consult your local travel medicine centre).

Vaccine administration

In this section we will examine the vaccines used against tuberculosis, diphtheria and tetanus oxides, pertussis, measles, poliomyelitis and rubella.

BCG (bacille Calmette-Guerin) vaccine 2000

The injection technique requires special training because if it is not done correctly an abscess could form.

The injection is given intradermally and causes a small mark, which looks like a mosquito bite, which can develop into a pimple-like structure. The injection site should not be rubbed nor should cream or ointments be applied. The site can take as long as three months to heal.

Note: BCG vaccine is affected by heat and light and should therefore be stored in a cool, dark place.

Diphtheria and tetanus toxoids

These are suspensions containing the toxins of the respective bacilli. Various methods are used to inactivate the toxins and render them harmless while allowing them to retain their antigenic properties.

Pertussis (whooping cough) vaccine

This is a suspension of dead pertussis bacilli. Diphtheria and tetanus toxoids are combined with pertussis vaccine to form a 'triple antigen'. This is administered by means of an intramuscular injection into the deltoid muscle after the skin over the area has been cleaned.

Note: After the age of two years only diphtheria and tetanus toxoid are administered because the whooping cough vaccine may cause serious reactions.

Measles vaccine

This is a freeze-dried vaccine containing attenuated, live measles viruses. A single dose is administered either intramuscularly or subcutaneously.

Note: Measles vaccine is sensitive to light and heat. It is inactivated by alcohol, ether and detergents. It is only effective for one year from the date of manufacture and for less than this period if it has not been stored under optimal conditions.

Poliomyelitis vaccine

This vaccine contains live but attenuated type 1, 2 and 3 poliomyelitis viruses. It is administered orally; three drops being squeezed into the infant's mouth from a dropper. It may also be given on sugar.

Note: An infant should not be breastfed for two hours before and two hours after the vaccine has been administered.

Rubella vaccine

The rubella vaccine is a freeze-dried, attenuated, live virus vaccine. One dose is administered subcutaneously.

Note: Reports received during recent measles and poliomyelitis epidemics indicate that many of the children who developed the infections had been immunised against them. There is no doubt that incorrect storage and faulty administration of the vaccines contribute to such failures.

It is important to remember the following when conducting immunisation campaigns:

- In the field, vaccines must be transported and kept in insulated cool bags.
- Expiry dates must be checked before administration.

- Any special precautions that must be taken in connection with the administration of a specific vaccine must be observed.
- The health workers should be proficient in the use of the correct techniques.

Conclusion

A basic understanding of microbiology is fundamental to understanding infection prevention and control. In this chapter we discussed the structure, characteristics and classification of single-cell microorganisms. We also looked at the methods that can be used to destroy pathogens, the reservoirs of infections, immunity, immunisation and vaccine administration.

Self-assessment

Match the causative organisms in column A with the diseases in column B.

Column A	Column B
Coronavirus SARS-CoV-2	COVID-19
Bacillus anthracis	whooping cough
Bordetella pertussis	syphilis
Yersinia pestis	anthrax
Treponema pallidum	pulmonary tuberculosis
Mycobacterium	thrush
Candida albicans	plague

Bibliography

COVID-19 Worldometer. nd. Available: https://www.worldometers.info/coronavirus/country/south-africa/ (Accessed 15 September 2020).

Department of Health (DOH). 1995. EPI manual SA. The expanded programme of immunisation (EPI). Available: www.health.gov.za (Accessed 11 September 2020).

South African Government. nd. Child immunisation. Available: https://www.gov.za/SERVICES/child-care/child-immunisation?gclid=CjwKCAjwzIH7BRAbEiwAoDxxTm P4CQslpRPQUwb0Te0dyNOT-6d20rcm53OFHKNLoFSM5UVGQp994BoC0igQAvD_BwE (Accessed 15 September 2020).

World Health Organization (WHO). 2019/2020. Coronavirus. Available: https://www.who.int/health-topics/coronavirus#tab=tab_1 (Accessed 15 September 2020).

World Health Organization (WHO). nd. Vaccinations and immunizations. Available: https://www.who.int/health-topics/vaccines-and-immunization?gclid=CjwKCAjwzIH 7BRAbEiwAoDxxTnbADBKKD_ICYI2dVkMAdGsdx-qtGwGwrBzKlnU9rdN_12gAvqV VHRoCq7sQAvD_BwE#tab=tab_1 (Accessed 15 September 2020).

Infection prevention and control

Joy Cleghorn

Learning outcomes

After studying this chapter, you should be able to:

- Describe what a healthcare-associated infection is.
- List the links in the chain of infection.
- Discuss the importance of hand hygiene.
- Discuss the 'five moments for hand hygiene'.
- Demonstrate the steps of hand washing and hand rubbing.
- Discuss factors that increase the risk of transmission.
- Discuss roles and responsibilities of the nurse and unit manager in infection prevention.
- Describe the term 'outbreak'.
- Describe the concept of 'bundles of care'.
- Describe the importance of antimicrobial stewardship.

Key terms

Antimicrobial stewardship: The practice of constant vigilance and countermeasures against microbial spread and infection.

CAI: Community-associated infection.

HAI: Healthcare-associated infection.

Vector: A mobile carrier of infection, such as a bird or an insect.

Introduction

Infection prevention and control refers to the prevention of infection from occurring, the identification of infection when it does occur, and the implementation of control measures to ensure that the infection does not spread to other patients or staff. Infections that manifest in healthcare facilities can be divided into:

- healthcare-associated infections (HAIs)
- community-associated infections (CAIs).

In this chapter, we are going to discuss HAIs, which are infections that were neither present nor incubating at the time of admission into the healthcare facility. These infections are sometimes referred to as 'nosocomial' infections (from the Greek 'nosus', which means disease, and 'komeion', which means to take care of).

HAIs also relate to staff and therefore the infection prevention and control programme should cover areas such as vaccination programmes for hepatitis B and the management of needlestick injuries and exposure to body fluids.

According to the World Health Organization (WHO), each year hundreds of millions of patients around the world are affected by HAIs. Although an HAI is the most frequent adverse event in healthcare, its true global burden remains unknown because of the difficulty in gathering reliable data.

Surveillance

Surveillance refers to the systematic collection and analysis of organism/disease data. The important function of surveillance is that it causes action to take place to stop further spread. There are various types of surveillance, for example:

- kardex/patient notes review
- routine ward/unit visits
- hospital-wide (comprehensive) surveillance
- laboratory-based surveillance
- targeted surveillance
- resistance surveillance.

Until recently, surveillance has predominantly been done manually; however, automated surveillance systems are becoming more popular and are less time consuming.

Preventing spread or 'breaking the chain' of infection

In order for infections to spread, all links in the chain of infection must be connected. In the prevention and control of infections, techniques used to break the link are referred to as 'breaking the chain of infection'.

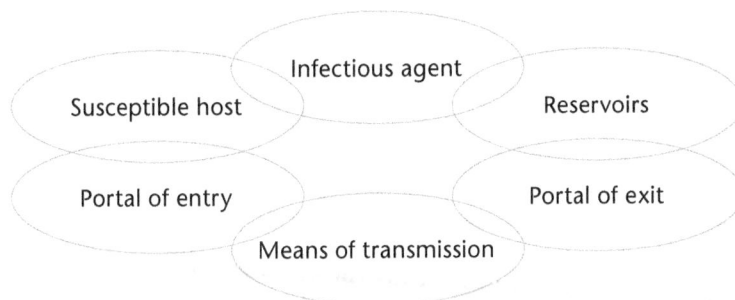

Figure 8.1 The chain of infection

Routes of infection

Routes of infection include:

- contact
- droplet
- airborne
- vector and common vehicle.

Risk factors for healthcare-associated infections

Factors that increase the risk of getting HAIs include the following:

- The microorganism involved as well as its strength (virulence), anti-microbial sensitivity or resistance.
- Patient risk factors, including:
  - length of patient stay
  - extreme age; that is, very young or very old
  - immunity levels
  - underlying disease/s such as diabetes
  - presence of a foreign body, as in joint replacement
  - disruption of host barriers, for example by central venous catheter.

Hand hygiene

Hand hygiene is the action of cleaning hands. There are two ways to clean hands – using an alcohol-based hand rub (ABHR) or, when hands are visibly soiled, washing with soap and running water.

Why is hand hygiene so important?

Keeping your hands clean through improved hand hygiene is one of the most important steps you can take to avoid spreading infections to one another. Most illnesses are spread when people do not clean their hands with soap and running water. If soap and water are not available, use an alcohol-based hand rub that contains 70 per cent alcohol to clean your hands.

When should hand hygiene be done?

The 'five moments for hand hygiene' approach defines the key moments when healthcare workers should perform hand hygiene, as presented by the WHO. See the WHO presentations on hand hygiene in Figure 8.2.

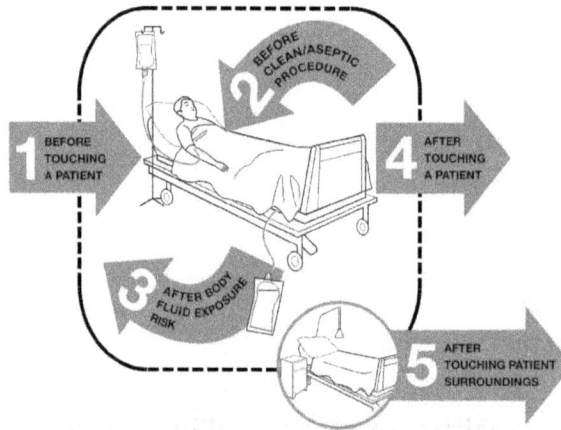

Your 5 moments for hand hygiene

1	Before touching a patient	WHEN?	Clean your hands before touching a patient when approaching him or her.
		WHY?	To protect the patient against harmful germs carried on your hands.
2	Before clean/aseptic procedure	WHEN?	Clean your hands immediately before performing a clean/aseptic procedure.
		WHY?	To protect the patient against harmful germs, including the patient's own, from entering his or her body.
3	After body fluid exposure risk	WHEN?	Clean your hands immediately after an exposure risk to body fluids (and after glove removal).
		WHY?	To protect yourself and the healthcare environment from harmful patient germs.
4	After touching a patient	WHEN?	Clean your hands after touching a patient and his or her immediate surroundings, when leaving the patient's side.
		WHY?	To protect yourself and the healthcare environment from harmful patient germs.
5	After touching patient surroundings	WHEN?	Clean your hands after touching any object or furniture in the patient's immediate surroundings, when leaving – even if the patient has not been touched.
		WHY?	To protect yourself and the healthcare environment from harmful patient germs.

Figure 8.2 The five moments for hand hygiene

Source: World Health Organization (nd (b))

The sequence used when cleaning hands with ABHR is important as this will ensure that all the surfaces of the hands have been covered with alcohol.

How to handrub?

Rub hands for hand hygiene! Wash hands when visibly soiled

⏱ **Duration of the entire procedure: 20–30 seconds**

1a / **1b** / **2**

Apply a palmful of the product in a cupped hand, covering all surfaces;

Rub hands palm to palm;

3 / **4** / **5**

Right palm over left dorsum with interlaced fingers and vice versa;

Palm to palm with fingers interlaced;

Back of fingers to opposing palms with fingers interlocked;

6 / **7** / **8**

Rotational rubbing of left thumb clasped in right palm and vice versa;

Rotational rubbing, backwards and forwards with clasped fingers of right hand in left palm and vice versa;

Once dry, your hands are safe.

How to handwash?

Wash hands when visibly soiled! Otherwise, use handrub

⏱ **Duration of the entire procedure: 40–60 seconds**

0 / **1** / **2**

Wet hands with water;

Apply enough soap to cover all hand surfaces;

Rub hands palm to palm;

3 / **4** / **5**

Right palm over left dorsum with interlaced fingers and vice versa;

Palm to palm with fingers interlaced;

Back of fingers to opposing palms with fingers interlocked;

6 / **7** / **8**

Rotational rubbing of left thumb clasped in right palm and vice versa;

Rotational rubbing, backwards and forwards with clasped fingers of right hand in left palm and vice versa;

Rinse hands with water;

9 / **10** / **11**

Dry hands thoroughly with a single use towel;

Use towel to turn off faucet;

Your hands are now safe.

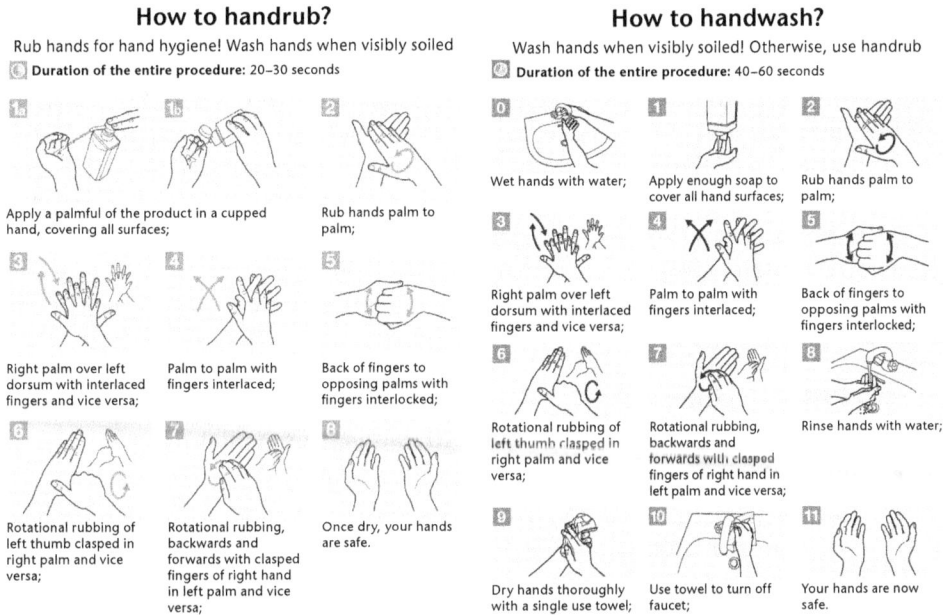

Figure 8.3 WHO guidelines on how to hand rub and hand wash

Source: World Health Organization (nd (a))

Infection prevention and control: Roles and responsibilities

Infection prevention and control is the responsibility of everyone, but we will focus on the roles and responsibilities of the ward/unit/clinic manager.

Infection prevention and control is the manager's direct responsibility and it falls within his or her scope of practice to ensure a safe environment that is clean and the risks of infection are minimised. This is done in close liaison with the infection prevention and control specialist/practitioner.

The unit manager is responsible for the safe practice of staff under her or his supervision and everyone who comes into the ward, including doctors, radiographers, physiotherapists, cleaning staff, catering staff and visitors. The unit manager must insist on compliance.

Other responsibilities include staff training to ensure safety and minimise the risk of infection through protective measures, correct technique, correct approach to injury on duty, and standard precautions that are used as standard practice.

The unit manager has a legal responsibility to ensure the availability of suitable protective clothing in keeping with the type of risk.

Bundles of care

A bundle of care is a grouping of best practices with respect to a disease process that individually improves care, but when applied together results in substantially greater improvement. The science behind the bundle is so well established that it should be considered as the standard of care. Bundles eschew the piecemeal application of proven therapies in favour of an 'all or none' approach.

In the healthcare context, a bundle is a set of evidence-based practices (generally three to five) which, when practised reliably on every patient every time (the meaning of bundled), have been shown to improve outcomes. Some examples of bundles of care are described below.

Surgical site infections (SSIs)

- If hair is removed, it is only done with clippers or depilatory cream.
- Antibiotics are given at the correct dose, within an hour of incision.
- Glucose is maintained above 4 and below 10 mmol/l for major surgical procedures on admission to ICU.
- Temperature is maintained at ≥ 35.5 for colorectal and major abdominal surgeries.

Ventilator-associated pneumonia (VAP)

- The head of the bed is elevated between 30° and 45°.
- Sedation vacation is done daily.
- Deep vein thrombosis (DVT) prophylaxis is given, or foot pumps are used.
- Mouth care is done at least six hourly using an antiseptic mouth wash.

Central line-associated bloodstream infections (CLABSIs)

- Hand washing procedure is followed.
- Maximal barrier precautions are used by the doctor.
- Chlorhexidine and alcohol skin preparation is done and allowed to dry before insertion.
- Central line is preferably sited in the subclavian vein for adults and the umbilical vein in neonates. (The femoral site should be avoided.)
- A daily review is done of the need to keep the line.
- The line is properly secured, for example with a dressing or special device, or it is stitched.
- The dressing is visibly clean and intact.

Catheter-associated urinary tract infection (CAUTI)

- Avoid the unnecessary use of catheters.
- Insert the catheter using aseptic technique.
- Maintain catheters based on recommended guidelines for daily care.
- Review the necessity for the catheter daily.

Outbreaks

An outbreak of a communicable disease or infection can be defined as the incidence of disease above that which is normally expected. Usually this means that there are two or more linked cases of the same illness or symptoms. An example of an internal outbreak spread within a hospital may be MRSA; an example of an external outbreak may be a number of people with foodborne illness from a mass sporting event.

In cases where a disease has spread across the world it is known as a pandemic, for example coronavirus disease 2019 (COVID-19) or SARS-CoV-2.

In some instances, only one case of significant risk may be sufficient to fulfil the definition, for example as is the case with an outbreak of Ebola.

The importance of antimicrobial stewardship

Antimicrobial resistance is a major public health crisis and there is very little development in the world with newer and better antibiotics. A call to action was made by the WHO in 2013 for urgent interventions to alleviate the problem.

HAIs, caused by organisms such as multi-drug resistant *Pseudomonas aeruginosa*, *Clostridium difficile*, *Klebsiella pneumoniae*, carbapenemase-producing organisms and MRSA, etc, are not only responsible for significant morbidity and mortality in healthcare facilities but also for an increase in healthcare costs. Resistant organisms have arisen due to a multitude of reasons and it is well documented that an important cause is due to the misuse and abuse of antibiotics. Strategies such as antimicrobial stewardship (AMS) have been implemented to discourage the over-prescription of antibiotics. Stewardship includes aspects such as ensuring that the correct dose is given at the right time for the right duration, de-escalating as soon as possible, for example intravenous to oral treatment; an awareness of regional and hospital resistance trends in order to guide empiric therapy; microbiologist-/physician-led ICU rounds; having a leading doctor who champions AMS, and so on. Although prescribing is a doctor-driven process, nurses, pharmacists and microbiologists all play a vital role in guiding the safe prescription of medicine in southern Africa by way of reminders and recordkeeping, ensuring availability of laboratory results, monitoring hospital resistance patterns, and so on.

Conclusion

Infection control is the responsibility of every person working in the healthcare environment and should not be reserved solely for the infection control specialist. Research has shown that by adhering to a set of simple measures it is possible to reduce the number of HAIs significantly.

Self-assessment

1. List the links in the chain of infection.
2. Why is antimicrobial stewardship so important?
3. Define an 'outbreak' in the healthcare context.
4. List the elements for the CLABSI bundle.

Bibliography

Centres for Disease Control and Prevention. 2020 (last updated). Transmission dynamics of COVID-19. Available: https://www.cdc.gov/mmwr/volumes/69/wr/mm6937e3.htm (Accessed 15 September 2020).

International Society for Infectious Diseases (ISID). 2018. Guide for infection control in hospital. Available: https://isid.org/wp-content/uploads/2018/02/ISID_InfectionGuide_Chapter16.pdf (Accessed 15 September 2020).

World Health Organization (WHO). 2015. Clean care is safer. Available: www.who.int/gpsc/5may/en (Accessed 10 March 2020).

World Health Organization (WHO). nd (a). How to handwash; How to handrub. Available: https://www.who.int/gpsc/tools/GPSC-HandRub-Wash.pdf (Accessed 11 September 2020).

World Health Organization (WHO). nd (b). My 5 moments for hand hygiene. Available: https://www.who.int/infection-prevention/campaigns/clean-hands/5moments/en/ (Accessed 15 September 2020).

Communicable diseases

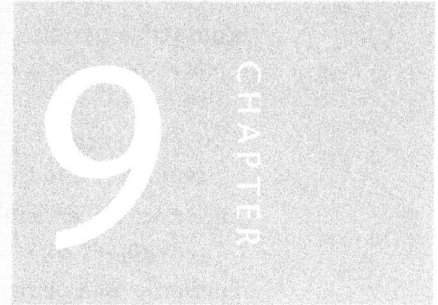

Joy Cleghorn

Learning outcomes

After studying this chapter, you should be able to:

- Define the terminology associated with communicable diseases.
- Identify the different types of rash associated with communicable diseases.
- Explain how a triad of host factors can influence the transmission of a communicable disease.
- Describe the different stages of a communicable disease.
- Explain what the 'triad' of factors in communicable disease means.
- Identify and share ways in which communicable diseases can be prevented and controlled in the community.
- Explain the term 'notifiable disease'.
- Name the communicable diseases that are common in Africa and identify ways to prevent them.
- Name the diseases spread by parasites that are common in Africa and identify ways to prevent them.

Key terms

Carrier: A person or animal that hosts a specific infective agent while not showing any clinical manifestation of the disease but who has the ability to spread the disease. The condition may be temporary or permanent and is dependent on the disease.

Communicable diseases: A group of infectious diseases caused by specific microorganisms that are readily transmissible from an infected person to a susceptible host. A rash accompanies some of these diseases.

Contact: A person who has been in contact with an infected person or animal or exposed to a contaminated object or infected agent. A contact can be a source of infection for other people.

Convalescence: This is the time elapsing between the total disappearance of all symptoms and the patient's restoration to full health.

Endemic: An endemic disease is one that is constantly present in a defined geographic area.

Epidemic: A large number of cases of a disease in a community, in excess of the expected number.

Isolation period: This is the length of time for which persons known to be ill with an infectious disease must be kept away from contact with other people, or must be isolated, so that they do not infect others. Isolation-period times vary for different diseases.

Quarantine: Applies to those who have been exposed to a contagious disease but who may or may not become ill. The quarantine period applies to the period of time persons have to be isolated to ensure that they are not harbouring and spreading the disease. The quarantine period is usually a day or two longer than the incubation period of the given disease.

Sporadic: An occasional instance or scattered instances of a disease.

Terminal disinfection: The application of disinfection measures after the patient has died or been transferred to a hospital, or after the patient has ceased to be a source of infection.

Terms used in connection with rashes:

Erythema: From the Greek *erythros*, meaning red, it is redness of the skin or mucous membranes, caused by hyperaemia (increased blood flow) in superficial capillaries. Examples of erythema not associated with pathology include nervous blush.

Macule: A discoloured area or spot that is not raised above the level of the skin.

Papule: A solid, circumscribed lesion that is raised above the level of the skin.

Pustule: A small, raised lesion of the skin that contains pus.

Vesicle: A raised lesion of the skin that is filled with a clear fluid and resembles a blister. It can occur with any skin injury, infection or inflammation.

Introduction

A communicable disease can be defined as an illness that arises from the transmission of an infectious agent or its toxic product from an infected person, animal, or reservoir to a susceptible host, either directly or indirectly through an intermediate plant or animal host, vector or environment. As the spread of these diseases can be linked with environmental conditions and with poverty, they pose a serious threat to under-developed areas such as those found in sub-Saharan Africa. The situation has been exacerbated in the area because of natural disasters caused by floods and droughts, geographic factors and political problems such as conflict and wars.

The spread of communicable or infectious diseases is preventable and there is evidence that these diseases can be controlled, even in the poorest countries. Such control can be achieved with an integrated approach that focuses on the underlying causes such as the socioeconomic, cultural and physical environment, as well as issues relating to the disease condition itself. Note that the terms 'infectious' and 'communicable' diseases can be used interchangeably.

Epidemiology of communicable diseases

In this section we examine the triad of host factors in the spread of communicable diseases, and the prevention and control of communicable diseases.

The triad of host factors in communicable disease

The triad, or triangle, of communicable disease shows that if the environment brings together a susceptible host and a causative organism, this will result in an infectious disease. The terms *agent*, *host* and *environment*, as used in this context, are defined as follows:

- **Agent**: The causative organism or the toxin the organism produces.
- **Host**: The susceptible individual or population linked to factors such as predisposing disease, and his or her level of immunity to the disease, or his or her state of nutrition.
- **Environment**: Factors including poverty and living conditions such as overcrowding or lack of sanitation, social exclusion and limited or no access to healthcare.

A healthy host is a person who has a high natural state of immunity and therefore can more easily resist infection. The person's immunity against a specific infective agent can be either natural or acquired. This was discussed in more detail in Chapter 7.

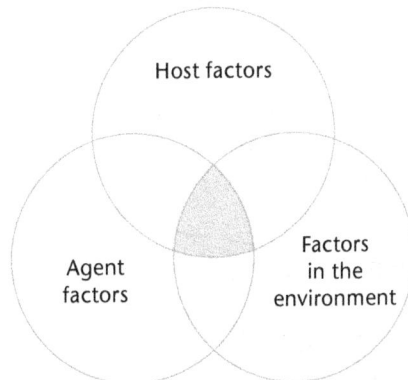

Figure 9.1 The epidemiology of communicable diseases

As the disease develops in the host, it passes through a number of stages:

- **Incubation period**: The time elapsing between initial infection and the onset of the first symptoms of the disease. The organisms multiply in the body during this period. The actual period of time differs from disease to disease and is usually characteristic of the specific disease (the person can be infectious during this period).

- **Prodromal**: Non-specific complaints (infectious).

- **Acme**: Symptoms characteristic of disease and marked by the period of highest temperature readings (most contagious).

- **Convalescence**: Regaining normal function (possibly still contagious).

The prevention and control of communicable diseases

Communicable diseases are preventable, but should they occur they can be controlled if certain procedures are followed. The following actions are important in the prevention and control of communicable diseases:

- **Early diagnosis**: The most infectious time is before the disease is diagnosed, when no steps are being taken to isolate the patient or to disinfect fomites or discharges.

- **Prompt and effective treatment**: This will reduce the risk of infection because the patient is frequently rendered non-infectious shortly after the commencement of treatment with adequate doses of the appropriate antibiotic, or other suitable medication, has decreased the number of microorganisms in the body.

- **Notification of diseases**: The Health Act 61 of 2003 makes it mandatory to report the listed conditions. This must be done verbally immediately and followed up in writing within 24 hours, by e-mail. The following information must be included:
  - name, age, gender, identity number and date of birth
  - residential address, place of employment or educational institution
  - information regarding the communicable condition, including information on where the disease may have been acquired, and possible contacts.

The latest Act separates tuberculosis (eg tuberculosis of the bones and joints, tuberculosis of the meninges and tuberculosis of other organs). The report should be sent to the district and provincial offices responsible for communicable disease control.

Notification is an important step in the control of the communicable disease because it sets in motion a series of steps designed to trace the source of the infection and to prevent its spread.

Certain diseases must be reported to the World Health Organization (WHO); some examples of these are cholera, plague, smallpox, polio, typhus and yellow fever as well as 'formidable epidemic diseases' such as viral haemorrhagic fevers like Lassa, Ebola, etc.

Table 9.1 Notifiable communicable diseases (Regulation R703 of 1993)

• Acute flaccid paralysis	• Plague
• Acute rheumatoid fever	• Poliomyelitis
• Anthrax	• Rabies (specify whether human case or human contact)
• Brucellosis	
• Cholera	• Smallpox and any smallpox-like disease, excluding chickenpox
• Diphtheria	
• Food poisoning (outbreaks of more than four persons)	• Tetanus
	• Tetanus neonatorum
• Haemorrhagic fevers of Africa (Congo fever, Dengue fever, Ebola fever, Lassa fever, Marburg fever and Rift Valley fever)	• Trachoma
	• Typhoid fever
	• Typhus fever (endemic louse-born typhus fever, endemic flea-borne typhus fever)
• Legionellosis	
• Leprosy	• Tuberculosis (pulmonary and other forms)
• Malaria	
• Measles	• Viral hepatitis A, B, non-A, non-B, and undifferentiated
• Meningococcal infections	• Whooping cough
• Paratyphoid fever	• Yellow fever

Source: Department of Health, KwaZulu-Natal (nd)

Note: Coronavirus disease 2019 (COVID-19) will be added to this list.

The management of various factors are crucial in the containment of infectious diseases:

- **Isolation:** The infectious patient must be isolated until regarded as not infectious. While the patient is infectious it is important to carry out:
  - rigorous hand hygiene
  - concurrent disinfection of all infective discharges and excretions and of fomites
  - terminal disinfection of the room and all the effects of the patient when the infectious period is over.
- **Contacts:** These must be traced and managed as follows:
  - Immune contacts may return to work or to school once they have been removed from the source of infection.
  - Susceptible contacts may be medically examined, immunised, placed in quarantine and, in some cases, placed on prophylactic chemotherapy.
- **Immunisation:** For a description of immunisation, see Chapter 7.

- **Improvement of environmental hygiene**: This is especially important where sanitation and water supplies are contaminated.
- **Control of the insect vectors**: The insect vectors responsible for the transmission of the microorganisms must be controlled.
- **Improved ventilation**: Adequate housing and the prevention of overcrowding are essential for the control of airborne infections.
- **Improvement of nutritional status**: Improving the nutritional status of community members will do much to increase resistance to infection.
- **Improved standards of personal hygiene**: Cleanliness and a clean, hygienic environment will help to eliminate the risk of communicable diseases to a great extent.
- **Health education**: Informing people about the early signs and symptoms of a disease, its mode of transmission and measures that can be taken to prevent it will assist the members of the community to prevent the disease and to seek medical help early.

An integrated approach is needed to control communicable diseases. One or more preventative interventions on their own will not reduce the incidence of communicable diseases.

Communicable diseases in Africa

Tables 9.2 and 9.3 show the most common communicable diseases, categorised by mode of spread.

Table 9.2 Mode of spread: Droplet infection or inhalation

Disease	Causative organism	Incubation period	Clinical signs	Source
Influenza	Types A, B and C and other serotypes	2–3 days	Rigors, sore throat, headache and aching muscles	Humans, birds, primates, mammals
SARS-CoV-1	Coronavirus	3–10 days	Rigors, sore throat, headache, aching muscles and very high temperature	Inconclusive

➤

Disease	Causative organism	Incubation period	Clinical signs	Source
SARS-CoV-2 causing coronavirus disease (COVID-19)	Coronavirus disease 2019 (COVID-19)	2–14 days	Cough, sore throat, shortness of breath, anosmia (loss of sense of smell) or dysgeusia (loss of sense of taste), with or without other symptoms (which may include fever, weakness, myalgia or diarrhoea). COVID-19 generally causes mild to moderate illness although patients with co-morbidities become more ill and may require oxygen therapy or ventilation and may die.	Believed to have zoonotic origin COVID-19 was first discovered in an animal market in Wuhan, China, in late 2019, and in 2020 swiftly spread across the globe, causing a large-scale global pandemic
Pulmonary tuberculosis	*Mycobacterium tuberculosis*	2–4 weeks (can be shorter or longer)	Chronic infection characterised in the later stages by a cough; there may be haemoptysis, night sweats and loss of weight. TB can affect other organs, but the rate of infection from other areas is low.	Humans and primates
Legionnaires' disease	*Legionella pneumophila*	2–14 days	Cold-like symptoms progressing to shortness of breath, fatigue, chest pain, loss of appetite and gastrointestinal symptoms	Water inhaled through air conditioning, waterfalls, etc
Anthrax	*Bacillus anthracis*	2–7 days	Cough, temperature with pneumonia and toxaemia that is often fatal, or it can present as skin lesions known as malignant pustules with a central black area surrounded by inflammation.	Animals (meat and hides), biological warfare

➡

Disease	Causative organism	Incubation period	Clinical signs	Source
Leprosy (Hansen's disease)	*Mycobacterium lepromatosis; M. leprae*	2–10 years in susceptible hosts	Manifestation is slow. First presents as skin lesions that change colour and are painless. Muscle weakness and loss of sensation in the feet and hands usually result in accidents and patients present with burns or other injuries.	Humans, but not highly infectious after treatment
Mumps	Paramyxovirus	14–21 days	Pyrexia, anorexia, malaise and headaches. Within 24 hours pain is experienced near the ear lobe and on swallowing. Swelling of the glands occurs. Swelling of both sides does not occur simultaneously and may only affect one side.	Humans
Rubella (German measles)	Rubella virus	14–21 days	Mild pyrexia, malaise, enlarged cervical and often occipital glands. An irregular pink and red macular rash appears on the first day on the face and torso, spreads to the limbs on the second day and disappears within 3–5 days. (It has serious risks for the pregnant mother in the first trimester.)	Humans

➡

Disease	Causative organism	Incubation period	Clinical signs	Source
Whooping cough	*Bordetella pertussis*	7–12 days	Disease occurs in three stages: *Catarrhal stage*: 1–2 weeks with malaise, anorexia and symptoms of a common cold. *Paroxysmal stage*: Lasts about three weeks and consists of bouts of coughing that become severe spasmodic repetitious coughing attacks that are followed by a 'whoop' as the patient sucks in air, and vomiting. *Recovery stage*: Lasts 3–4 weeks	Humans
Scarlet fever	*Streptococcus pyogenes*	2–5 days	Onset is sudden with a severe sore throat, tonsils are red, swollen, tongue is coated white and temperature is high 39–40°C. A red papular rash appears on the second day starting on the neck and chest and then spreads to the rest of the body. After 2–3 days the tongue peels and a red raw tongue known as strawberry tongue occurs. A pale circle around the mouth also appears.	Humans

Disease	Causative organism	Incubation period	Clinical signs	Source
Polio or Poliomyelitis	3 serotypes of poliovirus	6–20 days	Can present as a sub-clinical, non-paralytic or a paralytic disease. All present with pyrexia, headache, vomiting, sore throat and nausea. Followed in a minority of cases by a flaccid paralysis of certain muscles, most commonly the legs. All flaccid paralysis is notifiable to eliminate the possibility of it being poliomyelitis.	Oral–oral and oral–faecal – highly contagious
Ebola/Marburg	Filoviridae	2–21 days	Flu-like symptoms with muscle and joint pain. Followed by nausea, vomiting, laryngitis and chest pains. Maculopapular rash occurs over the whole body and can be followed by haemorrhages in skin, liver and kidneys, causing necrosis. Destroys lymphocytes.	Unknown, possibly primates and other mammals

Table 9.3 Mode of spread: Ingestion of infected water, milk and food

Disease	Causative organism	Incubation period	Clinical signs	Source
Cholera	Vibrio	2–3 days	Sudden onset of abdominal cramps with severe diarrhoea (rice-water stools), vomiting and results in very rapid dehydration. Patient can lose 15 litres or more in 24 hours, which can lead to renal failure, vascular collapse and shock.	Contaminated water/food (oral–faecal spread)
Typhoid fever	*Salmonella typhi*	8–14 days	Infected bile causes an inflammation of the small intestine causing 'pea-soup' stools after about a week. The patient becomes pyrexial and often has a slow pulse during the second week.	Contaminated water/food (oral–faecal spread)
Hepatitis A	Picornavirus	28–30 days	Fatigue, nausea, vomiting, dark urine, low-grade fever, yellowing of the skin and eyes	Oral–faecal spread
Food poisoning	Salmonella species	12–36 hours	Signs and symptoms of food poisoning	Poultry, meat, eggs
	Clostridium perfringens	22–36 hours	Signs and symptoms of food poisoning	Raw meat, dehydrated products
	Staphylococcus aureus	1–6 hours	Signs and symptoms of food poisoning	Dairy products
	Campylobacter	1–10 days	Signs and symptoms of food poisoning	Poultry, water, meat
	Bacillus cereus	1–6 days	Signs and symptoms of food poisoning	Cereals, rice

Table 9.4 Mode of spread: Sexual intercourse, infected blood and blood products including the placenta, also needles and sharp instruments through inoculation

Disease	Causative organism	Incubation period	Clinical signs	Source
HIV and AIDS	Retrovirus HIV-1, HIV-2	1–3 months	Asymptomatic for many years, then fatigue, loss of weight; recurrent infections, most commonly respiratory, such as pneumonia occur. Affects the auto-immune system and results in those infected being subject to secondary infections.	Sexual contact or through healthcare worker exposure to body fluids, eg through needle-stick injury
Hepatitis B	Hepadnavirus	45–180 days	Weakness and fatigue, abdominal pain, nausea, vomiting, dark urine, fever, joint pain, yellowing of the skin and eyes	Sexual contact or through healthcare worker exposure to body fluids, eg through needle-stick injury
Hepatitis C	Flaviviridae	2 weeks–6 months	Fatigue, fever, nausea or poor appetite, muscle and joint pains, tenderness in liver region	Sexual contact or through healthcare worker exposure to body fluids, eg through needle-stick injury and blood transfusions where the blood has not been tested for HCV
Chancroid	*Haemophilus ducreyi*	3–7 days	Affects men more than women. A papule, usually Singular, appears, and becomes necrotic forming a painful ulcer. It can occur in the genitalia or pharynx.	Sexual contact

➡

Disease	Causative organism	Incubation period	Clinical signs	Source
Granuloma inguinale	*Klebsiella granulomatis* (previously known as *Calymmato-bacterium granulomatis*)	8–80 days	Chronic infection of the genital organs with ulcers that cause scarring. Discharge can have offensive smell.	Sexual contact
Genital warts	Human papillomavirus	Months to years	Papulae that develop into pink warts. Can become large and obstructive and bleed easily. May progress to the cervix and anus.	Sexual contact
Gonorrhoea	*Neisseria gonorrhoeae*	2–14 days	Painful passing of urine followed by a yellowish-white discharge, pyrexia and swollen groin lymph glands. In men it is accompanied by a swollen, painful prostate and scrotum. Women complain of signs and symptoms related to pelvic inflammatory disease.	Sexual contact
Herpes genitalis or genital herpes	Herpesvirus HSV-1 and HSV-2	4–7 days	Vesicles form on the genital organs. They are painful and later rupture to form small ulcers that become itchy when healing.	Sexual contact
Chlamydia trachomatis infection	*Chlamydia trachomatis*	7 days to several months	The disease can cause urethritis, proctitis and pelvic inflammatory disease and is the single most important infectious agent associated with blindness.	Sexual contact

➡

Disease	Causative organism	Incubation period	Clinical signs	Source
Syphilis	*Treponema pallidum*	4–12 days	Primary syphilis presents with a chancre or ulcer on the genital organs forming erosion that will heal within 6 weeks. If untreated, latent syphilis develops within 2–20 years.	Sexual contact. Syphilis can be spread through healthcare worker exposure to body fluids, eg through needle-stick injury
Trichomoniasis	*Trichomonas vaginalis*	5–28 days	Women experience itching and a foul-smelling discharge. Men may be without symptoms.	Sexual contact

Table 9.5 Mode of spread: Bite of an infected (or carrier) interim host (vector). Once the patient is infected most of these conditions can be transmitted from person to person by droplet infection

Disease	Causative organism	Incubation period	Clinical signs	Source
Malaria	*Plasmodium falciparum; P. malariae; P. ovax; P. vivax.*	7–30 days	Moderate to severe rigors, chills, fever and then rigors as the fever breaks. Other signs may include headache, nausea, vomiting, diarrhoea.	Mosquito
Ebola	Filoviridae (mononegavirales). Reservoir is thought to be the fruit bat	2–21 days after coming into contact with the virus	Bleeding, vomiting, bloody diarrhoea, body pains, fever (common to other less serious illnesses). You cannot get Ebola from healthy people who have travelled to West Africa, or through air, food or water.	Contact with wild animals such as bats, monkeys and forest antelope (especially organs and blood) – in areas with endemic infection. Unprotected contact with people infected with Ebola, via blood, vomit, saliva and diarrhoea.

➡

Disease	Causative organism	Incubation period	Clinical signs	Source
Lassa fever	Arenavirus	6–21 days	General malaise, anorexia, diarrhoea, with pyrexia. This is followed by oedema of the face, pharyngitis and conjunctivitis. Haemorrhages occur in body tissues with myocarditis, often results in heart failure.	It is transmitted through food or fomites contaminated with rodent excreta. Highly contagious from person to person
Crimean-Congo fever	Nairovirus	1–12 days	Sudden onset with rigors, acute headaches and epigastric pain. Haemorrhages occur in the tissue and organs that can result in organ failure, shock and death.	Tick
Dengue fever	Flavivirus	3–14 days	Endemic in many African countries. Presents as a flu-like illness. Complications are caused by high fever, haemorrhagic phenomena, often with enlargement of the liver, and in severe cases circulatory failure.	Mosquito
Yellow fever	Flavivirus	3–6 days	Symptoms can be mild to severe. Fever and headaches, muscle aches (particularly back of knees) dizziness, red face, tongue and eyes	Mosquito

➡

Disease	Causative organism	Incubation period	Clinical signs	Source
Bubonic plague	*Yersinia pestis*	2–7 days	Enlarged and painful lymph glands (bubo), usually in the groin and pyrexia. Bacteraemia occurs resulting in purulent, necrotic and haemorrhagic lesions in the lymph nodes and later in the skin. Gives rise to the name of 'black death'.	Transmitted by an infected flea from an infected animal, usually rodents. Can be spread by droplet infection when the lungs are infected.
Rift Valley Fever	Virus transmitted by the mosquito or contact with infected animals, milk	3–7 days	Viraemia and pyrexia with rigors develop followed by capillary damage. This results in the loss of plasma and erythrocytes. During the acute stage, which lasts for up to two weeks, headaches, diarrhoea, vomiting and muscle weakness occur. Organ failure and haemorrhages can result in shock and death.	Virus transmitted by the mosquito or contact with infected animals, milk
Trypanoso-miasis Sleeping sickness	*Trypanosoma rhodesiense or gambiense*	2–6 months	The site of the bite is characterised by oedema and enlarged lymph glands. The spleen and the liver may be enlarged and palpable and if untreated results in neurological symptoms, including meningo-encephalitis, apathy with slow speech and later with a shuffling gait and tremor affecting the tongue.	Tsetse fly

Parasitic diseases common in Africa

Most parasitic conditions occur in places where basic standards of environmental hygiene are poor. Poor environmental sanitation, the accumulation of refuse and the unsatisfactory disposal of human excreta and other waste offer ideal breeding grounds for parasites. There are different types of parasite:

External: These parasites are usually associated with overcrowding and poor environmental hygiene. They include:

- lice (pediculosis)
- fleas
- flies
- mites (scabies)
- mosquitos.

To prevent diseases caused by parasites, a control programme needs to be implemented. Such a programme will consist of the following components:

- eradication of the parasite
- protection of individuals from the parasite
- chemoprophylaxis – the use of appropriate drugs where available.

Success of the control programme is dependent on community participation and acceptance of the activities. It is important, therefore, that community members be involved from the planning stage of these disease-control programmes.

Fungi: The forms of fungi that cause disease in humans are mostly mycelia such as *Candida albicans*, which causes thrush. *Candida auris* causes mainly bloodstream, wound and ear infections. The other group that causes conditions of the skin, such as ringworm and athlete's foot, is known as dermatomycosis.

Table 9.6 Infections caused by fungi

Disease	Causative organism	Clinical picture	Specific prevention
Ringworm	Trichophyton and Microsporum are common causes	Presents with itchy ring-shaped patches that have raised borders. If untreated the patches grow bigger and the centres heal with a silvery sheen. Some of the well-known diseases caused are: Tinea pedis (athlete's foot), Tinea corporis (affects arms, legs and trunks) and Tinea capitis (affects the scalp).	Avoid sharing clothes, towels and other toiletry articles. Avoid being barefoot in communal showers.

➡

Disease	Causative organism	Clinical picture	Specific prevention
Thrush (Candida)	*Candida albicans*	Grows in warm, moist areas of the body and can affect the skin and the mucous membranes, by being itchy. Skin infections appear as red patchy areas with white scaly edges to the lesions. Common sites are in skin creases and on the vulva or penis. Mucous membrane infections have a white milk curd appearance and the affected area bleeds easily.	Keep skin clean and dry. Avoid sharing clothes, towels and other toiletry articles. Maintain good personal hygiene and avoid taking unnecessary antibiotics.
Bloodstream, wound and ear infections	*Candida auris*	Bloodstream, wound and ear infections	Stringent cleaning of the environment and hand hygiene. Maintain good personal hygiene.

Helminthic infections: Worm infestation is very common in Africa. Infestation is mainly intestinal but can affect other organs. Children are principally affected, and the condition contributes to malnourishment in children who are already vulnerable as the result of poverty and poor environmental hygiene.

Table 9.7 Helminthic infections

Disease	Causative organism	Clinical picture	Specific prevention
Hookworm	*Ancylostoma duodenale*	Abdominal discomfort, bloody stools and bloody sputum, loss of appetite, pale skin. Cough and diarrhoea	Improve sanitation. Stop children playing in sand that may be contaminated by faeces.

➡

Disease	Causative organism	Clinical picture	Specific prevention
Roundworm (Ascariasis)	*Ascaris lumbricoides*	Long whitish/pink worms that grow to approximately 35 cm in length. Infestation is often associated with a cough and a painful distended abdomen. Intestinal obstruction can occur. Adult worms live in the small intestine of humans. Eggs passed in human faeces. Eggs swallowed. Larvae set free. Larvae carried to lung via bloodstream, then migrate to intestine via trachea.	Improve sanitation, environmental and personal hygiene.
Tapeworm	*Taenia saginata* (cattle) and *T. solium* (pigs)	Cysts are present in the muscle of the infected animal. The human host ingests the cyst through eating infected meat. The worm emerges from the cyst in the small intestine and attaches itself to the wall. It develops new flat white segments and the worm grows through this process. The *Taenia saginata* reaches 5–10 m while the *T. solium* reaches 2–4 m. Signs and symptoms are often not present.	Improve sanitation and environmental hygiene where animals graze. Inspect meat and ensure adequate cooking.
Threadworm	*Enterobius vermicularis*	White thread-like worms often seen in the stools. Anal itching occurs especially at night when the females lay their eggs. Eggs containing larva carried to human mouth by fingers. Adults live in small intestine of humans. Fertilised female migrates to rectum. Eggs deposited on peri-anal skin at night. Larva develops in egg. Spread by hand to mouth and through contaminated fomites.	Improve environmental and personal hygiene, including the management of sewage.

Rickettsia: These diseases are transmitted to humans by the bite of bloodsucking insects such as fleas, ticks and lice.

Table 9.8 Diseases caused by rickettsia

Disease	Causative organism	Clinical picture	Specific prevention
Tickbite fever	*Rickettsia conorii*	Incubation period can be 10–18 days. Bite is characterised by a black centre that may suppurate. Pyrexia and headaches will be present and the patient will develop a maculopapular skin rash.	Protection from tick bites
Typhus	*Rickettsia prowazekii* (spread by body lice)	The microorganisms enter and multiply in the small blood vessels, causing vessels to leak and thrombi to form. The patient will suffer from headaches and will present with a maculopapular infection over the whole body except on the palms of the hands and the soles of the feet.	Disinfestations of body lice

Protozoa: These single cells vary in shape, size and structure and cause disease if introduced to the human body.

Table 9.9 Diseases caused by protozoa

Disease	Causative organism	Clinical picture	Specific prevention
Amoebic dysentery	*Entamoeba histolytica*	Occurs mostly in tropical areas through the contamination of vegetables. The disease can cause abdominal pain and discomfort with intermittent diarrhoea that contains mucus and blood.	Practise good environmental and personal hygiene. Avoid contamination of vegetables and food with faeces.

➡

Disease	Causative organism	Clinical picture	Specific prevention
Bilharzia	*Schistosoma mansoni, S. haematobium,* and *S. japonicum*	The human host becomes infected when the skin comes into contact with cercariae in infected water. Penetration of skin occurs. The snail is the vector. Symptoms occur within 4–6 weeks. At the site of the bite there is an itchy papular rash for 24 hours. Within 4–8 weeks the person will present with pyrexia, rigors, headaches, joint pains and a rash. Haematuria or bloody stools occur.	It is spread by a freshwater snail found in rivers and dams. Educate people to discourage urination into rivers and dams and swimming in infected water. Control snails by removing vegetation along the shores of rivers and dams and promoting birdlife. Provide toilet facilities.
Giardiasis	*Giardia lamblia*	Infection may be asymptomatic or may cause acute or chronic diarrhoea with bulky, greasy offensive-smelling stools. Fatigue and weight loss can occur.	Practise good environmental and personal hygiene. Avoid contamination of vegetables and food with faeces.
Toxoplasmosis	*Toxoplasma gondii*	Transmitted via the oral-faecal route. Can cause spontaneous abortion, stillbirths and congenital abnormalities in pregnant women.	It is spread by domestic pets, infected meat and rodents. Maintain healthy domestic animals, especially cats. Wash hands after handling pets, especially cats and cat sandboxes.

The six major communicable diseases

Six major communicable diseases cause 90 per cent of the deaths currently caused by communicable diseases. They are HIV and AIDS, malaria, tuberculosis, lower respiratory conditions, diarrhoeal disease and measles. The first three will be dealt with briefly.

1. HIV and AIDS

HIV and AIDS continue to be a major health crisis, both globally and in South Africa. According to UNAIDS data (2019), as of 2018 South Africa's statistics reflected the following:

> 7.7 million people living with HIV; 20.4 per cent adult HIV prevalence (ages 15–49); 240 000 new HIV infections; 71 000 AIDS-related deaths, with many of these deaths caused by a secondary infection, such as tuberculosis. Globally, there were approximately 37.9 million people living with HIV at the end of 2018 (WHO, 2020a).

The disease has left many millions of children orphaned.

There is currently no cure for HIV or AIDS, though research is being conducted to develop a vaccine against the disease. However, prevention is better than cure and preventative programmes advocating the use of condoms have been implemented with moderate success.

Unprotected sexual contact with persons known to have, or who are suspected of having, HIV or AIDS should be avoided; so should casual sexual contact with multiple, anonymous partners. Health education with regard to safe sex and monogamy is therefore important. Other factors to be remembered, include the following:

- The use of condoms will decrease the risk of infection.
- All blood donors should be screened and tested. Heat treatment of pooled blood products such as Factors VIII and IX will inactivate the virus and render these products safe.
- Sufferers and carriers should be asked not to donate blood, sperm or organs.
- Only sterile and disposable needles, syringes and other equipment should be used. Many countries in Western Europe are issuing free disposable needles and syringes to drug abusers to avoid the spread of the condition to this group of people.
- Razors, toothbrushes and similar equipment that could become contaminated by blood should not be shared.

Healthcare staff must protect themselves when handling any bodily fluids by wearing protective goggles and gloves and by the careful handling of all material and specimens. All patients are treated as if they are infected.

Everyone should know their HIV status and must be encouraged to undergo testing. There are a number of methods used for testing but the most common is the rapid finger-prick test, which gives a result within 15 minutes. If the result is positive, it needs to be confirmed with an Elisa test, when blood will be drawn and sent to a laboratory for testing. Every person undergoing an HIV test must receive counselling, regardless of the outcome.

If infected, the person should be encouraged to lead a healthy lifestyle to keep their immunity intact to prevent HIV from developing into AIDS. It is important to note that keeping healthy and taking treatment, if necessary, can lead to a full and happy life lived with the disease. There are two stages of the disease:

- **HIV (human immunodeficiency virus):** The person is infected with the HI-virus but shows no signs and symptoms of the disease. This period of time can extend from two to ten years. As good preventative strategies are being identified, the period of infection with the HI-virus, without it becoming full-blown AIDS, is increasing.

- **AIDS (acquired immune deficiency syndrome):** This is the progressive form of the disease that affects the body's immune system and as a result its ability to fight certain infections. The reduction of resistance results in the person contracting a secondary infection that can be fatal.

The HIV and AIDS pandemic directly or indirectly affects all southern African regions. It has the potential to destroy the country's economy and the labour force while at the same time being both a medical and a political crisis. Combating this crisis will require a multisectoral, multifaceted approach. Prevention strategies need to be continued and improved. These include voluntary counselling and testing (VCT), psychosocial support, palliative care, addressing social stigma, home-based care and prevention of mother-to-child transmission (PMCT). Good management needs to be implemented in the form of early diagnosis and treatment of opportunistic infections and by ensuring the availability of antiretroviral (ARV) treatment to those who need it. ARVs must continue to be introduced in a well-structured programme that will ensure that people living with AIDS can live longer, more productive, healthier lives. If the process is managed properly, then the effect of AIDS can be managed like any other chronic disease.

2. Malaria

According to the National Institute for Communicable Diseases (NICD), 90 per cent of the world's approximately 440 000 annual malaria deaths occur in Africa. In the last few years (2015–2019) South Africa has had between 10 000 and 30 000 notified cases of malaria per year.

Malaria is caused by Plasmodium parasites, transmitted exclusively through the bite of an infected *Anophelese* mosquito. Almost half of the world's population is at risk of malaria, with sub-Saharan Africa being the most vulnerable. According to a WHO report (2020b), 97 countries around the world, including those in Asia, Latin America and some parts of the Middle East and Europe are susceptible to malaria transmission.

It should be remembered that malaria is both preventable and curable. To prevent transmission, vector control (killing mosquitos and their larvae) is most effective. The WHO recommends one of two methods:

1. Providing insecticide-treated nets to those at risk.
2. Spraying indoors with a residual insecticide.

These two methods have largely been responsible for the decrease in infection rates.

In addition, antimalarial drugs can be taken to prevent infection. However, a new problem has developed, with mosquitos developing a resistance to one of the commonly used classes of insecticides – the pyrethroids – and to common antimalarial medication.

The WHO is very active in the area of malarial research. Through various programmes the WHO aims to totally eradicate the disease. The Global Malaria Programme is responsible for charting the course for malaria elimination through:

- setting, communicating and promoting the adoption of evidence-based norms, standards, policies, technical strategies and guidelines
- keeping independent score of global progress
- developing approaches for capacity building, systems strengthening and surveillance
- identifying threats to malaria control and elimination as well as new areas for action.

The WHO is also the co-founder and administrator of a programme called Roll Back Malaria (RBM). The RBM is a global initiative for coordinated action against malaria, with more than 500 partnerships from around the world. This is another organisation that works consistently to look for solutions to the global malaria problem.

One of the goals of the RBM partnership is to reduce malaria-related deaths through:

- early detection
- rapid treatment
- multiple means of prevention
- well-coordinated action
- dynamic global movement
- focused research.

The success of the RBM partnership will continue to depend on the commitment of all concerned. All healthcare workers will need to play an active and meaningful role in the process.

3. Tuberculosis

Globally, tuberculosis (TB) is one of the biggest killers, with South Africa having one of the highest TB burdens in the world. The WHO annual tuberculosis report (2019) estimated that Africa has 24 per cent of the global burden of tuberculosis. The estimated incidence of 301 000 cases of active TB in South Africa in 2018, and an estimated 63 000 deaths from TB. Of the 63 000 people estimated to have died, an estimated 42 000 were HIV positive. South Africa has committed to the global plan to end TB by implementing the 90-90-90 strategy. Three main targets have been set:

- Target 1 is that 90 per cent of all TB patients are traced and treated.
- Target 2 is that 90 per cent of patients are both traced and given effective treatment.
- Target 3 is that there is a 90 per cent treatment success identified in people needing treatment (including resistant TB).

As detailed in the preceding tables, TB is caused by bacteria (*Mycobacterium tuberculosis*) that most often affect the lungs. The bacteria are spread from person to person through the air when the ill person coughs, sneezes or even spits. Only a few of the germs need to be inhaled to become infected. People who are ill with TB can infect up to 10 to 15 other people through close contact over the course of a year. Without proper treatment, up to two-thirds of people ill with TB will die.

About one-third of the world's population has latent TB, which means that many people have been infected with the TB bacteria but are not (yet) ill with the disease and cannot transmit it. Those infected with TB bacteria have a lifetime risk of falling ill with TB of 10 per cent. However, those with a compromised immune system, such as people living with HIV, malnutrition or diabetes, or people who use tobacco, have a much higher risk of falling ill.

When a person develops active TB (disease), the symptoms (cough, fever, night sweats, weight loss etc.) may be mild for many months. This can lead to delays in seeking care, and results in transmission of the bacteria to others.

However, TB is both curable and preventable. If the disease is diagnosed early and medication is taken correctly, then complete recovery is possible. If preventative measures are taken, such as covering the nose and mouth when coughing or sneezing, then transmission can be prevented. The following steps can be taken in the home environment to prevent infection:

- Separate the patient from other members of the household and visitors if possible.
- Prevent the spread of secretions from coughs and sneezes by covering the nose and mouth.
- Wash hands frequently, particularly after coughing or sneezing.
- Ensure a clean and well-ventilated environment.

Everyone with TB should take an HIV test.

Conclusion

As outlined in this chapter, South Africa has a high burden of communicable diseases. However, these diseases are preventable and can be controlled if diagnosed early and treated promptly.

Self-assessment

1. You are working in a community where malaria is common. How will you develop a preventative programme in your district to reduce the incidence of malaria?
2. Define the following:
   - Carrier
   - Communicable diseases
   - Contact.
3. List the signs and symptoms for COVID-19.
4. What is the causative organism for Crimean Congo Fever?

Bibliography

Centres for Disease Control. 2019. Coronavirus disease (COVID-19): Frequently asked questions. Available: https://www.cdc.gov/coronavirus/2019-ncov/faq.html (Accessed 17 September 2020).

Department of Health, KwaZulu-Natal. nd. Notifiable medical conditions. Available: http://www.kznhealth.gov.za/cdc/notifiable.htm (Accessed 17 September 2020).

UNAIDS (Joint United Nations Programme on HIV and AIDS). 2019. Data: Country fact sheets. Available: https://www.unaids.org/en/regionscountries/countries/southafrica (Accessed 17 September 2020).

World Health Organization (WHO). 2019. WHO global tuberculosis report 2019. Available: https://apps.who.int/iris/bitstream/handle/10665/329368/9789241565714-eng.pdf?ua=1 (Accessed 17 September 2020).

World Health Organization (WHO). 2020a. HIV/AIDS fact sheet. Available: https://www.who.int/news-room/fact-sheets/detail/hiv-aids (Accessed 17 September 2020).

World Health Organization (WHO). 2020b. Malaria fact sheet. Available: https://www.who.int/news-room/fact-sheets/detail/malaria (Accessed 17 September 2020).

World Health Organization (WHO). 2020c. Tuberculosis fact sheet. Available: https://www.who.int/tb/publications/factsheets/en/ (Accessed 17 September 2020).

Genetic factors in health and disease

10

Colleen Aldous

Learning outcomes

After studying this chapter, you should be able to:

- Understand basic concepts of genetics.
- Broadly describe congenital abnormalities.
- Explain the relationship between genetic factors and disease.
- Discuss some of the different types of genetic disorder.
- Outline the guidelines for genetic counselling.

Key terms

Congenital: Any abnormality of structure or function that is present from birth (of genetic cause or not).

Genotype: The genetic code that a person carries, which determines his or her genetic make-up.

Heredity: The transmission of genetic characteristics from parent to child.

Phenotype: The observable characteristics of a person as a result of the genotype, or genotype and environment.

Syndrome: A group of signs that are typical of a particular condition.

Trait: The characteristic resulting from the expression of a gene.

Introduction

Congenital disorders are anatomical or physiological abnormalities that are present from birth. The defect may, or may not, be inherited, meaning that it may be genetic or may be caused by other factors. A congenital defect could be mild, eg colour blindness, or it could be more serious, eg haemophilia. In some cases the abnormality is lethal and the infant dies soon after birth, eg with some chromosomal trisomies. Although these abnormalities may be present from birth, they may only manifest later in life, sometimes a few months after birth.

Sometimes they will only manifest in adult years, eg Huntington's disease, which is due to a single defective gene that affects the person after the age of 30. An anatomical abnormality can be diagnosed easily by looking at the patient, but sometimes the congenital defect cannot be seen and is only discovered on thorough examination of the patient, such as with cardiac defects.

The South African National Department of Health has identified certain priority birth defects for attention. They are Down syndrome, neural tube defects, foetal alcohol syndrome, albinism, cleft-lip and -palate, club feet, congenital infections (TORCH viruses) and genetic deafness, blindness, physical handicap and mental retardation. Many, but not all of these, have a genetic component to their cause. Congential abnormalities may be attributed to:

- chromosomal defects
- single gene defects
- multifactorial inherited defects, which is a combination of genetic and environmental causes
- teratogenic or specific environmental agents such as the TORCH diseases, drugs, some antibiotics, alcohol and radiation.

In this chapter we will look at these causes in more detail. In order to understand them, we will first look at basic genetics concepts. We will also look at the various patterns of inheritance, the effect of teratogens, and genetics counselling for those affected by a genetic disorder.

Basic genetics concepts

In this section we will examine the topics of chromosomes, cell division, sex determination and genes.

Chromosomes

If we study a typical cell under a microscope during its resting stage, we will see a mass of darkly stained material in the nucleus. This is the *chromatin*. It consists of the chromosomes, which are spread out, unwound and intertwined with each other. During cell division these chromosomes coil up, become packaged with proteins and take on their compact characteristic X-like structure, with individual chromosomes becoming more visible under the microscope. Each chromosome consists of two chromatids joined together by a centromere. Each chromatid is a long strand of DNA, which carries the genetic code.

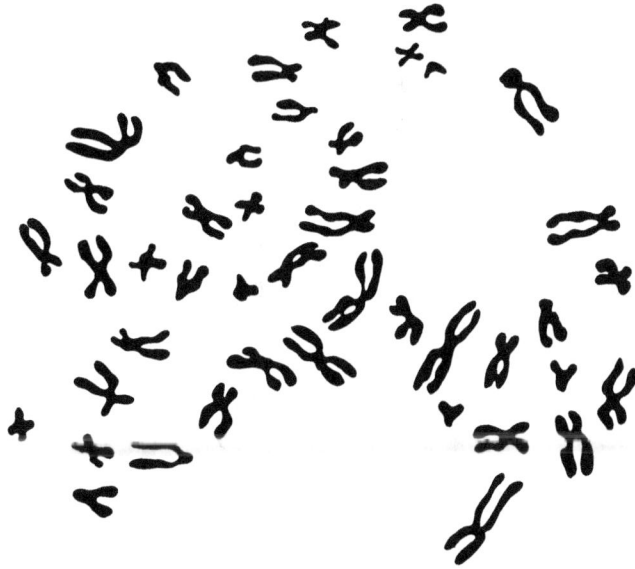

Figure 10.1 Chromosomes in a somatic cell during cell division

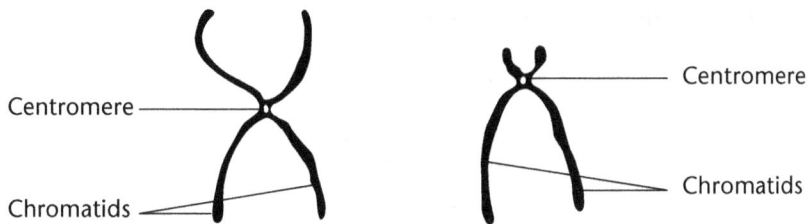

Figure 10.2 Chromosomes of different shapes and sizes

A *karyotype* is a diagrammatic representation or photomicrograph of the 23 pairs of chromosomes showing the chromosomes arranged according to their shape and size from biggest to smallest. Chromosome 1 is the biggest chromosome and chromosome 22 is considered the smallest. Karyotypes enable a geneticist to detect any structural or numerical abnormality in an individual's chromosomes.

In humans there are 23 pairs of chromosomes. Twenty-two pairs of chromosomes are the same in both males and females and are known as *autosomal* chromosomes. The twenty-third pair, the sex chromosomes, differs from the others, with the female having two X chromosomes and the male having one X and one Y chromosome.

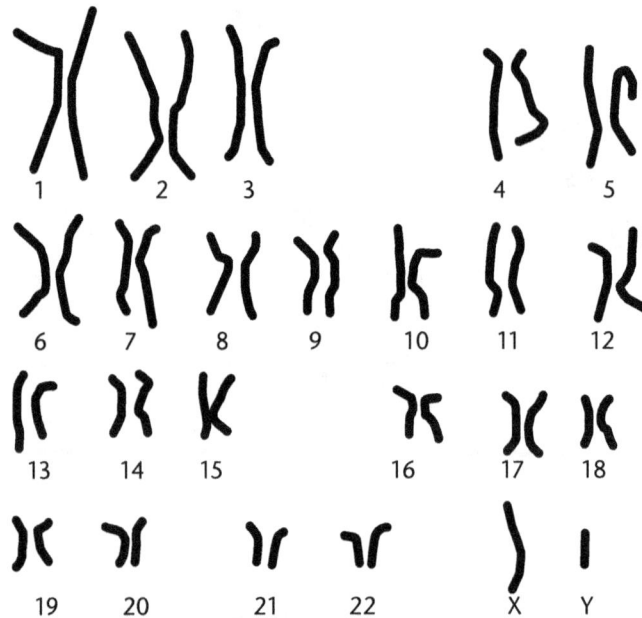

Figure 10.3 Karyotype of a normal male

Cell division

In order for organisms to continue to grow, heal themselves and live healthily, cells need to reproduce themselves. For life to go on, cells must be created to ensure the continuance of the same number of chromosomes from one generation to the next. Two different cell-division processes therefore need to take place.

Mitosis

In normal body cell or *somatic* cell division, the cell divides to reproduce daughter cells that are identical to the original cell, with 46 chromosomes in each. This process is known as *mitosis*. The chromosomes need to double themselves so that one cell with 46 chromosomes will give rise to two new cells, also with 46 chromosomes.

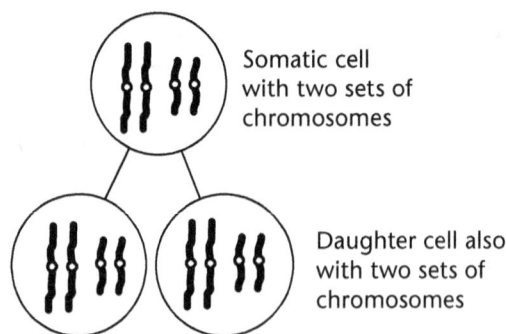

Somatic cell with two sets of chromosomes

Daughter cell also with two sets of chromosomes

Figure 10.4 Mitosis

Meiosis

For organisms to reproduce themselves sexually, there must be a mechanism whereby the pairs of chromosomes are separated to form gametes that have only one set of chromosomes each. This mechanism is called *meiosis*. Meiosis takes place only in the development of the ova and the spermatozoa. During meiosis, the chromosome pairs separate, with one chromosome of a pair going to each cell, halving the number of chromosomes but ensuring that each cell has at least one copy of each chromosome.

Each gamete has 23 chromosomes, and will merge with another gamete from the opposite sex, which also has 23 chromosomes, to form a zygote. The zygote will then have two pairs of each chromosome again, one from each gamete, to have 46 chromosomes. Meiosis is a process of *reduction division* and is necessary for the number of chromosomes to remain constant (ie 46) in each generation.

Figure 10.5 shows that the offspring receives 23 chromosomes from the mother and 23 from the father. Every child, therefore, receives a full set of chromosomes from each parent.

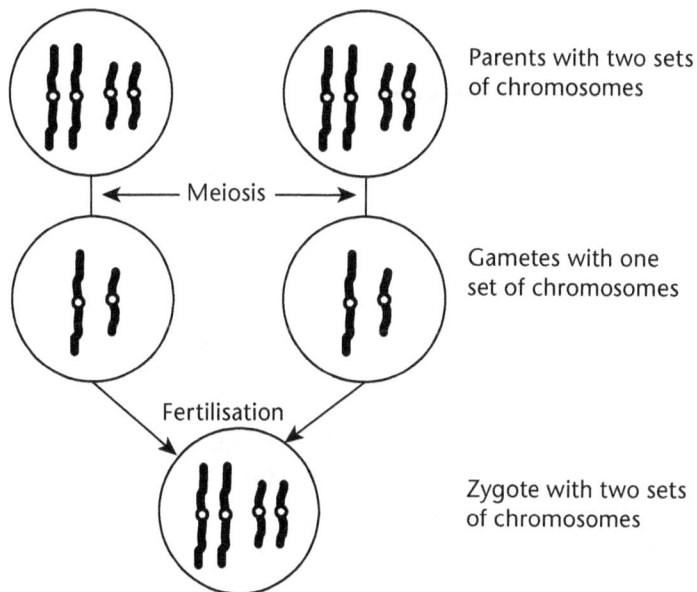

Figure 10.5 Meiosis

Sex determination

Because a female has two X chromosomes, all her ova contain one X chromosome. A male has one X and one Y chromosome. Therefore, half his spermatozoa will contain an X chromosome and the other half will have a Y chromosome. If an ovum is fertilised by a spermatozoon carrying an X chromosome, the offspring will be XX, ie female. If it is fertilised by a spermatozoon carrying a Y chromosome, the offspring will be XY, ie male.

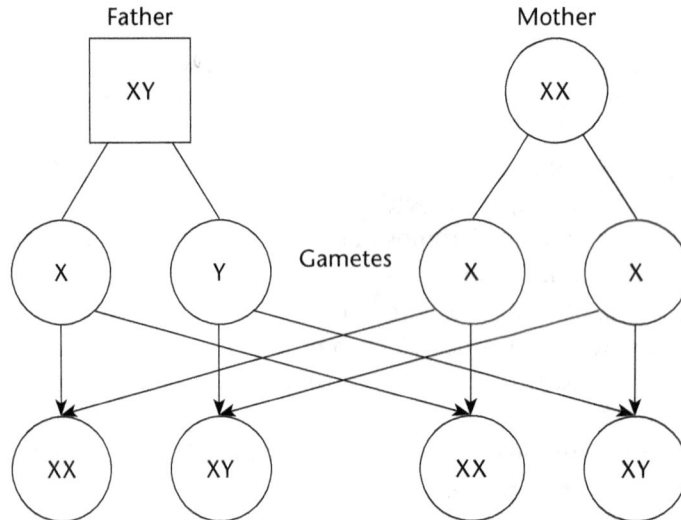

Figure 10.6 Sex determination

Note:

- It is the sex chromosome composition of the male gamete that determines the sex of the offspring.
- On average, equal numbers of male and female offspring are conceived.

Genes

It is estimated that we have about 25 000 genes in our chromosomes. Each gene holds the genetic code for some product that the body needs to make for itself to grow, heal itself and in general to allow it to perform well. Some genes play a big role in what we look like. Often someone will look at a baby and say 'He looks just like his dad!' This is because some of the genes that the dad has also now exist in his little boy. These genes that they both have make them look alike.

The growth and development of a normal, healthy individual from a single cell, the zygote, is a complex process requiring thousands of genes working cooperatively and synchronously. In the zygote only some genes work to start off with. As the zygote divides and an embryo forms, some of those genes switch off and others switch on. As some genes are needed they are brought into play and as soon as their products are no longer needed, they are stopped. In a fully grown adult, of the 25 000 genes he or she has, only some of them will be working some of the time. Others will be switched off never to work again, such as those that produced the special type of haemoglobin that a foetus has. Some will work every now and then, like those required to make digestive enzymes. Others keep working all the time.

Genes are the units of inheritance and are arranged along the chromosomes much like beads on a string. All 25 000 genes we have are placed on our chromosomes. The position that a gene occupies on a chromosome is known as its locus. Chromosomes occur in pairs and in each pair of chromosomes there are genes governing the same characteristic (eg eye colour). These genes are situated at the same position on each of the chromosomes.

A person who carries two identical genes for a certain characteristic (bb), is said to be a *homozygote*. In this case the person got one b gene from the father and the other from the mother to give him or her the *genotype* bb. Someone with two different genes (Bb) is said to be a *heterozygote*. Here, one parent's gamete had a B and the other had a b, so the person now has the genotype Bb.

If the person with only one gene for a certain characteristic (Bb) manifests that trait, the gene is said to be *dominant*. This means that the *phenotype* will be that of B. When two similar genes (bb) are necessary before a trait manifests itself, then the gene is said to be *recessive*.

Table 10.1 Examples of characteristics that are transmitted by dominant or recessive genes

Dominant genes	Recessive genes
Brown eyes	Blue eyes
Dark hair	Blond or red hair
Curly hair	Straight hair
Abundant body hair	Sparse body hair
Rh positive blood	Rh negative blood
Group A blood	Group O blood

The genetic make-up of the person and its interaction with the environment also influence the health status and the diseases that may occur during that person's lifespan. Many genetic defects give rise to *syndromes*. Syndromes are a specific group of symptoms that usually occur together in a disorder, eg Down syndrome where the patient has characteristic facial and anatomical features, mental retardation and sometimes cardiac defects.

We will look at how whole chromosome abnormalities may cause birth defect syndromes such as Down syndrome and how single defects in genes might cause diseases such as albinism. We will also look at multifactorial diseases where the genes and the environment work together, such as in some central nervous system (CNS) birth defects.

Chromosomal abnormalities

There are two kinds of chromosomal abnormalities: those in which the chromosomal number changes (known as numerical abnormalities) and those in which the chromosomes lose, gain, or invert some chromosomal material (known as structural abnormalities).

Numerical abnormalities

These are common. It is estimated that one in 200 infants is born with a chromosomal abnormality, while nearly half of all miscarriages are thought to be the result of chromosomal defects in the foetus. Mistakes in meiosis may result in an individual having either too many autosomal or sex chromosomes (resulting in trisomies) or too few. Usually the foetus will not survive unless it has the normal number of chromosomes, but a small number of syndromes are compatible with life.

Down syndrome (Trisomy 21)

This condition is due to the presence of an extra number 21 chromosome, so the affected child has 47 instead of 46 chromosomes. This most commonly happens because the two number 21 chromosomes did not separate during meiosis. A child suffering from Down syndrome has a characteristic appearance, some level of mental retardation and numerous other congenital defects. The frequency is about two to three in 1 000 live births in developing countries. The risk of producing a child with Down syndrome increases with increasing age of the mother. The condition can be detected before birth by screening under ultrasound. If a nuccal fold is seen on the back of the neck of the foetus on the ultrasound, the mother will be offered a blood test. If the blood test confirms the suspicion that the foetus has Down syndrome, an *amniocentesis* will be carried out. Amniotic fluid that contains foetal cells is extracted from the womb and these cells are examined to confirm a diagnosis of Down syndrome.

Table 10.2 shows other common numerical chromosomal syndromes that can occur in liveborns.

Table 10.2 Common numerical chromosomal syndromes

Syndrome	Chromosome number affected	Symptoms
Patau syndrome	Trisomy 13	Infant has a small head, deformed hands, cleft palate and sometimes a single umbilical artery. Infants often die soon after birth.
Edwards' syndrome	Trisomy 18	Infant has a small head, abnormally small jaw, upturned nose, widely spaced eyes and rockerbottom feet. Infants die soon after birth.
Klinefelter syndrome	An extra X chromosome in a male	Taller than average with weak muscle tone. Can have reduced fertility or be infertile. Developmental milestones may be delayed, but can be ameliorated with occupational therapy and remedial teaching.
Turner syndrome	Only one X chromosome in a female	Short stature with a webbed neck. Women suffer from amenorrhoea and are often infertile.

Structural abnormalities

These abnormalities are the result of breaks that occur in the chromosomes that may lead to a part of a chromosome being lost, or rejoining in an abnormal way. These structural defects can be the cause of several physical and mental abnormalities. *Microdeletions* occur when small pieces of the chromosome are lost. An example of a microdeletion disease is Prader Willi syndrome where a piece of chromosome 15 is missing. *Translocations* occur when pieces of the chromosome break off and rejoin in the wrong place. A form of schizophrenia has been identified where a piece of chromosome 14 becomes included into chromosome 1.

Gene defects

Sometimes there are changes in the DNA sequence of a gene. These changes are known as *mutations*. Many mutations occur spontaneously, without influence from outside, but certain environmental factors such as radiation may increase the mutation rate. Mutations may be beneficial, neutral or harmful. Beneficial mutations are important in the evolution of a species. Neutral mutations merely add variety, like hair colour and hair straightness. We are concerned about the harmful mutations. These are the ones that cause disease.

If mutations occur in the gametes, the changes can be transmitted to succeeding generations, but a mutation occurring in a gene in a somatic cell cannot be transmitted. All genetically inherited diseases are a result of a mutation that occurred in the gametes in an ancestor. Cancers are often a result of a mutation that occurs in a somatic cell.

Preconception care and counselling

Sometimes, congenital disorders may be prevented. If a pregnancy is planned, a woman can prepare for a healthy pregnancy from about six months before she plans to become pregnant. Steps that she can take to minimise the risk of having a child with a congenital disorder include: to stop smoking and drinking alcohol, find out if chronic medications she takes could have a teratogenic effect if there are any inherited diseases from either side of the family, and take supplements such as folic acid which will contribute to a healthy pregnancy. Pre-conception counselling is important if there is any history of an inherited disorder.

Inheritance patterns

Genetic abnormalities often run in families. By understanding how a particular genetic abnormality is transmitted through the generations, you will be able to give parents some information about the generations to come and their chances of getting and transmitting the disease.

Autosomal-dominant inheritance

The following are some of the conditions transmitted by dominant genes:
- Huntington's chorea
- porphyria variegata
- some types of achondroplasia (dwarfism)
- tuberous sclerosis and senile cataracts.

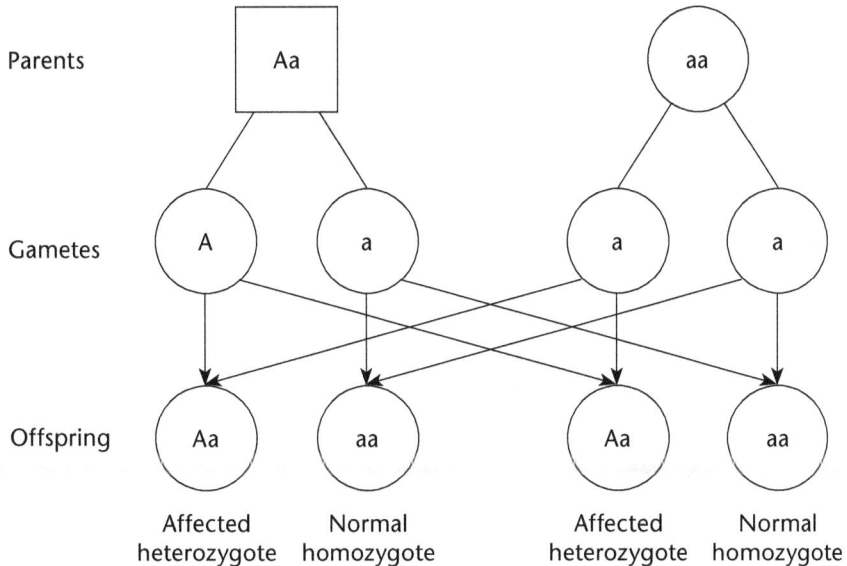

Figure 10.7 Diagram illustrating autosomal-dominant inheritance

In general, dominant inheritance has the following characteristics:

- Each affected person usually has an affected parent and so the pattern of inheritance is vertical, ie from generation to generation. If an affected person reproduces with one who is not affected, then the chance of their children being affected is one in two.

- If both parents are affected, then there is a probability of three in four of their children being affected.

Autosomal-recessive inheritance

The following are conditions that are transmitted by autosomal-recessive genes:

- albinism
- Tay-Sachs disease
- cystic fibrosis
- phenylketonuria.

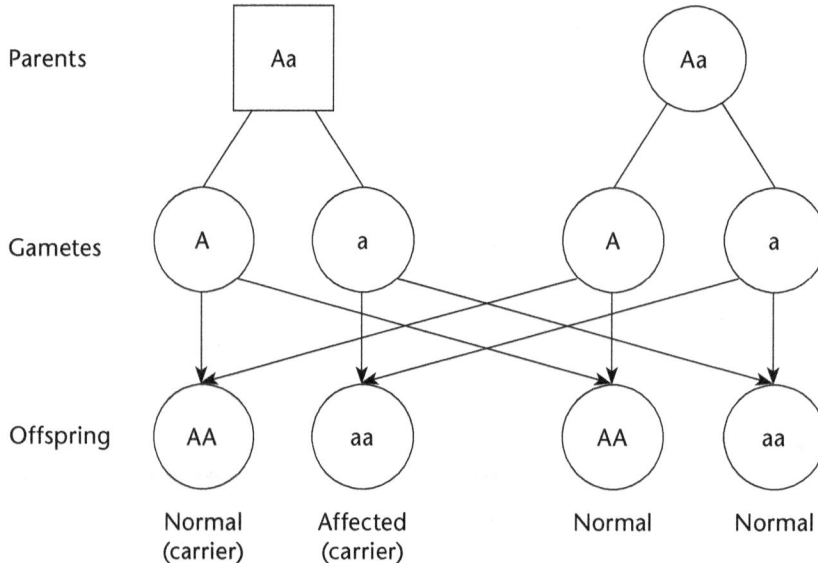

Figure 10.8 Diagram illustrating autosomal-recessive inheritance

This type of inheritance has the following characteristics:

- The condition does not generally occur in successive generations.
- Affected children have unaffected parents.
- If one child is affected there is a probability that some of the brothers or sisters may also be affected.
- If two carriers of a condition reproduce, then on average one in four of the offspring will manifest the trait, one in four will be unaffected, and one in two will appear unaffected but will be carriers of the harmful gene.

Consanguinity

When closely related family members such as cousins have children together, there is an increased risk of their offspring getting rare recessive disorders. A recessive gene will have a higher frequency within a family than outside the family. It is unlikely that a person who is heterozygous for a recessive gene will reproduce with another heterozygote for the same disorder outside the family. But if cousins, for example, have offspring, the chances are increased for the offspring to be affected with the disorder.

X-linked inheritance

Females have two X chromosomes. In the case of a recessive disease gene on one X chromosome it will not be expressed in the female if there is a normal gene on the other X chromosome. This heterozygote female will be a carrier of the condition or characteristic.

Because the male has only one X chromosome, the trait determined by this harmful recessive gene will manifest itself in him if he receives the recessive disease gene and not the other healthy one from his mother. An affected male will transmit this gene to all his daughters, who receive his X chromosome, but to none of his sons, who receive only a Y chromosome from him. The carrier daughters will in turn transmit the gene to half their sons, in whom the trait will be expressed, and to half their daughters, who will be carriers. *Partial colour blindness, haemophilia, certain types of deafness* and *Duchenne muscular dystrophy* are conditions that are transmitted by defective genes on the X chromosome. To summarise:

- X-linked traits are more commonly manifested in males than in females.

- Healthy females who are mothers of affected sons are carriers of the harmful gene. Daughters of affected males will be carriers of the harmful genes and daughters of carrier mothers have a 50 per cent chance of being carriers of the harmful gene.

- This condition may appear to skip generations if girls are carriers and only healthy boys are born in one generation.

- The gene is transmitted from an affected male through his daughters, who will be normal, but they will be carriers.

- In rare cases a female who has an affected father and a carrier mother will suffer from the condition.

Multifactorial inheritance

Genes do not all work in isolation. Sometimes the action of a gene is affected by something the person requires (eg folic acid) or is exposed to (eg a teratogen) from the environment. For example, if a mother does not get enough folic acid in her diet, the foetus's genes may be affected and the baby could be born with a cleft-lip and -palate. For the genes involved in lip and palate formation to work perfectly, they need folic acid. We will look at teratogens in the next section of this chapter.

Numerous traits such as intelligence, skin colour and height are determined by the action of several genes working together, each of which contributes a small amount of the characteristic seen in the individual. In multifactorial inheritance, there is some influence from the environment on the characteristic, but it is difficult to say how much of each trait is determined by genetic factors and how much is due to the influence of the environment. *Diabetis mellitus, hypertension, spina bifida, cleft-lip* and some cases of *clubfoot* are a few of the conditions that may be influenced by multifactorial inheritance.

Precision/personalised medicine: In this chapter we have looked at the basics of genetics as a science that affects people. Most of our knowledge about genetics was developed in the 20th century. We have carried our understanding of chromosomal, single gene and multifactorial disorders with us into the

21st century. Since 2005, we have been able to look at the entire genome of humans to find these and other disorders. New technologies have allowed scientists to look closer at the genetics of people and communities, and now, in some cases, treatments can be tailored to specific genetic causes. This science is still in development and will be more widely available in the future.

The effect of teratogens

If the mother is exposed to one of the TORCH viruses early on in her pregnancy, the foetus's genes will be affected. They will not function as intended and the foetus can become deformed and disabled. The TORCH viruses are teratogenic. Other teratogens, such as heavy metals, radiation, some medications and toxic chemicals, may have the same effect on the developing foetus. Whether or not the developing foetus will be affected depends on the stage of development of the foetus when the mother is exposed to the teratogen. The first 12 weeks of pregnancy, when the various organ systems are developing, seems to be the most critical period.

Genetic counselling and referring people who may be at risk

There is a growing interest in, and demand for, information about genetic abnormalities. Genetic counselling services should form an integral part of a comprehensive health service. The people most likely to ask for such information are:

- couples who have already had an affected child
- two people who are blood relations, for instance first cousins, and who wish to have children
- members of a family in which there is a history of congenital defects, or a disease with a familial incidence
- a woman who has had repeated miscarriages
- a middle-aged couple who wish to have children.

Note: It is important that an individual or couple should voluntarily seek help and not feel pressured to go for genetic counselling.

Genetic counselling is the provision of information on the nature and implications of a specific birth defect. It involves giving psychological support and referring the family to appropriate facilities. The process should allow the couple or individual seeking information to make an informed decision. A team approach is the most effective in successful genetic counselling. Ideally the team should consist of the family doctor, a medical geneticist, a professional nurse, a social worker and a clinical psychologist. However, these services are not available at all community clinics and patients should be referred to get the assistance they need.

Who should seek genetic counselling?

According to the *Fact sheet on birth defects* (DOH, nd) it is advisable for a couple to seek advice before determining whether they should conceive a child if:

- either of the couple has a birth defect
- they have a child with a birth defect
- either of the couple has a family history of a genetic disorder
- the woman has a series of miscarriages or a stillbirths for no medical reason
- they are close relatives
- the woman is in her late thirties and planning a pregnancy
- the pregnant woman is exposed to an infection or harmful chemical, especially during the first three months of pregnancy, such as alcohol, irradiation and infections like German measles.

Once the person or the couple has an accurate indication of the probability of producing an affected child, the various options should be presented to them and they must be allowed to make their own decision. Psychotherapy and emotional support should be given where necessary.

If a woman is already pregnant, but is regarded as high risk, an amniocentesis should be done to determine whether the foetus is affected. Certain biochemical tests may also be carried out. A large number of genetic, congenital and chromosomal abnormalities, such as meningomyelocele and Down syndrome, may be diagnosed in this way. If the foetus is severely affected the mother will be offered elective termination of pregnancy (TOP). Once again, it is important that she be allowed to make her own decision concerning the TOP.

The ultimate aim of genetic counselling is to prevent, if possible, the birth of severely affected children. However, for those who have a child with a birth defect there are support groups. Rare Diseases South Africa (RDSA) is a non-profit organisation (NPO) that works to ensure that people living with rare diseases and congenital disorders in South Africa experience better recognition and support, improved health services, and a better life overall. RDSA members include patients, patient support groups, healthcare professionals, researchers, academics and industry partners. RDSA may be contacted at:

Block 7 Stratford Office Park
Valley Road, Broadacres
Johannesburg 2191
Tel: +27 10 594 3844 or email: hello@rarediseases.co.za
Website: www.rarediseases.co.za

Where can genetic counselling be obtained?

Genetic counselling for patients can be obtained in the private health sector or at government tertiary hospitals. Some district and regional hospitals have nurses who have undergone basic training in genetic counselling. Local primary healthcare services should have the necessary information available to be able to refer patients when necessary. As a qualified nurse, you could receive basic training in genetic counselling by contacting:

> The Directorate: Women's Health and Genetics
> Sub-Directorate: Human Genetics
> Civitas Building
> Cnr of Thabo Sehume & Struben Streets
> Pretoria 0001
> Tel: (012) 395 9357 or (012) 395 8364

Conclusion

It is hoped that the information in this chapter has raised awareness of the topic of genetics and that this will lead to awareness of the importance of genetic counselling for those in need.

Self-assessment

A middle-aged couple – a woman aged 37 years and a man of 40 years – visits your clinic. They have been together for a year and wish to start a family. They are blood relatives as their fathers are brothers. They are aware of the risk involved with having children but do not fully understand the challenges they may encounter. As a nurse in the clinic, outline the information you will give to the couple using the following headings:

- Possible genetic risks involved
- Older women and pregnancy
- Counselling, advice and referral.

Bibliography

Department of Health (DOH). 2001. Human genetics policy guidelines for the management and prevention of genetic disorders, birth defects and disabilities. Pretoria: Department of Health.

Department of Health (DOH). nd. Fact sheet on birth defects. Pretoria: Department of Health.

Gardner, E.J., Simmons, M.J. & Snustad, D.P. 1991. *Principles of Genetics*. New York: Wiley.

Health needs through the lifespan

Sharon Vasuthevan

Learning outcomes

After studying this chapter, you should be able to:

- Understand the stages, milestones and associated healthcare issues in the lifespan of an individual in South Africa with regard to:
    - maternal and child healthcare
    - adolescent-friendly healthcare
    - child-spacing services, benefits and methods available
    - family healthcare
    - men's health issues
    - care of the elderly.

Key terms

Anorexia nervosa: A psychosomatic disorder characterised by an aversion to food, leading to atrophy of the stomach and emaciation.

Bulimia nervosa: An uncontrollable urge to overeat followed by induced vomiting or purging.

Chronological: The arrangement of events or dates in the order of occurrence.

Crude birth rate: The number of births per 1 000 people per year.

Homeostasis: The state of relative stability or equilibrium of the internal environment of the body.

Incontinence: Inability to control the urge to urinate or defecate.

Kyphosis: An excessive backward convex curvature of the spine, usually in the thoracic region.

Parasuicide: Apparent attempted suicide without the actual intention of killing oneself.

Introduction

Maintaining our health throughout our lifespan is an important goal for everyone. At each chronological milestone, the body becomes vulnerable to different diseases and external influences. It is therefore important to have a health system that addresses the differing age-related needs of the population as these needs change throughout a person's lifespan. The third sustainable development goal (SDG 3) of 'Good Health and Well-being', as outlined by the United Nations in the 17 life-changing goals, is applicable to a number of areas in this chapter.

The objectives for this chapter are to introduce the most important aspects of health needs through the lifespan of a person and the associated services that are available to meet these needs.

Maternal and child health

Maternal and child health services are an essential part of the healthcare system in any country, but in the less developed countries of the world, such as those in Africa, they are of particular importance. In African countries crude birth rates are high – in the region of 35 per 1 000 (much higher in some southern African countries such as Angola and Malawi); infant mortality rates are also very high and may reach 200 per 1 000 live births in some areas; the under-five death rate is even higher than the infant mortality rate; and nearly half the children die before reaching the age of five years. Maternal mortality rates are also unacceptably high.

Owing to the lack of strong reporting systems in a number of countries, it has been difficult to assess accurately the progress towards achieving the SDGs. However, the World Health Organization (WHO) estimates that global maternal deaths decreased by 45 per cent between 1990 and 2013, and under-five mortality levels dropped by 49 per cent during the same period (WHO, 2014). The original millennium development goal (MDG) was to reduce under-five mortality by 66 per cent, which regrettably has not been met.

Mothers and children therefore not only make up a large proportion of the population, but also form a particularly vulnerable group; therefore effective maternal and child health services could have a profound influence on the health of the community. Maternal and child health services should be comprehensive and include promotive, preventative, curative and rehabilitative care. The following are essential components of such a service:

- prenatal care
- services for delivery
- postnatal care
- child spacing
- child health services
- adolescent health services.

Prenatal care

All women should receive adequate supervision during pregnancy and particular attention should be paid to 'high-risk' mothers, such as women:

- under the age of 16 years or over the age of 35
- who are pregnant for the first time
- who have had three or more pregnancies
- suffering from hypertension, renal disease, cardiac conditions, diabetes mellitus or other systemic diseases
- who are unmarried mothers
- whose previous obstetric history gives cause for concern, for example if they have had a previous caesarian section, stillbirth or postpartum haemorrhage
- from lower socioeconomic levels
- who are HIV positive.

The basic objectives of prenatal care are to ensure the delivery of a live and healthy baby without any injury or harm to the mother, and to promote a healthy relationship between the mother and the infant. In order to achieve these objectives, the following steps must be taken:

- The mother should be examined early in her pregnancy and at regular intervals thereafter so that any abnormalities may be detected and treated, and complications avoided.
- The first visit is the most important one; at this visit a detailed history should be taken and a thorough examination carried out.
- Signs of infection should be looked for, and if any infections such as tuberculosis are present, these should be treated vigorously.
- The mother should be tested for HIV.
- The possibility of systemic diseases such as diabetes mellitus or cardiac conditions should be excluded.
- Blood should be taken so that the blood group, rhesus factor and haemoglobin levels can be established.
- The urine should be tested for sugar and albumin.
- The size of the pelvis should be assessed and any abnormality noted. In areas where nutritional standards are poor, occurrence of contracted (small) pelvis is fairly common.
- Where there is a high incidence of neonatal tetanus, two doses of tetanus toxoid should be administered to the mother during the third trimester.
- Health education includes testing for HIV and AIDS. A pregnant mother who is infected with HIV can pass on the virus to her infant during pregnancy and childbirth. Once it is established that the mother is HIV positive, depending on her CD4 count, she could commence on antiretroviral (ARV) therapy.

- Opportunities for effective health education are greatly increased during pregnancy, as most women are eager to do what is best for their babies.
- Education in nutrition is essential and the mother should be encouraged to eat a balanced diet, as pregnancy makes extra demands on her. Where necessary, vitamin supplements and iron should be provided.
- The importance of sufficient exercise, rest and sleep should be stressed.
- The pregnant woman should be advised to avoid contact with those suffering from infections, and to refrain from taking medications that have not been prescribed, while the dangers associated with smoking and the use of alcohol and other drugs should be brought to her attention.
- Preparation for breastfeeding commences during the prenatal period and all possible steps should be taken to encourage it.
- The mother should be educated in various aspects of childcare, particularly in infant feeding and hygiene, and psychologically sound childrearing practices should be encouraged.
- The mother should be prepared for delivery: she should be told what to expect and what is expected of her during the various stages of labour.

HIV-positive mothers

If a pregnant woman is infected with HIV, she can transmit the virus to her baby during pregnancy, labour, delivery or breastfeeding. Without treatment, around 15 to 30 per cent of babies born to HIV-infected women will become infected with HIV during pregnancy and delivery. A further 5 to 20 per cent will become infected through breastfeeding.

Available drugs are highly effective at preventing mother-to-child transmission of HIV. When combined with other interventions, including formula feeding, a complete course of treatment can cut the risk of transmission to below 2 per cent.

A woman who knows that she or her partner is HIV positive before she becomes pregnant can find out about interventions that may be able to protect her, her partner and her baby from becoming infected with HIV. Doctors will be able to advise which interventions are best suited to her situation and whether she should adjust any treatment she is already receiving if she is HIV positive.

In July 2010, the WHO issued new HIV and AIDS guidelines on the prevention of mother-to-child transmission (PMTCT) and on HIV and breastfeeding. South Africa adopted these guidelines, which state that all HIV-positive mothers identified during pregnancy should receive a course of specified ARV drugs to prevent mother-to-child transmission. All infants born to HIV-positive mothers will receive a course of ARVs for the duration of breastfeeding.

Ideally, newborns of HIV-positive mothers should not be breastfed. However, in low-resource settings such as some of the rural areas in southern Africa, prevalence of the disease and the availability of clean drinking water to make up formula feeds influence breastfeeding choices. Whether to breastfeed and for how long to breastfeed will be negotiated with the mother and managed by the nurse practitioner. The nurse practitioner will be guided by current South African guidelines.

Breastfeeding and the prevention of mother-to-child transmission of HIV

All confirmed HIV-positive pregnant women are eligible for immediate initiation with lifelong ARVs, irrespective of CD4 count. Initiate lifelong ARVs in all pregnant or breastfeeding women on the day of diagnosis regardless of CD4 count. The emphasis is on exclusive breastfeeding for the first six months, after which complimentary feeding can be introduced. Breastfeeding should continue for at least 12 months.

Mother taking ARVs

A mother taking ARVs for her own health should take a combination of ARVs as recommended by current guidelines. Once the mother has commenced with ARVs (known as highly active antiretroviral therapy or HAART) she will take this medication for life. Optimal adherence will be negotiated with the practitioner.

Mother not taking ARVs

The child of a mother who has not started ARV treatment but who will be breastfed, will need medication in the form of a daily dose of nevirapine. The dosage of the nevirapine will be calculated according to the baby's weight. The baby will stay on nevirapine for the duration of breastfeeding. If the HIV-positive mother chooses not to breastfeed, then the child will be given nevirapine for the first six weeks of life.

> Because guidelines for the care of HIV-positive mothers and babies change frequently, it is extremely important to consult your unit's policy and the most recent guidelines for PMTCT of HIV.

Infants

As discussed above, all infants born to HIV-positive mothers should receive a course of medication for PMTCT, which is linked to the drug regimen that the mother is taking.

Services for delivery

The immediate aims during delivery are prevention of injury to the infant and establishment of respiration, and prevention of damage to the mother. Arrangements for delivery should be made during pregnancy. In towns and cities in South Africa most deliveries take place in hospitals and nursing homes and are conducted by medical practitioners and/or registered midwives. The mother remains in hospital for a variable time after delivery. In rural areas, expectant mothers are encouraged to attend prenatal clinics and to arrange for their delivery to take place at the rural health clinic where there is always a midwife available. However, there are still many women in such areas who deliver their babies themselves at home or who are assisted by friends and relatives.

Blood, and any equipment that may be needed for dealing with an emergency, should be available. In the case of rural health clinics, it should be possible to transfer the mother to the district hospital without delay, should the need arise.

Antenatal, delivery and postnatal services are free in the public sector.

Postnatal care

In the immediate postnatal period relatively minor complications such as retention of urine and, later, painful breasts, may occur in the mother and these should be dealt with promptly and effectively. The mother should also be observed for the early signs of more serious complications such as infection and deep-vein thrombosis, and these should be treated vigorously if they occur.

It is important to remember, however, that the puerperium does not end when the mother is discharged from hospital but that it takes about six weeks for a woman's organs to return to a normal non-pregnant state. During this time, she should be encouraged to continue the exercises that she has been taught, as these will assist the processes of recovery.

A woman has to make many adjustments during the postnatal period, especially if she has had her first baby. She has to adjust to breastfeeding, to attending to the infant's physical needs and to disturbed sleep. She also has to establish a relationship with her baby. Psychological problems may also arise at this time, such as depression, which can be severe. The mother may also feel anxious and uncertain about handling the baby. It is an important period and adequate services for helping the mother should be available.

Once the mother returns home, she may use the services of a private midwife or home health nurse if she lives in an urban area. The midwife or nurse enquires about the mother's health as well as that of the baby and is always willing to discuss any problems that the mother may have. In rural areas the mother should be encouraged to visit the health centre where all the necessary services are available.

Six weeks after delivery a physical examination is carried out and the position and size of the uterus, the condition of the cervix and the presence of any vaginal discharge are noted. This visit is probably a suitable time to introduce the subject of family planning.

Counselling in family planning can form a valuable part of postnatal care, with most women being receptive to family planning advice at this time.

Child spacing and family planning

Child spacing makes it possible for couples to have the number of children they desire, to space them sufficiently and to limit the size of their family if necessary.

However, it is always the right of the mother/father to make their own informed decisions regarding child spacing and contraception. Men and women have the right to be informed; to have access to safe, effective, affordable and acceptable contraceptive methods of their choice, as well as fertility regulation that is not against the law; and the right to access appropriate healthcare service that will enable women to proceed safely through pregnancy and childbirth and provide couples with the best chance of having healthy infants.

Contraception is also an important strategy in the struggle to achieve gender equality (SDG 5) and an intervention to prevent risky and unprotected sexual behaviour. We know that gender relations have a significant impact on people's lifestyles, reproductive lives and sexual health. Women and young people, particularly girl-children's lack of decision-making power and economic and social autonomy, is both a cause and a consequence of their limited power over their sexual and reproductive lives.

Health benefits of child spacing

- The mother has time to recover completely after delivery before she falls pregnant again.
- She is able to continue breastfeeding her baby for as long as she wishes.
- The mother is able to care for her baby adequately because she has both the time and the energy to do so. It has been well documented that large families with many young children are associated with poor childcare and high morbidity and mortality rates.

Financial benefits

- A young couple can choose to postpone having a family until they are financially stable.
- The parents will be able to provide their children with the material things necessary for their health and welfare, such as food, clothing, housing and medical care.
- Parents will be able to ensure that all their children are adequately educated.
- The quality of life of the entire family will be improved.

Benefits to the family

- Child spacing promotes a stable and harmonious relationship between the spouses. It is possible for them to enjoy a sexual relationship without the constant fear of another pregnancy.
- Because there are fewer children, the mother and father can devote more time to each child.
- The children benefit by being brought up in a home that is happy and free from marital strife.
- There is less likelihood of family disorganisation, and as the children are more likely to be properly socialised, they, in turn, will become good parents.

Benefits to society

- A stable family life is the foundation on which a strong, healthy society is built. Widespread family disorganisation leads to social disorganisation and increased social deviance.
- The rate of population increase is slowed down, and society is better able to provide basic services.

In South Africa, the state has assumed responsibility for family-planning services, which are rendered free of charge at many hospitals and clinics throughout the country. It is important to remember that family planning alone will not reduce fertility rates but must form part of a comprehensive primary healthcare system and be accompanied by opportunities for the education and employment of women, as well as improvement in their social and financial circumstances.

Methods of contraception

The methods described in this section include the rhythm method, coitus interruptus, the condom, diaphragms or caps, spermicides, oral contraceptives, injectable long-acting contraceptives and implants, intra-uterine devices (IUDS), sterilisation and termination of pregnancy.

Rhythm method or the safe period

Pregnancy can occur only if sexual intercourse takes place during the 24 hours that the ovum remains alive after ovulation. If one could determine exactly when ovulation took place, this would be the only method of contraception needed. Unfortunately, it is almost impossible to determine the date of ovulation with absolute accuracy, and if the rhythm method is practised, sexual intercourse has to be avoided for a week or more every month.

Nevertheless, this is the only method of contraception that is allowed by the Catholic Church.

In order to make use of the rhythm method a woman must keep a record of her menstrual cycle for about a year to determine the average length of her cycle. In a woman with a perfectly regular 28-day cycle, ovulation may occur anywhere between the 16th and the 12th day before menstruation. There is no way of determining the exact day of ovulation if only the 'calendar method' is used. She should therefore refrain from intercourse from the 18th to the 11th day before menstruation. This is far more complicated in women who have irregular menstrual cycles.

The effectiveness of this method may be improved by keeping a record of the basal body temperature. At the time of ovulation, the temperature falls slightly, to rise a day or two later by about 0.3 or 0.4 °C. A woman should take her temperature every morning before she gets out of bed, and before she has anything to eat or drink, or smokes. Sexual intercourse should be avoided until the temperature has been at this higher level for three days. The reliability of this method depends on the accuracy with which the woman takes and records her temperature and, as we all know, many factors may affect this. It must be pointed out that this method can be very useful for sub-fertile women who wish to have children, for they should have sexual intercourse on the first day the temperature rises, as this will be the time at which they will be most likely to fall pregnant.

Coitus interruptus or withdrawal

This method also requires the fullest cooperation from the male if it is to be used as a means of family planning. It requires the withdrawal of the penis from the vagina before ejaculation takes place in order to prevent entry of the sperm. It has many advantages and will prevent pregnancy from occurring in a large number of instances, but it is not a reliable method of contraception.

The condom

This is still one of the most common methods in use in spite of the recent developments in contraceptive methods. The condom is a very thin latex rubber sheath that is drawn tightly over the erect penis before sexual intercourse takes place. It acts as a mechanical barrier to the passage of spermatozoa to the cervix. The condom has many advantages as it is easy to use, easily obtainable, cheap, harmless and very useful as a temporary measure, or when other methods cannot be used for various reasons. It is a fairly reliable method of contraception and its effectiveness can be greatly increased if it is used in conjunction with a spermicide.

If correctly used, a condom will prevent the spread of sexually transmitted infections (STIs) such as syphilis, gonorrhoea and AIDS because it acts as a mechanical barrier to transmission of the causative organisms of such diseases.

Use of the condom has increased dramatically as part of the prevention of HIV transmission. Condoms are available free of charge from clinics. Many companies also make them available in their toilets in the workplace.

Female condoms are also available, and their use should be encouraged.

Diaphragms or caps

These consist of shallow dome-shaped cups made of thin rubber, with a flexible metal ring around the circumference. They fit into the vault of the vagina and so cover the cervical os and prevent entry of the sperm into the uterus. They have to be fitted by a medical practitioner or suitably trained person to ensure that they are the correct size, and they must be refitted after the woman has had a baby. They have to be inserted before intercourse and not be removed for at least six hours afterwards.

Diaphragms have many advantages as they are harmless, clean and hygienic and simple to introduce. They can be a fairly effective contraceptive method if used properly and if they fit properly. Their effectiveness is greatly enhanced if they are used in conjunction with a spermicide.

Spermicides

These are chemicals that destroy the spermatozoa and so prevent them from reaching the ovum. Spermicides must be inserted high into the vagina before intercourse. An applicator is supplied with the spermicide. Although these chemicals are useful when used together with other methods such as condoms or diaphragms, they cannot be relied upon to prevent pregnancy from occurring when used alone. From time to time burning, itching or tenderness is reported. This is the result of a sensitivity to the chemicals.

Oral contraceptives

The pill is the most effective method of contraception available today. In cases where pregnancy does occur, it is probably due to failure to use the method correctly rather than due to failure of the method as such.

Many different types of oral contraceptive are available, but, basically, they all contain synthetic hormones similar to the female sex hormones oestrogen and progesterone. Some pills contain only oestrogen and some only progesterone, while others are a combination of both hormones. Different types of the pill are suitable for different women and if the first one used causes unpleasant side-effects, then it should be changed to another type.

There is not yet absolute certainty about the way in which these pills prevent pregnancy, but it is known that they inhibit ovulation, prevent the development of the endometrium and bring about changes in the cervical mucus.

The use of oral contraceptives has many advantages:

- The pill is a reliable method of contraception with a success rate of 98 per cent and higher.
- It is a method that is acceptable to most women.

Taking the pill is not connected directly with the sexual act.

Injectable long-acting contraceptives and implants

There are a number of these available: Depo-Provera is a progesterone derivative, while Nur-Isterate is a derivative of 19-nortestosterone. Administration is by means of an injection; this has to be repeated at intervals of 8 or 12 weeks depending on the preparation used. These products are particularly useful for women who cannot be relied upon to take a contraceptive pill regularly or in situations where regular attendance at clinics is not possible.

Table 11.1 Advantages and disadvantages of long-acting contraceptives

Advantages	Disadvantages
They are effective.	Treatment cannot be discontinued once the injection has been given.
They do not require continuous motivation on the part of the woman.	Disturbances of the menstrual cycle are common.
The cooperation of the male partner is not necessary.	Most women gain weight.
In some cases, prolonged periods of amenorrhoea may be beneficial.	

In most cases, there is a delayed return to fertility, although the literature reports that 75 per cent of women who wish to conceive do so within 18 months and 95 per cent within two years.

Intra-uterine devices

These are small structures of various shapes and sizes that are made of polythene. They have to be inserted by a medical practitioner or a suitably qualified nurse. Intra-uterine devices (IUDs) are useful for women who are not highly motivated or reliable about using other methods, or for those who for some reason cannot use the contraceptive pill. They are very effective and once they have been inserted they require no further action to be taken by the user, apart from a yearly visit to the clinic for a check- up, or to have the device replaced if necessary. IUDs act by interfering with the implantation of the fertilised ovum.

Because IUDs may be expelled, become displaced or migrate into the peritoneal cavity, the threads attached to the device should be checked regularly to ensure that they are still in position.

IUDs should not be used in the presence of the following: abnormal vaginal bleeding, pelvic inflammatory disease, cervical or vaginal infection, menorrhagia, valvular heart disease because of the danger of subacute bacterial endocarditis, previous ectopic pregnancy, HIV and AIDS.

Disadvantages of IUDs are:

- persistent vaginal discharge
- heavy and prolonged menstrual bleeding
- pelvic infections (these are important because they can be the cause of tubal damage and occlusion and may result in infertility or ectopic pregnancies)
- vaginal and cervical infections.

Sterilisation

Either the male or the female may be rendered permanently sterile by means of a surgical procedure. In males this is a relatively minor operation and may be carried out in an out-patient department or clinic. It involves tying off the vas deferens, which carries the spermatozoa from the testes to the penis, on either side of the scrotum. In females an abdominal operation is involved and the fallopian tube on either side of the uterus is severed and tied off. The results of these operations are irreversible, and care should be taken to ensure that the man or woman considering sterilisation has given the matter serious attention and fully understands the implications.

Sterilisation may be the method of choice in cases where there is a high risk of producing a child with a serious genetic defect, where the woman is suffering from a disease that makes a pregnancy inadvisable, or where a couple have a number of children and feel strongly that they do not wish to have any more.

Termination of pregnancy

According to the health legislation in South Africa, a termination of pregnancy or abortion is allowed on request up to 14 weeks' gestation, and in certain specified circumstances and for specific reasons, from 14 to 24 weeks' gestation.

The fact that termination of pregnancy or abortion is now available on request should not impede efforts to promote more conventional methods of contraception. The Choice on Termination of Pregnancy Amendment Act of 2004 allows nurses and midwives to be trained to conduct the terminations. The Act clearly outlines that the function of the nurse is to inform the patient of her rights and the choices she can make – not to force her own beliefs on the patient.

Sexually transmitted infection management

The Department of Health believes that many unwanted pregnancies, STIs and HIV and AIDS can be prevented through the provision of reproductive health services and youth-friendly services, in conjunction with other strategies to advance the position of women and youth in society. It has been demonstrated that the provision of reproductive health services and contraceptives to sexually active youth and women greatly reduces the incidence of unwanted pregnancies, STIs, HIV and AIDS, and the incidence of unsafe termination of pregnancies. However, success of these services is dependent on the quality of care provided at health services and the promotion of healthy lifestyles. Hence, quality of care is an important area of focus for the respective health departments.

One of the key concerns about reproductive health services is that there is a gap between the services offered and the clients' needs. All too often, an unintended pregnancy occurs because of incorrect or irregular use of contraception, inadequate information and lack of choice on the method. Many pregnancies are unplanned and/or unwanted, so are repeated terminations of pregnancy. Termination of pregnancy should not be seen as a contraceptive method and should not be used as such.

Well baby clinics

In the urban areas 'well baby' or 'child health' clinics supervise the health and development of children from birth to the age of two years. In the less-developed rural areas where child death rates are high, these clinics alone are not sufficient to protect the health of children, which is why 'under-five' clinics are an essential part of the child health services. In some countries, such as India, a register is kept of all children under the age of five years as they are an 'at risk' group.

Mothers should be told of the health benefits associated with regular attendance at such clinics. If a mother is not bringing her infant to the clinic, the community health nurse should visit the home to establish the reason for non-attendance.

Child health clinics provide promotive, preventative and curative services and should be equipped to meet the daily needs of the children in a community.

The following aspects of child health are attended to at child health clinics:

- *Growth and development are monitored.* The infant's height and weight are recorded at regular intervals, and if these are not within normal levels the reason for this should be established. If nutritional factors are responsible, it may be necessary to ensure that the child receives food supplements.

- *Health education and counselling* of the mother can do much to improve the child's health and to prevent disease. Health education in all aspects of child nutrition and hygiene is particularly important.

- *Regular medical supervision* is provided for the early detection and treatment of disease.

- *Immunisation* is vital in the prevention of the communicable diseases and is supplied free of charge at these clinics. The importance of immunisation should be impressed upon the mother.

- *Breastfeeding* is promoted at these clinics. In the economically deprived sections of the community breastfeeding can mean the difference between life and death to the child, and two years should be the absolute minimum age of weaning in these communities. In many of the developing countries the most serious problem is the lack of suitable weaning foods and few infants can survive on the food that is available to the adults.

Breastfeeding

Before discussing breastfeeding with a client, you should familiarise yourself with the latest guidelines on recommendations for HIV and breastfeeding, as these change from time to time. The advantages of breastfeeding are set out below:

- The milk of all mammals is designed to meet the particular needs of their young, so it stands to reason that breast milk is the perfect food for the human baby and contains all the nutrients that it requires in the correct proportions.

- Breast milk contains fewer saturated fatty acids than cow's milk and it is thought that breastfed infants are less likely to develop atherosclerosis in later life.

- The breastfed baby takes only as much milk as he or she requires, which means that overfeeding and obesity are less common in breastfed babies than in those who are bottle fed.

- Hygienically, it is the best method of feeding as breast milk is unlikely to contain pathogenic organisms.

- Breastfeeding is labour saving as no preparation or sterilisation of equipment is required.

- It is economical, as not only does the breast milk not cost anything but the mother does not have to buy bottles and teats.

- The risk of infection in the infant is reduced because the mother's milk contains antibodies against many infectious diseases. The acidic stools of breastfed babies also discourage the growth of pathogens and so the risk of gastrointestinal infections is reduced.

- Breastfeeding is of psychological value to both the mother and the infant.

Weaning

Weaning is the term used for the introduction of mixed feeding. It can be started at the age of 12 weeks or even earlier, but if suitable weaning foods are not available, or if poverty and unsatisfactory environmental conditions exist, it should be delayed for as long as possible.

The following are some of the important points to be observed when introducing the infant to mixed feeding:

- New foods should be introduced in small amounts, and only one new food should be added to the diet at a time.
- The aim should be to ensure that the infant receives a balanced diet, ie one that contains all the food constituents in the correct proportions.
- Infants have small stomachs and cannot take a lot at one feed, so one must not use 'high-bulk' foods that will fill the stomach without providing sufficient kilojoules.
- The baby should still continue to receive sufficient quantities of milk, for there is no other food that can replace it in an infant's diet.
- The food must be hygienically prepared.

Integrated management of childhood illnesses

Integrated management of childhood illnesses (IMCI) is an integrated approach to child health that focuses on the well-being of the whole child. IMCI aims to reduce death, illness and disability, and to promote improved growth and development among children under five years of age. IMCI includes both preventative and curative elements that are implemented by families and communities as well as by health facilities. The strategy includes three main components:

- improving case management skills of healthcare staff
- improving overall health systems
- improving family and community health practices.

In health facilities the IMCI strategy promotes the accurate identification of childhood illnesses in outpatient settings, ensures appropriate combined treatment of all major illnesses, strengthens the counselling of caretakers and speeds up the referral of severely ill children. In the home setting it promotes appropriate care-seeking behaviours, improved nutrition and preventative care, and the correct implementation of prescribed care.

Adolescent health

Adolescence is the period of physical, psychological and social transition between childhood and adulthood. This transition involves biological, social and psychological changes, although those that are biological are the easiest to measure objectively.

Frequently occurring problems experienced by adolescents include:
- teenage pregnancy
- substance abuse
- suicide and parasuicide
- anorexia nervosa and bulimia.

A number of outreach programmes and community organisations are available to support parents with their adolescents. Counselling services and referral to community organisations that specifically manage adolescent problems are available at health clinics and schools.

The government has reintroduced school health nurses in the re-engineered primary healthcare services in South Africa.

The National Adolescent-friendly Clinic Initiative

In 1999, as part of the SDG 5, the Wits University Reproductive Health Research Unit, Chris Hani Baragwanath Hospital and Love Life, coordinated the National Adolescent-friendly Clinic Initiative (NAFCI), which grew to about 350 clinics by 2005. The following is their published list of health rights to which adolescent children are entitled.

Any young person, irrespective of age, sex, race, religion, culture, social status and mental and physical ability, has basic health rights (NAFCI, 2000), which include:
- the right to information on health
- the right to a full range of affordable health services
- the right to privacy when receiving healthcare
- the right to be treated with dignity and respect when receiving healthcare
- the right to be assured that personal information will remain confidential
- the right to be given an explanation of the processes that the young person goes through when receiving healthcare
- the right to be treated by people who are trained and knowledgeable about what they do
- the right to continuity of services
- the right to be treated by a named provider
- the right to express views on the services provided and to complain about unsatisfactory health services
- the right to gender equality
- the right to a healthy and safe environment
- the right to make free informed choices in matters relating to sexual expression, sexual pleasure and sexual orientation.

Men's health

The specific needs of this group are not addressed adequately in current health services, although some changes are occurring. Contraception has traditionally focused on women. Increasingly, however, we are recognising men's influence in reproductive health. Men play a key role in supporting women's health, preventing unwanted pregnancies and slowing the transmission of STIs including HIV and AIDS. Furthermore, we have realised that men also need access to clinical services and information on contraception.

Men often exert a strong influence over their partners. Men determine the timing and conditions of sexual relations, family size and access to healthcare. Men's reproductive health directly affects their partners, although it has taken the HIV and AIDS epidemic to bring this reality into focus. Men usually decide whether to use a condom or not.

Health of the elderly

It is a known phenomenon that people are living longer because of better care, preventative health and advances in medical science. In South Africa, many working people retire from 60 years onwards and depend on good healthcare services.

According to predictions made by the UN, the current demographic revolution will continue well into the future. The major features of this trend are listed below:

- One out of every 10 people is 60 years or older; by 2050, one out of five will be 60 years or older and by 2150, one out of three people will be 60 years or older.

- The older population itself is ageing. The oldest old (ie 80 years or older) is the fastest-growing segment of the older population. They currently make up 11 per cent of the 60+ age group and this will grow to 19 per cent by 2050. The number of centenarians (aged 100 years or older) is projected to increase 15-fold, from approximately 145 00 in 1999 to 2,2 million by 2050.

- The majority of older people (55 per cent) are women. Among the oldest, 65 per cent are women.

- Striking differences exist between regions. One out of five Europeans, but one out of 20 South Africans, is 60 years or older.

- In some developed countries, the proportion of older people is close to one in five. During the first half of the 21st century that proportion will reach one in four and in some countries one in two.

- The impact of population ageing is increasingly evident in the old-age dependency ratio – the number of working-age persons (15 to 64 years) per older person (65 years or older) – that is used as an indicator of the 'dependency burden' on potential workers. Between 2000 and 2050, the old-age dependency ratio will double in more developed regions and triple in less developed regions.

More than half of the world's elderly live in developing countries, of which a large proportion live in Africa where they experience declining family support and low standards of living.

The demographic trends discussed above have resulted in the rapid development of two relatively new sciences, namely gerontology and geriatrics.

- *Gerontology* is the science that studies the processes of ageing.
- *Geriatrics* is the branch of medicine that studies the diseases of the elderly; it includes all levels of prevention, namely primary, secondary and tertiary prevention.

In South Africa, legislation is in place to protect the elderly: the Older Persons Act 13 of 2006 states as its objective 'to deal effectively with the plight of older persons by establishing a framework aimed at the empowerment and protection of older persons, and at the promotion and maintenance of their status, rights, well-being, safety and security; and to provide for other matters connected with the same' (RSA, 2006). The main features of the Act include:

- programmes for the development of older persons
- ensuring an enabling and supportive environment for older persons
- protection for older persons.

Services for the elderly are provided by the following authorities or organisations:

- The Department of Health, which provides health services at community, regional and teaching hospitals
- Departments of Health, provincial and local, including the district health services, which provide services at community and primary healthcare clinics, as well as community nursing services
- Local authorities that provide preventative geriatric services and housing for the aged and other low-income groups. The larger local authorities play an important role in providing recreation and adult education at their many recreational centres
- Voluntary welfare organisations – such as the National and Regional Councils for the Care of the Aged, various religious bodies and social clubs and organisations like the Red Cross – play a vital role in the provision of services and facilities for the elderly. They provide housing; institutional care; financial aid; social, psychological and spiritual support; adult education, recreation and counselling; and advice on various matters.

It should be mentioned that the majority of elderly people will be able to remain reasonably active in the community if the necessary facilities and services are available.

> You should be familiar with the services that are available in your area so that you can help older people with information and advice when they are in need. Make time to research more about services in your community.

The process of ageing

Ageing is a natural and inevitable process that takes place gradually. It affects the whole organism, leading to anatomical and physiological changes that make increasingly greater demands on the homeostatic mechanisms that enable a living organism to adapt to its environment.

Because these changes are universal, they may be considered 'normal'. Some of them are listed below:

- The hair turns grey and becomes sparse.
- The skin loses its elasticity and becomes wrinkled.
- There is some reduction in height, mainly due to atrophy of the vertebra discs, and a thoracic kyphosis may develop.
- Muscle power diminishes and muscle tone decreases.
- Physiological changes include decreased cardiac output, diminished capacity of the lungs and reduced respiratory efficiency.
- Changes occur in the mucous membrane of the gastrointestinal tract and there is a decreased secretion of digestive juices and decreased absorption of nutrients, especially vitamins.
- There is nearly always sensory loss, a decrease in visual acuity and hearing loss, while a diminished sense of taste and smell are common.
- Psychological changes also occur. It is said that sometimes there is a narrowing of interests and the elderly tend to become self-centred, selfish, withdrawn and introspective.
- There is some reduction in learning skills and in memory – at one time it was a widely held belief that there was a 'normal' decline in intelligence with advancing age. It has now been shown that intellectual impairment is not an inevitable consequence of ageing. An individual's previous intellectual ability and the type of work in which he or she is engaged are important variables. Where a person is engaged in an occupation that requires intellectual activity, any decrease in intelligence is minimal.
- Anxiety and depression are common.

Factors affecting the ageing process

There is no doubt that many of the psychological traits that are said to be characteristic of the aged are the result of the social and economic situation in which they find themselves and not to psychological factors.

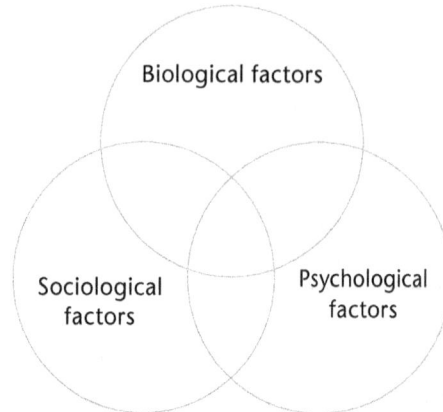

Figure 11.1 Factors affecting the ageing process

The rate at which these changes occur varies greatly from person to person and there may be little correlation between a person's chronological age (age in years) and his or her biological age. Ageing, and the rate of ageing, is the result of the interaction between biological, psychological and social factors.

Biological factors

Biological factors include genetic endowment, presence or absence of disease, obesity and smoking.

- **Genetic endowment:** There is evidence to suggest that longevity is genetically determined and there is a marked similarity in the age at which death occurs in the members of different generations of a family.
- **The presence or absence of disease affects rate of ageing:** Those suffering from diseases such as diabetes mellitus or hypertension usually die younger than those who do not have such conditions.
- **Obesity:** Diseases such as diabetes mellitus, hypertension, gout, arthritis and gall-bladder disease, which are more common in obese people, decrease life expectancy.
- **Smoking:** The dangers of smoking are well known, but it is appropriate to mention here that smoking accelerates ageing and hastens death.

Social factors

These factors include socio-economic level, integration in society and level of social interaction:

- **Socioeconomic level**: The role that socio-economic status plays in death and disease has been well researched and documented. It is clear that those from higher socioeconomic levels live longer and age more slowly than those from lower socioeconomic levels. Better nutrition, better medical care, a safer environment and less hazardous occupations all contribute to the lower death rates in this group, while death rates are highest in the most deprived sections of the community. However, the concept of social categories is a complex one in which educational, occupational and economic factors play a part and it is therefore difficult to establish specific deciding factors.
- **Social integration and social interaction**: The more social contacts a person has and the more closely he or she is integrated into the community, the more slowly the person will age.

Psychological factors

These factors include the following:

- **Personality**: It has been said that old age is the true test of personality. Personality does not change during ageing, but certain traits, or personality features, become more pronounced. Optimism, enthusiasm and an interest in life will facilitate adaptation to the inevitable changes of ageing.
- **Motivation**: Those who are motivated to remain young, and those whose careers depend upon their doing so, age more slowly. This is probably the result of continuing mental and physical activity.

The family and the aged

In traditional societies, such as African tribal society, where the dominant family form is the extended family, elderly people remain important members of the family; they suffer no loss of status and their roles are clearly defined. They are looked upon as a wise and all-knowing authority, are consulted and asked for advice about all important matters. They play a major part in the education and socialisation of children in the family. They are well integrated into the community and have fewer social and psychological problems than their counterparts in urban industrialised societies.

In modern society the nuclear family is the dominant family form. This is essentially a two-generation family and for various reasons such families find it unsatisfactory to have elderly parents or relations living with them.

Problems of the elderly

Old age is not a disease, but it does result in many problems with which the elderly person has to cope.

Physical problems

While it is wrong to think that all elderly people are ill, bedridden, incontinent, institutionalised and/or senile, it is true that the incidence of disease and disability increases with increasing age, and a large percentage of elderly people suffer from some physical condition that requires treatment.

Among the more common conditions are the following:

- diseases of the cardiovascular system, ischaemic heart disease, congestive cardiac failure, atherosclerosis and hypertension
- diseases of the cerebrovascular system, cerebral thrombosis and cerebral haemorrhage
- malignant neoplasms
- diseases of the respiratory system, chronic bronchitis, pulmonary emphysema and pneumonia
- diseases of the musculoskeletal system, rheumatism, osteoarthritis and rheumatoid arthritis.

In addition to those mentioned above, a large number of less serious conditions are often present that nevertheless cause a considerable amount of ill health, increase disability and detract from quality of life. These include diabetes mellitus, anaemia and hypothyroidism. Unfortunately, these are often undiagnosed as the clinical picture is vague and poorly defined, and symptoms such as lassitude and breathlessness are often attributed to 'old age' by both the client and the practitioner. This leads to the conclusion that nothing can be done about the symptoms and so the condition is left untreated. This is unfortunate as nowhere is early diagnosis and prompt treatment more important than in geriatrics. Simple treatment often leads to a dramatic improvement in health and well-being.

Elderly people often suffer from multiple pathology that makes diagnosis difficult and complicates treatment, while multiple medication may give rise to drug interactions and unpleasant side-effects. Non-compliance – that is, failure to take prescribed medication or taking it incorrectly – is another problem with which those who care for the elderly have to deal.

Accidents, particularly domestic accidents, contribute heavily to death and disability in the elderly and are dealt with in Chapter 12.

A more detailed discussion of the diseases of the elderly is beyond the scope of this chapter, but we would like to emphasise the basic principles, or 'eternal truths', of geriatric medicine:

- Vigorous treatment, coupled with a positive attitude, will cure or improve many of the diseases from which the elderly suffer.

- Avoid putting an elderly person to bed rest, as there is a good chance that he or she may never get out of bed alive and will die from the complications of bed rest.
- Never institutionalise an elderly person unless there is no other option. Hospitalisation often leads to disorientation, mental confusion, incontinence and a rapid deterioration of health.
- Nowhere is rehabilitation more important than in the treatment of the elderly patient.

Financial problems

In modern industrial societies both men and women have to retire on reaching a certain age – usually 60 or 65 years. This results in some loss of income, unless the person has managed to save adequately for his or her retirement. However, most South Africans who do not have an income or do not own property qualify for an older person's grant (this used to be called the old age pension). The South African Social Security Agency (SASSA) is responsible for paying this grant.

> **Further reading**
>
> To read more about the older person's grant, go to www.services.gov.za.

Psychological problems

Elderly people may also suffer from the following:

- **Anxiety and depression**: These are common in the aged and are often due to bereavement, physical illness and sensory loss such as failing eyesight or increasing deafness, social isolation and loneliness. Suicide rates, especially among males, show a marked increase with increasing age.
- **Sleep disturbances**: Changes in sleep occur and may increase anxiety. The habit that elderly people have of having 'cat naps', may contribute to disorientation and confusion, especially if the person finds him- or herself in an unfamiliar environment.
- **Acute confusional states**: Confusion occurs and may result from cerebral anoxia, which can be due to any of the following conditions: infections, especially respiratory infection; anaemia; a fall in arterial blood pressure; hypotensive drugs; or small 'strokes'. Acute mental confusion may also result from the toxic effects of certain drugs such as digitalis, barbiturates and antidepressants, while social isolation and sensory deprivation also play a role.
- **Chronic conditions**: Conditions such as senile dementia, are the result of degenerative changes in the cerebral blood vessels and also result in mental confusion.

Social problems

Abuse of the elderly is a widespread problem. Several socio-demographic factors contribute to abuse of the elderly:

- **Intra-family stressors**: With the incidence of HIV and AIDS and the number of young people dying, elderly grandparents are now often responsible for raising their grandchildren on their old-age pensions. Some adult children take advantage of their elderly parents living in rural areas and leave the grandchildren in their care while the parent works in the urban areas.

- **Decreasing importance of traditional age roles, including ageism and loss of respect for aged persons**: African culture has always been characterised by respect for elderly people, including the ancestors. With more children moving away from rural homes and adopting Western cultures, the inherent lack of respect for their elderly, uneducated rural parents is becoming increasingly prevalent. The financial situation in most families where children are earning much more than their parents and are living a different lifestyle in the urban suburbs also contributes to a loss of respect for the elderly parents who are now dependent on their children for support.

- **Increased life expectancy**: The elderly are living much longer and this further increases the demand on their families, communities and nations as a whole.

- **Advances in pharmaceuticals and medical technology that prolong years lived with chronic disease**: In the past, with the poor management of chronic diseases, many elderly people died early due to complications or mismanagement of chronic diseases. Today, with improved drugs and access to monthly chronic medications, their diseases are better managed, thus prolonging their lives (Levine, 2003:37).

Conclusion

South Africa has limited infrastructure to provide for its citizens' health needs throughout their lifespan. We also know that this infrastructure faces many challenges, particularly with the shortage of dedicated healthcare professionals, the continuing burden of HIV and AIDS and the care that the ageing population requires. It is hoped that the implementation of the National Health Insurance (NHI) will improve care for the citizens of South Africa.

Self-assessment

1. Describe the maternal and child services available in South Africa at primary care level.
2. Outline child spacing methods and benefits.
3. How can we make health services more adolescent-friendly?
4. Describe the physical and social services that can positively influence care of the elderly.

Bibliography

Clarke, M. (ed.). 2014. *Vlok's Community Health.* 6th edition. Cape Town: Juta.

Eliopoulos, C. 1993. *Gerontological Nursing.* 5th edition. Philadelphia: Lippincott.

Goodburn, E.A. & Ross, D.A. 1995. *A picture of health: A review and annotated bibliography of the health of young people in developing countries.* World Health Organization and UNICEF.

Health Systems Development Unit. 2001. *Primary Clinical Care.* Volume 3. Cape Town: Heinemann.

Iipinge, S.N. 2001. Capacity building for home care in rural Namibia. Doctoral research thesis, p. 107.

Levine, M.J. 2003. Elder neglect and abuse: A primer for primary care physicians. *Geriatrics,* 58(10):37–44.

National Adolescent-friendly Clinic Initiative (NAFCI). 2000. Adolescent sexual and reproductive health rights document. Reproductive Research Unit, Chris Hani Baragwanath Hospital.

Orb, A., Davis, P., Wynaden, D. & Davey, M. 2001. Best practice in psychogeriatric care. *Australian and New Zealand Journal of Mental Health Nursing,* 10(1):10–19.

Republic of South Africa (RSA). 1997. White Paper on Social Development. *Government Gazette.* Pretoria: Government Printer.

Republic of South Africa (RSA). 2004. The Choice on Termination of Pregnancy Amendment Act 38 of 2004. *Government Gazette.* Pretoria: Government Printer.

Republic of South Africa (RSA). 2006. Older Person's Act 13 of 2006. *Government Gazette.* Pretoria: Government Printer.

United Nations (UN). 1998. World population prospects, the 1998 revision. Volume II: Sex and age. The Population Division, Department of Economic and Social Affairs, United Nations Secretariat.

United Nations (UN). 2013. World population aging. Available: http://doi.org/10.18356/e59eddca-en (Accessed 4 October 2020).

United Nations (UN). nd. Sustainable development goals (SDGs). Available: https://www.afro.who.int/media-centre/infographics/sustainable-development-goals (Accessed 4 October 2020).

United Nations Development Programme (UNDP). 2015. Post-2015 sustainable development agenda. Available: http://www.unsdg.un.org (Accessed 4 October 2020).

Van Vuuren, S. & Groenewald, D. 1998. The living conditions of elderly black people in a typical rural area in the Free State. *Curationis*, September 1998:77–90.

World Health Organization (WHO). 2013. Trends in maternal mortality 1990–2013. Available: http://apps.who.int/iris/bitstream/10665/112697/1/WHO_RHR_14.13_eng.pdf?ua=1 (Accessed 14 September 2020).

World Health Organization (WHO). 2014. Child mortality estimates. Available: http://www.who. int/mediacentre/news/releases/2014/child_mortality_estimates/en/ (Accessed 14 September 2020).

World Health Organization (WHO). 2016. National consolidated guidelines for on the use of antiretroviral drugs for treating and preventing HIV infection: Recommendations for a public health approach. Available: https://www.who.int/hiv/pub/arv/arv-2016/en/ (Accessed 14 September 2020).

Home accidents

Sindi Mthembu

Learning outcomes

After studying this chapter, you should be able to:

- Give a concise definition of home accidents.
- Explain the demographic factors related to home accidents.
- Categorise and describe the different types of home accidents.
- Outline the preventative measure(s) that can be taken for each potential home accident.

Key terms

Accident: An unfortunate incident that happens unexpectedly and unintentionally, typically resulting in damage or injury.

Injury: A damage or bodily harm suffered by a person and caused by physical hurt.

Poison: Any substance that is harmful to your body. You might swallow it, inhale it, inject it, or absorb it through your skin.

Trauma: Injury that can potentially lead to serious outcomes.

Introduction

Your home is supposed to be your 'safe place'. However, the majority of injuries to children occur in and around their own home. An accident may be defined as an unanticipated or unexpected event that results in death or injury to someone and/or damage to property. This definition reflects the commonly held belief that nobody is to blame for an accident because it could not have been foreseen, whereas, in fact, most accidents are a result of someone's carelessness and negligence of safety at home, which could have been prevented if certain obvious steps had been taken.

Home or domestic accidents, this context, include all the accidents that take place in and around the home. These accidents are prominent among the causes of death and disability in South Africa and contribute substantially to potential years of life lost. The most common accidental deaths at home are caused by falls, burns from fire and flames and traumatic injuries caused by sharp instruments. Poisoning, drowning, choking and asphyxia also contribute heavily to the accident incidence rates.

The objectives of this chapter are to raise awareness about home accidents, to explain how some accidents can be prevented and to advise on some first-aid techniques.

Demographic factors in home accidents

According to the World Health Organization (WHO), nearly half of all accidents occur in the home. Far from being the haven of safety that we imagine it to be, the home is filled with potential dangers. The kitchen is said to be the most dangerous room in the house as more accidents take place there than anywhere else in the home. The annual incidence of home accidents from hospital admissions has been reported in many studies; low-income countries have more morbidity and mortality associated with home accidents. Some possible causes of home accidents include:

- large families or child-headed households, resulting in inadequate care
- carers being under the influence of alcohol, resulting in negligent care
- uneven flooring or electrical wires trailing on the floor, causing a trip hazard
- cold-drink bottles containing poisonous substances, such as paraffin, resulting in accidental poisoning
- candles or paraffin stoves being knocked over, resulting in burn injuries.

Young children and elderly people are the two groups at greatest risk of home accidents and the extremes of age are periods of particularly high incidence. Toddlers are most vulnerable as they are curious, adventurous and fearless, but lack the experience and judgement necessary to look after themselves. The incidence of home accidents in this age group is directly related to the quality of supervision that the child receives and accidents are often the result of negligence on the part of child carers.

Types of home accidents

There are three main categories of home accidents:

- **Impact accidents**: Including falls, being hurt by falling objects and general 'bumping-into' type of accidents.
- **Heat accidents**: Including burns and scalds.

- **Ingestion/inhalation and foreign-body accidents**: These include accidental poisoning, suffocation, choking and objects stuck in the ear, nose and eye.

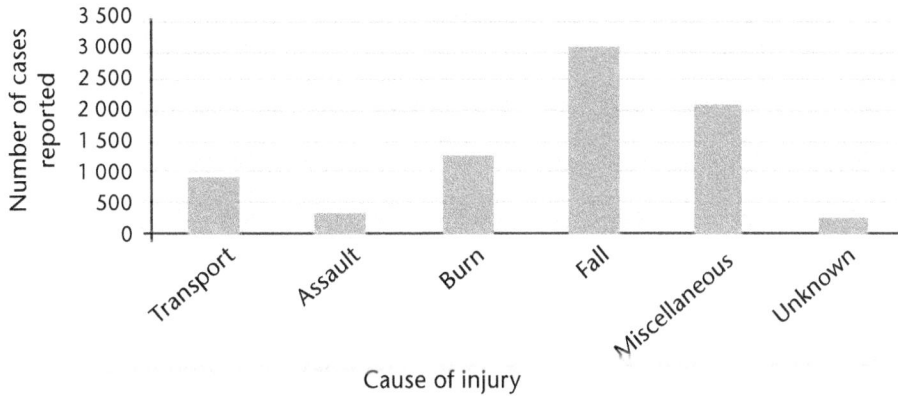

Figure 12.1 Main causes of injury in South Africa for 2013

Source: Adapted from Red Cross War Memorial Children's Hospital Trauma Unit Statistics (2013)

Falls

Falls are the accidents most frequently suffered by the elderly and often result in death either directly or as a result of the complications that occur. It has been estimated that over half the accident fatalities in people over the age of 65 years are the result of falls. Poor vision, unsteady gait, dizzy spells, postural hypotension and blackouts all contribute to the high frequency of serious falls in the elderly. Falls are the main cause of admission to hospital for both children and the elderly.

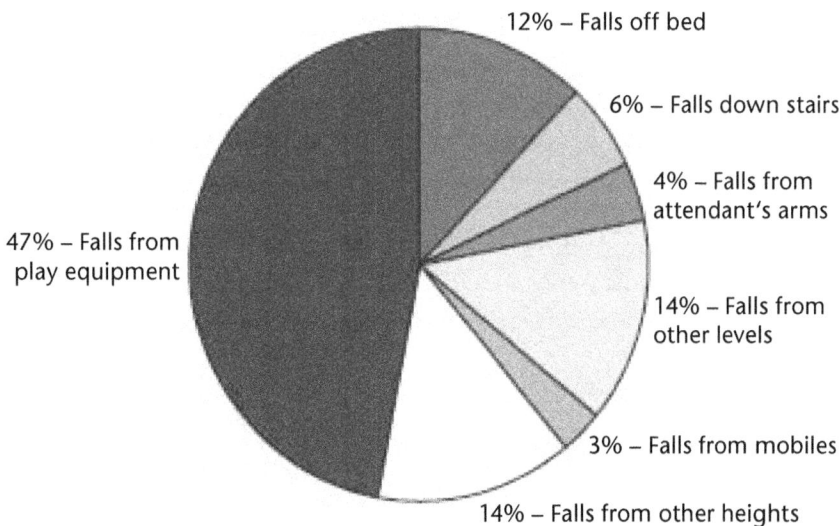

Figure 12.2 Main causes of falls in South Africa

Source: Adapted from Red Cross War Memorial Children's Hospital Trauma Unit Statistics (2013)

Preventative measures

Floor safety tips:

- Clean up spills, such as water or any liquid, as soon as they happen, and keep floors dry.
- Pick up shoes, newspapers, clothes, toys and other potential obstacles from the floor.
- Repair uneven floor surfaces.
- Clear all pathways of any obstructions to prevent the chance of falling.
- Remove or secure any electrical wires lying on the floor.
- Exercise close supervision when a toddler learns to walk.
- Ensure that the bed rail of the baby cot is raised when the baby is in the cot.
- Avoid placing 'step-stones' such as a chair next to a window.
- Use a securely fitted safety harness in a pram, pushchair or highchair.
- Lock windows and doors to avoid misadventure by children.

Stair safety tips:

- Ensure that lighting is good so that stair edges are well lit. In public buildings, paint the edge of the stairs in a contrasting colour.
- Install handrails on both sides of the stairs.
- Repair uneven or damaged stairs.
- Repair or remove torn or worn carpets.
- Avoid carrying loads that reduce vision when using stairs.

Burns

Most fatal burn accidents occur in the home, although industrial fires also contribute to the statistics. All such accidents are preventable. Burn injuries can cause lifelong scarring that requires long-term medical treatment, usually resulting in years of physical, psychological and occupational therapy. Harmful practices that may result in burns include:

- smoking cigarettes while working with flammable substances such as petrol, paraffin and benzene
- smoking in bed where there is a danger of falling asleep with a burning cigarette in one's hand
- the use of open fires and naked flames such as candles, oil lamps and primus stoves for cooking, heating and lighting in homes
- leaving potentially dangerous items such as matches and cigarette lighters lying around the house and within the reach of children
- allowing children to play in the kitchen while cooking is taking place
- leaving hot liquids or hot objects such as irons where children can reach them or pull on the electrical cord.

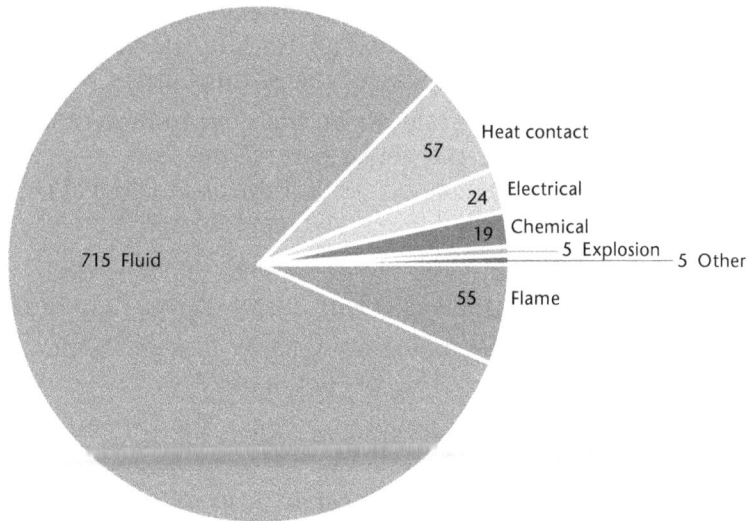

Figure 12.3 Burn injuries in South Africa

Source: Adapted from Red Cross War Memorial Children's Hospital Trauma Unit Statistics (2019)

Preventative measures

- Education in fire safety is important. Everyone, particularly the parents of young children, should be made aware of the dangers that may result from the careless use of fire.

- Smokers should exercise great care when smoking. Lighted cigarettes should not be left to smoulder. Smoking indoors affects the health of everyone in the room/house and should be avoided at all costs.

- Smoking in bed must be discouraged.

- Ensure that matches and cigarettes have been properly extinguished before discarding them. Cigarette butts should be fully extinguished and discarded in a suitable container – not in the road or garden as this can start a fire.

- No one should smoke while working with flammable liquid and/or while with children.

- Smokers must make use of ashtrays.

- Where it is necessary to use open fires for domestic purposes, the fire should be adequately guarded. Children should be kept away from it and taught that the fire is hot and dangerous.

- Place candles firmly in suitable candle holders and away from flammable items such as curtains that may catch alight.

- Never run hot water into the bath first and never leave the child alone in the bath as he or she may open the hot water tap.

- Never place hot liquids and foods near the edges of cupboards and tables where children can reach or pull on a tablecloth and in so doing pull the hot substances over onto themselves and getting burned.
- Turn pan and pot handles inwards on the stove to prevent a child from reaching up and pulling the pot or pan off the stove onto themselves. Never put a pot with hot food such as porridge on the floor as children can put their hands into it or fall into it and scald themselves.
- Replace worn-out electric cords or broken plugs immediately.
- Do not overload an electric socket with adaptors as this can cause a fire.
- Disconnect all electrical appliances such as heaters, kettles, radios or televisions at night or when they are not in use.
- Keep domestic fire extinguishers or a container of sand in areas such as the kitchen, where fires are most likely to occur.
- Avoid wearing loose-fitting sleepwear or a loose scarf near the stove, fireplace or heater as they could easily catch alight while you are working.
- Do not carry a lighted gas heater around. Never move or fill a paraffin heater or stove when alight.
- Do not hang clothes over a heater or in an oven to dry. They may begin to burn when you are not around. Never dry clothes too close to open fires.
- Never go to sleep with a burning heater, candle, lamp or fire.
- Keep portable stoves out of reach of children and away from curtains.
- Never pull out the tank of a paraffin fridge while the flame is burning. To extinguish the flame, blow only from the top of the funnel.
- People prone to epileptic seizures should keep away from open fires as the flickering flames might precipitate an attack and they may fall into the fire.
- Use tag-less teabags if you have toddlers in the home, as they are attracted by the colourful tags on teabags and may pull the string and spill hot tea on themselves.
- Supervise and instruct older children on the correct use of matches (eg not to light matches near petrol or other flammable substances, or to be sure to place a candle in a secure holder on a firm surface before lighting it). Explain the correct uses and dangers to them; simply forbidding them without explaining the risks may tempt them to experiment.

Management of burns

Emergency action:
- If your clothing catches alight, drop onto the floor and roll over to smother the flames.
- If there is thick smoke during a fire, crawl on the floor to escape the smoke because smoke rises.

Emergency treatment for general burns:

- Run clean cold water over the burn area for at least 20 minutes.
- Cover the burned area with a clean, wet dressing. If the dressing becomes dry replace with a wet dressing.
- Seek medical assistance immediately if the burn is larger than the casualty's fist.
- Do not cool the burn area with ice as this may cause an ice-burn.
- Do not use oil, butter or soap on a burn.
- Do not attempt to remove clothing that may be stuck to a burn area.

Emergency treatment for chemical burns:

- Burns caused by acids – run clean cold water over the burn for at least 20 minutes.
- Burns caused by dry acid powder – brush the powder off the skin with a gloved hand or a cloth.
- Assist the patient to change any clothing that has been splashed with the chemical.
- Wash the clothing in cold running water.

Emergency treatment for electrical burns:

- Do not touch the person if he or she is still touching the source of the burn (ie still touching the faulty electrical point). First switch off the power at the mains.
- Once it is safe to touch the person , move them to a safe area, and cool the burn as you would any other burn.
- If the person is showing no signs of life, it may be necessary to commence cardiopulmonary resuscitation (CPR). This should only be done if you are trained in this procedure.
- Do not apply any substances such as oil or butter to the burn area.
- Do not attempt to remove any clothing that may be stuck to the burn.
- Treat any other injury (an electrical shock can throw a person across a room resulting in wounds, dislocations, fractures, etc).
- Call for assistance immediately.

Emergency treatment for fire burns:

- Extinguish clothes that are on fire by dropping to the ground and rolling.
- Remove hot or burned clothing immediately, if possible, or stop any contact with the fire, hot object, steam or liquid.
- Cool the burned area by running cold tap water over it for several minutes.
- Do not use ice as this may worsen the injury to the skin.
- Do not remove blisters.

- Do not attempt to remove clothing that has stuck to burned areas.
- Call for assistance immediately.

Poisoning

Accidental poisoning affects people of all ages. In children it peaks between the ages of one and four years and is primarily a result of ingesting medicines and household cleaning products. The elderly are susceptible to carbon monoxide poisoning from fires and flames and to accidental overdose because of poor management of medication.

Accidental poisoning in children is preventable. To safeguard against accidents, keep all poisonous substances out of reach of children, preferably in a locked cupboard. Pay particular attention to cleaning and other substances in the kitchen, bathroom and garage.

Refer to the poison emergency care card in Figure 12.4.

Preventative measures

- Keep all poisonous substances and medicines in the house and outbuildings under lock and key and out of reach of children.
- Teach children from an early age not to put anything except food into their mouths and not to eat or drink from bottles or cans left standing or lying around.
- Ask your local pharmacist how best to discard any unwanted toxic substances and medicine.
- Do not store poisonous substances in the kitchen where they might be mistakenly used or contaminate foodstuffs. Never decant poisonous liquid into cold-drink bottles.
- Clearly label all poisons and medicines and ensure that they have child-proof stoppers.
- Never allow children to play with medicine and other harmful containers, empty or full.

Management tips

First conduct an assessment of your own home or unit to establish which items may be a potential hazard.

> **Poison information centres**
>
> Tygerberg Hospital, Cape Town: +27 21 938 6084 (office hours),
> +27 21 931 6129 (24 hours)
>
> Red Cross War Memorial Children's Hospital, Cape Town: +27 21 689 5227

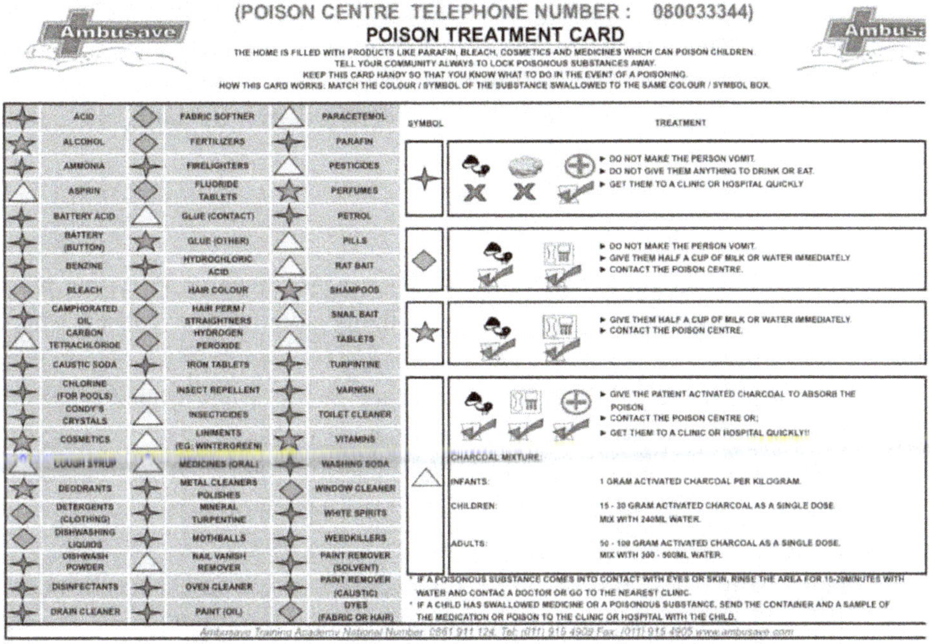

(POISON CENTRE TELEPHONE NUMBER : 080033344)

POISON TREATMENT CARD

THE HOME IS FILLED WITH PRODUCTS LIKE PARAFIN, BLEACH, COSMETICS AND MEDICINES WHICH CAN POISON CHILDREN.
TELL YOUR COMMUNITY ALWAYS TO LOCK POISONOUS SUBSTANCES AWAY.
KEEP THIS CARD HANDY SO THAT YOU KNOW WHAT TO DO IN THE EVENT OF A POISONING.
HOW THIS CARD WORKS: MATCH THE COLOUR / SYMBOL OF THE SUBSTANCE SWALLOWED TO THE SAME COLOUR / SYMBOL BOX.

Figure 12.4 Emergency card for poison treatment

Source: Ambusave (nd)

When caring for young children, constant vigilance is necessary, and the following should be taken into consideration:

- If poisoning does occur, obtain medical assistance as soon as possible.
- Treat all cases of poisoning as urgent.
- Take the victim to the hospital as soon as first aid has been administered. Advice on first-aid treatment can be obtained from the Poison Information Centre.
- In case of suspected poisoning, the container should not be discarded as it not only makes it possible to identify the poison but often carries useful information concerning the antidote.
- Take along the container, label, prescription, remaining tablets, the substance swallowed, vomited matter or whatever might help the doctor to identify and estimate the amount of poison taken.

Drowning

Many children and adults drown each year along South Africa's coastline and in rivers, dams and swimming pools. Any open water should be considered a hazard because an infant can drown even in a dog's drinking bowl.

Alcohol is often a contributing factor to a drowning – drinking alcohol will result in a lack of judgement and may cause a swimmer to take a risk, or it may lead to a lack of vigilance when caring for a child.

It is especially dangerous to leave infants unattended in the bath, no matter how little water it contains.

Preventative measures

Children should be taught about the potential dangers of water. However, most children love to play in water and extra vigilance should be exercised where water is concerned.

- Never leave small children alone in a bath or tub, even for a short time. Even answering the telephone or a knock at the door can result in a tragedy. Ignore the phone and doorbell or take the child along with you.
- Use a non-slip mat in the bath/tub. Hold the baby with your hand around the upper arm, with your other arm around the back.
- Empty baths, tubs and other containers after use; if full, keep the door shut or locked to keep young children away from the water.
- Always fit lids firmly on buckets of water as many children have drowned in buckets of water.
- Teach all children to swim at the earliest possible age. However, even if a child can swim, constant supervision is always necessary.
- Fence in all swimming pools and keep gates locked at all times, but do not allow the fact that a pool is fenced to create a false sense of security. Children can, and do, climb over swimming pool fences, and gates can, and often are, inadvertently left unlocked.
- Do not swim within about 60 minutes of eating a large meal or after drinking alcohol.
- Never go out on a boat, yacht or similar craft without life vests.
- The sea is unpredictable. Even in shallow water, it is necessary to supervise children constantly. Teach children never to turn their back to the sea – they should always face the sea.

Choking

It only takes a few seconds for a child to pop a small object into his or her mouth and choke. With a few simple precautions you can protect children against these accidents. Many young children die from choking and suffocation.

Preventative measures

For choking on food:

- Never leave a baby to drink his or her bottle unattended. The baby could vomit, inhale the milk and choke.
- Babies should not be given any food they cannot chew properly. Large chunks are easily breathed in and/or can stick in the throat.
- When preparing food, remove small bones such as those in fish or chicken.
- Never give children under five years of age peanuts because they frequently cause choking.
- Avoid giving children dried peas and beans to play with.
- Teach older children not to give anything, including hard biscuits or sweets, to a young child – let the parent/childminder do this.
- Keep strings and plastic bags out of reach of children.

For choking on small objects:

- Babies between the ages of five months and 18 months are particularly susceptible to choking, partly because they are at the hand-to-mouth age of development, where any object they touch goes straight into their mouth. It is important, therefore, to keep all small objects out of reach of the baby.
- Keep small toys or toys with small parts away from babies until they are old enough to handle them. Parts broken off toys and games should be thrown away or repaired. Also get rid of small pieces of crayons.
- Beware of soft or small dummies that may fit completely into the baby's mouth. Also be aware of parts separating and becoming lodged in the throat.
- Beware of letting small children play with beads, buttons, coins, bits of torn plastic or broken balloons. Make a habit or picking up these small items if they are lying around.

Suffocation

As with most accidents, a child can suffocate if certain simple rules are not followed. Consider the measures discussed below.

Preventative measures

Suffocation caused by plastic:

- Never leave sheets of plastic or plastic bags lying around. Cut them up before throwing them away or recycling.
- Teach children never to put plastic bags over their heads and do not allow little ones to play with them. Tie a knot in the bag for safety.

Suffocation caused by a cord or ribbon:

- Remove bibs or any clothing with ribbons or cords before putting the baby to sleep. A loose bib may cause suffocation.

- Do not attach a dummy to a string around the baby's neck.

- Most babies do not need pillows. If you have to use a pillow, make sure it is thin and firm, not soft. Pillows with ventilation holes are available.

- Take care that no dangling cords, like those of venetian blinds, are within the baby's reach.

- Children under five years should not be allowed to play with cords, string and ropes, etc unless an adult is watching.

- Do not put a baby to sleep on his or her stomach until the baby is able to roll over.

Note: An unusual form of suffocation occasionally happens when a child climbs inside an old-fashioned fridge. The locking mechanism on these old fridges does not allow them to open from the inside and refrigerators are airtight. It can happen that a child suffocates because no one knows the child is inside. It is therefore a necessary preventative measure to remove the entire door or locking device before discarding an old refrigerator.

Emergency treatment for suffocation or choking

- Do not panic if a child appears to be choking. His or her normal cough reflex will generally expel the object. If the child is small, hold the child up by the heels and give a firm slap on the back. If this is not successful, get the patient to a doctor immediately.

- Do not slap the child hard on the back while the child is sitting up as this may make the child gasp and suck the object further into the air passage.

- Do not try to remove the object with your fingers unless you can get a grip on it. This will only push it further down. If an older child is choking, stand behind the child, put your arms around the child's waist, and find the spot in the chest halfway between the waist and lower ribs. Gently press the clenched fist of your left hand as far as you comfortably can. Firmly clasp your right hand over your clenched fist and give short, sharp 'hugs' pushing inwards and upwards as far as you can. Repeat if necessary. Air pressure will cause the obstructing object to pop out. If you suspect that the child has inhaled an object or pushed beads or nuts up the nose or into his or her ears, get medical assistance as soon as possible.

- If a child develops a chronic cough or wheeze (breathing with difficulty), consider the possibility that the child may have inhaled a foreign body into the air passage, and take the child to the doctor.

- If the child cannot breathe spontaneously after removal of the foreign object, CPR may be necessary (only a trained first-aider should carry out CPR).

Objects in the ear, nose and eye

It is possible for a child to get a foreign object stuck in his or her ear, nose or eyes or any other body opening – usually as a result of playing. In such cases, the child needs to be taken to the doctor, hospital or clinic immediately. Parents are advised not to try to remove the object themselves as this may cause further injury.

Objects and foods to avoid

Children under four are most at risk of inserting or swallowing small objects. To keep children safe, avoid:

- foods such as popcorn, dried peas, watermelon (unless seeds are removed) and chocolate that contains nuts
- marbles, buttons, beads, pen lids and coins
- small batteries, which can leak acid and cause injury if swallowed
- toys with removable eyes, noses or other small parts
- needles, pins and safety pins – use pins with a safety catch and keep them closed when not in use.

Adults should avoid the habit of placing safety pins in the mouth, because children might copy them.

Preventative measures

- Supervise toddlers and small children while they eat, because they like to experiment and play with food, which can lead to injuries.
- Encourage the child to sit quietly when eating and drinking. The child should not lie down when eating solids, nor should fluids be given faster than the child can swallow.
- Avoid giving children popcorn or nuts (especially peanuts) until they are at least five years old. A thin layer of peanut butter or hazelnut spread on bread is a good alternative. Check for nut allergies.
- Cut all food into small pieces, and remove sharp or small bones from fish, chicken and meat before giving it to the child.
- Try to wait until the child is four years old before letting him or her eat small lollies, even as a treat.
- Avoid glitter, glue and small beadwork.
- Teach older siblings that a baby's ears and nose are delicate, and that they are not for poking things into.
- Check the floor and low tables for pieces of jewellery, beans or dried peas and other small objects.

Conclusion

It is clear that there are many dangers in the home and if reasonable care is not taken, an accident can and probably will happen. However, by exercising due care and following some simple rules, such as locking away poisons and medicines, not leaving open flames near children and by watching infants and young children at all times, most home accidents can be prevented.

Self-assessment

Read the following scenario and answer the assignment:

You are giving a group of young mothers at the clinic an educational talk on home accidents and what can be done to prevent them.

Prepare a health-education programme and highlight the content that will be covered in your health talk. Include a hazard- and risk-assessment chart and draw up a management plan to mitigate home accidents.

Bibliography

Ambusave. nd. Poison treatment card. Available: http://www.sundowner.org.za/SRA_Poison_Treatment_Card.pdf (21 September 2020).

Department of Health (DOH). 2000. National guidelines on prevention of falls in older persons. Available: https://www.westerncape.gov.za/Text/2003/falls.pdf (Accessed 11 September 2020).

Othman, N. & Kendrick, D. 2010. Epidemiology of burn injuries in the East Mediterranean region: A systematic review. *BMC Public Health*, 10(83):1 471–2 458.

Red Cross War Memorial Children's Hospital Trauma Unit. 2013. Child injury statistics. Cape Town.

Red Cross War Memorial Children's Hospital Trauma Unit. 2019. Child injury statistics. Cape Town.

World Health Organisation Organization (WHO). 2014. Injuries and violence: The facts. Available: https://www.who.int/violence_injury_prevention/en/ (Accessed 11 September 2020).

Social and mental health

Sharon Vasuthevan

Learning outcomes

After studying this chapter, you should be able to:

- Describe the principles of a healthy lifestyle.
- Identify self-destructive behaviours.
- Explain the effects of tobacco smoking and preventative measures.
- Describe the effects of alcohol consumption and preventative measures.
- Explain the factors contributing to obesity and preventative measures.
- Identify the warning signs of child abuse.
- Explain the process to follow in cases of intimate partner violence.
- Define the concept of mental health.
- Discuss the causes of mental illness.
- Outline the preventative measures for mental illness.

Key terms

Adipose: Pertaining to fat.

Aetiology: The science that deals with causation of diseases and their modes of introduction into the host.

Anoxia: No oxygen in the tissues, which occurs when blood supply to a part is cut off.

Ectomorph: An individual whose body build tends to be lean and fragile, with thin muscles and slightly underdeveloped digestive organs.

Endomorph: An individual whose body build differs from the normal in that the digestive viscera are large, there are accumulations of fat around the abdomen, the trunk and thighs are large, and the extremities are tapering.

Introduction

With the rising cost of healthcare and continued popular interest in health issues, preventative health measures are an increasingly important part of maintaining a healthy lifestyle. People are encouraged to:

- exercise regularly
- eat healthy foods
- drink alcohol in moderation
- reduce their stress levels
- enjoy plenty of rest and fresh air
- find work–life balance.

People are also becoming more conscious of self-destructive behaviours such as smoking, alcohol abuse and over-eating.

These behaviours are considered risk factors and contribute to major illnesses such as heart attack and diabetes. It is important to manage self-destructive behaviours to promote social and mental well-being. Below we discuss some of these self-destructive behaviours, and how to prevent them.

Self-destructive behaviours

Self-destructive behaviours include personal habits and behaviour patterns that are harmful to health, such as tobacco smoking, the excessive use of alcohol, dietary excesses and violent and aggressive behaviours, all of which influence the incidence, prevalence and distribution of certain chronic conditions such as carcinoma, ischaemic heart disease and hypertension. These conditions have also been described as 'culture-borne' diseases.

Tobacco smoking

Tobacco was introduced into Europe from tropical America during the 16th century and its use quickly spread across the continent. Tobacco has been, and still is, used in many forms: as snuff, in cigarettes, in pipes and in cigars. Today cigarette smoking is the most popular method of use. In recent years, there has been a decline in smoking in developed countries such as the United States of America but an unfortunate rise in smoking in developing countries, such as those in southern Africa.

Smoking and diseases

Although tobacco has been used for hundreds of years, it has only relatively recently been suspected of causing serious diseases. In the early 1950s a definite relationship between carcinoma of the lung and cigarette smoking was noted.

Today there is sufficient evidence to prove that there is an association between tobacco smoking and many extremely dangerous conditions.

Smokers are 10 times more likely to develop lung cancer than non-smokers. Because of the presence of carcinogens in cigarette smoke, a number of other malignancies are also more common in smokers, namely carcinoma of the mouth, larynx, oesophagus, pancreas and bladder. It has been estimated that cancer deaths would be reduced by 15 to 20 per cent if everyone stopped smoking.

There is an association between cigarette smoking and ischaemic heart disease. The carbon monoxide released by a cigarette increases atherosclerotic changes in the blood vessels, and also reduces the amount of oxygen reaching the heart muscle. Smokers are five times more likely to suffer from chronic respiratory diseases than non-smokers.

Smoking is particularly harmful in women of childbearing age. Smoking during pregnancy reduces the amount of oxygen reaching the foetus through the placenta, which retards its growth and results in a low birth weight and all the complications associated with it. Women who smoke while raising infants and young children are forcing their children to be 'passive smokers' and exposing them to all the dangers associated with smoking. Women who smoke and take a contraceptive pill are more likely to develop thrombi than women who do not smoke.

Smoking reduces life expectancy, and death rates for smokers are 70 to 120 times higher than in non-smokers, largely due to deaths from ischaemic heart disease and carcinoma of the lung.

These ill effects are directly related to the number of cigarettes smoked, the length of time the person has been smoking and the tar content of the particular brand of cigarette smoked. Smokers endanger their own health but also the health of those who come into contact with them.

Cigarette smoking creates a fire hazard and is responsible for many accidents. An aeroplane accident in which hundreds of people died was caused by a person smoking in one of the toilets. Smoking in bed is a particularly dangerous habit, as people often fall asleep while smoking and set the bed alight. The following three factors perpetuate smoking in our society:

- **Incitement**: Until recently, unrestricted advertising of tobacco was allowed. This took place through the medium of advertising in the mass media. In newspapers and magazines, at the cinema and on billboards we saw rich, manly, sophisticated men and wealthy, glamorous, sophisticated women smoking. The implications were clear: anyone who smoked that particular brand of cigarette would become rich, beautiful, brave and sophisticated.

- **Example**: Children who see their parents, teachers and other authority figures or community leaders smoking learn by example. Certain people have a moral obligation to set an example as non-smokers and should not allow themselves to be seen smoking in public. These include medical doctors, particularly those who hold public office, and hospital superintendents, nurses, teachers and other government officials.

- **Opportunity**: Cigarettes are too freely available. They should, for example, not be sold by canteens in hospitals, universities, tuck shops, military camps and similar institutions.

Smoking legislation

In South Africa, legislation is in place that protects non-smokers in public places and restricts smokers in terms of where they may smoke (Tobacco Products Control Amendment Act 63 of 2008, which came into effect on 21 August 2009). This legislation has been extremely effective in achieving its objectives. Some of the recent changes to the law governing smoking include the following:

- Fines are given for smoking or allowing smoking in a non-smoking area.
- Smoking is not allowed in 'partially enclosed' public places, such as covered patios, verandas, balconies, walkways and parking areas. Young children will be better protected from the harms of second-hand smoke, like asthma, wheezing, or bronchitis.
- Adults may not smoke in a car when a passenger under 12 years is present.
- Smoking is not allowed in premises (including private homes) used for commercial childcare activities, or for schooling or tutoring.
- No person under 18 may be allowed into a designated smoking area. The practice of parents taking babies into smoking areas of restaurants is outlawed.
- The tobacco industry can no longer hold 'parties' or use 'viral' marketing to target young people. Although tobacco advertising was banned in 2000, the cigarette companies found creative ways to promote cigarettes.
- Sale of tobacco products to and by persons under the age of 18 years is prohibited, as is the sale of confectionery or toys that resemble tobacco products.
- Cigarette vending machines must sell tobacco products exclusively and cannot be used to sell other products like crisps and chocolates. The vending machines may only be located in areas to which minors do not have access.
- Health warnings are mandatory on cigarette boxes.

The following advice may assist those who are trying to give up smoking:

- Do not buy cigarettes and do not carry any around with you. One cannot smoke if one does not have any cigarettes and it eventually becomes too embarrassing to ask others for a cigarette.
- Smoking is largely a conditioned reflex – that is, a response to a specific stimulus or set of stimuli – so try to avoid the stimuli that lead to smoking. If you always light a cigarette at the table after a meal then you should leave the table as soon as you have finished eating; if you always have a cigarette after a cup of coffee, then drink orange juice instead.

- Avoid people who smoke, if possible.
- Drink lots of fluids.
- Practise deep breathing exercises and relaxation.
- Keep yourself occupied.
- Reward yourself for any progress made towards not smoking, however slight it may be.

Alcohol consumption

The excessive use of alcohol is a socio-medical problem that requires urgent attention. The World Health Organization (WHO) considers that problems relating to the consumption of alcohol constitute one of the world's major public health challenges. Alcohol consumption is increasing in all countries, but particularly in the developing world where increase in its use has been accompanied by a change from traditional drinking patterns to the consumption of Western alcoholic beverages. This has been largely due to the vigorous and sophisticated marketing campaigns of multinational corporations.

A further trend that is giving cause for concern is the marked increase in the number of teenagers that drink alcoholic beverages. In South Africa a large percentage of the adult population consumes some form of alcohol daily and a small percentage of these regular users will become alcoholics in the true sense of the word. This means that they will reach a stage where they will no longer be able to control their drinking. The WHO defines alcoholics as: 'Those excessive drinkers whose dependence on alcohol has reached such a stage that they show a noticeable mental disease or an interference with their mental and bodily health, their interpersonal relations and their smooth social and economic functioning. They therefore require treatment' (WHO, 2018).

In our society drinking alcohol is considered to be socially acceptable behaviour and considerable pressure is brought to bear on people to 'have a drink, come on, just a small one' or the even more dangerous suggestion of 'come on, have one for the road'. Alcohol is freely available. In fact, some people consider that it is too freely available. Alcohol is a causal factor in many serious conditions; the list that follows is not intended to be exhaustive. Medical conditions include:
- abnormalities of the foetus if taken during pregnancy
- carcinoma of the mouth, oesophagus, stomach, pancreas and other organs
- cirrhosis of the liver
- chronic gastritis
- malnutrition
- peripheral neuritis
- vitamin deficiencies
- injuries caused by accidents.

Social problems include:
- assault and other crimes
- dysfunctional families
- homicide
- sexual promiscuity
- suicide.

Psychological conditions include:
- addiction to other drugs
- delirium and dementia
- personality deterioration
- psychotic reactions.

Preventative measures

Health education has an important role to play in the prevention of alcohol abuse. The ill effects of even moderate prolonged alcohol consumption should be emphasised.

The aim of health education should not be to promote absolute abstinence but rather to teach people, and particularly parents and adolescents, how, when and what to drink. The preservation of an intact and functioning family can reduce the risk of alcohol abuse since statistics show that those most likely to develop alcohol-related problems are people who are deprived of normal family relationships, for example single and divorced men, those living in dysfunctional families, and migrant workers. Psychologically, healthy child-rearing practices can do much to prevent the development of neuroses and stresses that may, in later life, lead to alcohol abuse.

Specific protection should involve some control over the advertising of alcoholic drinks and should exert pressure on all who are involved in the promotion of these products to present both sides of the picture instead of concentrating on the pleasurable effects of their products. However, in fairness to the advertisers, it should be pointed out that alcohol consumption is also high in countries such as Russia, where there is very little advertising. The prompt treatment of alcohol-related problems involves the early identification of those people who for various social and/or psychological reasons are likely to develop a drinking problem. During the acute phase of alcoholism, admission to a hospital for detoxification is necessary. Psychotherapy, particularly group psychotherapy, has proved useful in the rehabilitation of people who have decided to give up the use of alcohol. Manipulation of the environment, such as a change of occupation, may help in dealing with domestic problems, and giving financial advice may be all that is required in some cases to reduce a person's problems to manageable proportions.

Drink driving

Drink driving is one of the biggest threats to road safety in South Africa. Research indicates that 50 per cent of people who die on the roads have a blood alcohol concentration above the legal limit (Department of Transport, 2020).

The legal limit for alcohol in the blood is 0.05 g per 100 ml of blood.

However, this is also influenced by your fitness level, type of build, having eaten or not, medication intake, menstruation, etc. The South African government has proposed a zero-percentage alcohol consumption for all drivers with the inception of the Covid-19 pandemic.

Legal consequences

If you are found guilty of drunk driving in South Africa you could face up to six years in jail. You could also be liable for fines of up to R120 000 and your driver's license may be suspended. You will have a criminal record which can have serious ramifications for the rest of your life.

Example: On New Year's Eve an 18-year-old girl from Johannesburg drank two glasses of wine. Returning home in a rainstorm and driving at 60 km/h, a tyre burst, and she crashed into a house. She tested over the legal limit and her license was taken away for eight years.

Read more about organisations that help people living with alcoholism, such as Alcoholics Anonymous, available at: https://aasouthafrica.org.za/

Do some research on the internet and identify similar organisations.

Obesity

Obesity is a condition characterised by the accumulation of excessive amounts of adipose tissue in various parts of the body. Someone who is more than 20 per cent above the weight considered normal for his or her age, height and build is said to be obese. Obesity has become a global epidemic, with 13 per cent of adults being classified as obese worldwide (WHO, 2015). In South Africa, 69.3 per cent of women and 39 per cent of men are either obese or overweight (SAMRC, 2014).

Certain pathological conditions, such as metabolic and endocrine diseases, may be responsible for obesity, but these disorders are comparatively rare and account for only about 3 per cent of cases. Obesity is usually the result of a kilojoule intake that exceeds kilojoule expenditure. This occurs either where there is decreased energy expenditure due to under-activity, or where the diet contains an excessive amount of high-kilojoule foods.

Obesity reduces life expectancy and is associated with many serious diseases, such as diabetes mellitus, hypertension, cardiac diseases, arthritis, postural abnormalities, and accidents such as falls.

Factors associated with obesity

Here we will discuss the genetic, social and cultural, psychological, learning, exercise and dietary factors commonly associated with obesity.

Genetic factors

Body shape and size are largely genetically determined. Identical twins, who have the same genes, show marked similarities in body build even when they have been raised in different homes and exposed to different environmental influences.

The dissimilarities in build that are so noticeable between the tall, thin, fragile ectomorph and the soft, plump, rounded endomorph are the result of genetic endowment.

Nevertheless, nutrition can influence genetic factors and even an endomorph will lose weight if put on a low-kilojoule diet.

Social and cultural factors

All diets are culturally determined and influenced by the physical environment in which the society exists, the kind of food most easily obtainable, and the attitudes, values and beliefs of the society.

In affluent Western nations certain high-kilojoule foods and rich and elaborate dishes have status value and are eaten whenever possible. In such countries overnutrition is common and obesity rife.

Psychological factors

Some people tend to overeat when they are bored, anxious, depressed or stressed; food is used as a comfort and a crutch. There are also people with psychological problems who become compulsive eaters, unable to control their eating habits.

Learning

Early feeding practices and family dietary habits learned by a child are often responsible for obesity. The amount of food that is considered 'normal' varies from family to family, as does the type of food that is eaten and the frequency with which meals are taken.

Harmful practices such as eating high-kilojoule snacks between meals and a predilection for sweets and chocolates are transmitted from generation to generation of the family through the process of learning.

Research has found that some mothers and other caregivers never distinguish between a child's physical and emotional needs. Every time the baby cries or is restless, the mother/caregiver responds by giving the baby something to eat as a way of keeping them happy. Consequently, the child learns to equate food with comfort and affection and later throughout their life they eat whenever they are anxious or stressed.

Activity

There is considerable evidence to show that obese people are less active than those of normal weight, but it is difficult to determine what is cause and what is effect: is the person obese because he or she is inactive, or is the person under-active because the obesity makes him or her less mobile?

Dietary factors

Large meals consisting of high-kilojoule foods, and between-meal snacks, are the two dietary habits most often responsible for obesity in individuals and families. Ignorance of the kilojoule value of various foods is to some extent a contributory factor, as is poverty. Families with limited income have to buy cheap foods and as these usually consist of carbohydrates rather than protein, they are more likely to lead to overweight.

Preventative measures

Diet is a major determinant of health, but health education designed to promote healthier diets meets with considerable opposition from those who have a financial interest in the production, processing or marketing of certain foodstuffs, such as dairy farmers, sugar producers and meat producers. Once again, the 'sweet smell' of gain prevents certain preventative measures from being taken. Of course, parties with such vested interests usually argue that the evidence linking diet with certain diseases is inconclusive.

Primarily, health education aims at bringing about a change in the food habits of members of a community while changing their way of life as little as possible. Ideally, one should try to bring about a reduction in the consumption of red meat, saturated fats and refined sugars, and an increase in the consumption of fruits, vegetables and whole grains.

The use of processed foods should be discouraged; not only are they expensive but they contain various additives and have a high salt content.

Certain popular misconceptions should be dispelled: potatoes and whole-wheat bread eaten in moderation are not fattening and in fact make a valuable contribution to the diet as they contain useful amounts of vitamins, mineral salts and fibre.

More specifically, the prevalence of overweight and obesity in a community can be reduced by observing certain basic rules:

- During pregnancy a woman should be encouraged to eat a balanced diet and should be warned against 'eating for two' as there is some evidence to show that a tendency to overweight and obesity may start during foetal life.

- Breastfeeding must be encouraged as breastfed babies are less likely to be overfed than those who have been bottle fed.

- Weaning is an important period in an infant's development, as it is during this time that the foundations of the child's later dietary habits are laid. Once again, the importance of the child receiving a balanced diet should be stressed and the mother informed of the dangers of overfeeding.

- Where overweight and obesity are present, dietary modification is required and a reduction in kilojoule intake is necessary. A good reducing diet should be acceptable to the client, should be enjoyable, and should involve as little change in the person's way of life as is compatible with the aims of the diet.

- The reduction in food intake should be accompanied by an increased utilisation of kilojoules through increased exercise.

Social and psychological support is necessary during this time. Eating is a pleasurable and self-rewarding behaviour and it is not easy to persevere with a reducing diet. Organisations such as Weight Watchers offer group support and encouragement and so help to maintain a high level of motivation. Dietary aids, appetite suppressants and 'miracle machines' are best avoided.

Child abuse

There are many assumptions and myths about child abuse. People often assume that it is rare, that all abuse is sexual, that only girls are victims, that abuse does not happen in 'good families', that only strangers are abusers, and that abuse that happened many years ago no longer matters.

Recognising and preventing child abuse

Child abuse is more than bruises and broken bones. While physical abuse might be the most visible sign, other types of abuse, such as sexual or emotional abuse or even child neglect, also leave deep, long-lasting scars. By learning about common types of abuse and some of the warning signs that might indicate abuse, you can make a huge difference in a child's life. The earlier an abused child gets help, the greater chance they have to heal.

> For various reasons, the child will not always be willing to disclose the abuse. In particular, victims of sexual abuse have a strong tendency not to disclose.

Long-term consequences of child abuse

All types of child abuse and neglect leave lasting scars. Some of these scars might be physical, but emotional scarring has long-lasting effects throughout life, damaging a child's sense of self, ability to have healthy relationships and ability to function at home, at work and at school. Some effects include:

- **Lack of trust**: Abuse by a parent or primary caregiver damages the most fundamental relationship a child has – that he or she is safe and cared for in their own home. Without this base, it is very difficult to learn to trust people or know who is trustworthy. This can lead to difficulty maintaining relationships due to fear of being controlled or abused. It can also lead to unhealthy relationships because the adult does not know what a good relationship is.

- **Feelings of being 'worthless' or 'damaged'**: If the child is told over and over that he or she is stupid or no good, it is extremely difficult to overcome these negative feelings. Low self-esteem is most likely to result from this, which, in turn, has an effect on the child's development, emotional growth, health and personality. Sexual abuse survivors, with the stigma and shame surrounding the abuse, struggle especially hard with feelings of 'being damaged'.

- **Trouble regulating emotions**: Abused children cannot express emotions safely. As a result, the emotions are internalised, and come out in unexpected ways. Adult survivors of child abuse can struggle with unexplained anxiety, depression or anger. There is a possibility that they may turn to alcohol or drugs to numb their painful feelings.

- **Inappropriate sexual behaviour**: If sexual abuse was the child's only means of getting physical contact and love in childhood, it may happen that he or she confuses nurturing with sexual activity. He or she may then continue to look for nurturing and affection in sexual ways, which may lead to promiscuity.

Types of child abuse

There are several types of child abuse, but the core element that ties them together is the emotional effect on the child. Children need predictability, structure, clear boundaries and the knowledge that their parents are looking out for their safety. Abused children cannot predict how their parents will act. Their world is an unpredictable, frightening place with no rules. Whether the abuse is a slap, a harsh comment, a stony silence or not knowing if there will be dinner on the table tonight, the end result is a child who feels unsafe, uncared for and alone.

Emotional child abuse

Emotional abuse is particularly difficult to recognise and treat, as there are no visible scars. Emotional abuse can severely damage a child's mental health or social development, leaving lifelong psychological scars. Examples of emotional child abuse include:

- constant belittling, shaming and humiliating a child
- calling names and making negative comparisons to others
- telling a child he or she is 'no good,' 'worthless,' 'bad,' or 'a mistake'
- frequent yelling, threatening, or bullying
- ignoring or rejecting a child as a form of punishment, giving him or her the silent treatment
- limited physical contact with the child – giving him or her no hugs, kisses, or other signs of affection
- exposing the child to violence or the abuse of others, whether it be the abuse of a parent, a sibling, or even a pet.

Child neglect

Child neglect – a very common type of child abuse – is a pattern of failing to provide for a child's basic needs, whether it be adequate food, clothing, hygiene, or supervision. Child neglect is not always easy to spot. Sometimes, a parent might become physically or mentally unable to care for a child, such as when the parent has a serious injury, untreated depression, or anxiety. Other times, alcohol or drug abuse may seriously impair judgement and the ability to keep a child safe.

Older children might not show outward signs of neglect, as they become used to presenting a competent face to the outside world, and even taking on the role of the parent. However, ultimately, neglected children are not getting their physical and emotional needs met.

Physical child abuse

Physical abuse involves physical harm or injury to the child. It may be the result of a deliberate attempt to hurt the child, but not always. It can also result from severe discipline, such as using a belt to hit a child.

Many physically abusive parents and caregivers insist that their actions are simply forms of discipline – ways to make children learn to behave. However, the point of disciplining children is to teach them right from wrong; not to make them live in constant fear.

Sexual child abuse

Sexual abuse is an especially complicated form of abuse because of its layers of guilt and shame. It is important to recognise that sexual abuse does not always involve body contact. Exposing a child to sexual situations or material such as pornography is sexually abusive, whether or not touching is involved.

While news stories of sexual predators are scary, what is even more frightening is that sexual abuse usually occurs at the hands of someone the child knows and should be able to trust – most often a close relative or family friend. And contrary to what many believe, it is not just girls who are at risk. Boys and girls both suffer from sexual abuse. In fact, sexual abuse of boys may be underreported due to shame and stigma.

The problem of shame and guilt in child sexual abuse

Aside from the physical damage that sexual abuse can cause, the emotional component is powerful and far-reaching. Sexually abused children are tormented by shame and guilt. They may feel that they are responsible for the abuse or somehow brought it upon themselves. This can lead to self-loathing and sexual problems as they grow older – often either excessive promiscuity or an inability to have intimate relations.

The shame of sexual abuse makes it very difficult for children to come forward. They may worry that others will not believe them, be angry with them or that it will split their family apart. Because of these difficulties, false accusations of sexual abuse are not common, so if a child confides in you, take him or her seriously. Do not turn a blind eye!

Warning signs of child abuse and neglect

The earlier child abuse is identified and dealt with, the better the chance of recovery and appropriate treatment for the child. Child abuse is not always obvious. By learning some of the common warning signs of child abuse and neglect, you can catch the problem as early as possible and get both the child and the abuser the help they need.

Of course, just because you see a warning sign does not automatically mean a child is being abused. If you notice something peculiar, it is important to dig deeper, looking for a pattern of abusive behaviour and warning signs.

Behavioural and emotional indicators are difficult to identify and interpret; however, they are the best indicators for early detection. Have a high level of suspicion if you see any of the warning signs or unexplained injuries, as detailed in Table 13.1.

Table 13.1 Warning signs of child abuse

General signs	• Non-verbal cues from the parent when the child explains the injury. Does the child explain it freely, or does the child look for the parent's approval of the story? It may be that the child was instructed not to disclose information about the incident. • The child may blame him- or herself for the injury, for instance 'I was naughty, I did not listen'. This may be associated with disobedience and punishment. • The child may refer to his or her own abuse as that of a third person, for example 'I know a girl whose uncle …' • The parent may delay reporting an injury and may give an inconsistent report of what happened. • The parent may appear over-anxious or stressed, or project anger and behave aggressively. Ask yourself if it is appropriate behaviour under the present circumstances.
Emotional abuse	• Excessively withdrawn, fearful, or anxious about doing something that may be considered wrong. • Shows extremes in behaviour (extremely compliant or extremely demanding; extremely passive or extremely aggressive). • Does not seem to be attached to the parent or caregiver. • Acts either inappropriately adult (taking care of other children) or inappropriately infantile (rocking, thumb-sucking, tantrums).
Physical abuse	• Frequent injuries or unexplained bruises, welts or cuts. • Is always watchful and 'on the alert', as if waiting for something bad to happen. • Injuries appear to have a pattern, such as marks from a hand or belt. • Shies away from touch, flinches at sudden movements or seems afraid to go home. • Wears inappropriate clothing to cover up injuries, such as long-sleeved shirts on hot days.
Neglect	• Clothes are ill-fitting, filthy or inappropriate for the weather. • Hygiene is consistently bad (unbathed, matted and unwashed hair, noticeable body odour). • Untreated illnesses and physical injuries. • Is frequently unsupervised, left alone or allowed to play in unsafe situations and environments. • Is frequently late or missing from school.

➡

Sexual abuse	• Trouble walking or sitting.
	• Displays knowledge or interest in sexual acts inappropriate for his or her age, or even seductive behaviour.
	• Uses inappropriate-for-age sexual language.
	• Makes strong efforts to avoid a specific person, without there being an obvious reason.
	• Does not want to change clothes in front of others or participate in physical activities.
	• A sexually transmitted infection or pregnancy, especially under the age of 14.
	• Runs away from home.

Source: HelpGuide.org (2019)

Risk factors for child abuse and neglect

While child abuse and neglect occur in all types of families – even in those that look happy from the outside – children are at a much greater risk in certain situations, which include the following:

- **Domestic violence**: Witnessing domestic violence is terrifying to children and emotionally abusive. Even if the mother does her best to protect her children and keeps them from being physically abused, the situation is still extremely damaging. If you or a loved one is in an abusive relationship, getting out is the best thing to do to protect the children.

- **Alcohol and drug abuse**: Living with an alcoholic or addict is extremely difficult for children and can easily lead to abuse and neglect. Parents who are drunk or high are unable to care for their children, make good parenting decisions, and control often-dangerous impulses. Substance abuse also commonly leads to physical abuse.

- **Untreated mental illness**: Parents who suffer from depression, an anxiety disorder, bipolar disorder or other mental illness have trouble taking care of themselves, much less their children. A mentally ill or traumatised parent may be distant and withdrawn from his or her children, or quick to anger without understanding why. Treatment for the caregiver means better care for the children.

- **Lack of parenting skills**: Some caregivers never learned the skills necessary for good parenting. Teen parents, for example, might have unrealistic expectations about how much care babies and small children need. Or parents who were themselves victims of child abuse may only know how to raise their children the way they were raised. In such cases, parenting classes, therapy and caregiver support groups are great resources for learning better parenting skills.

- **Stress and lack of support**: Parenting can be a very time-intensive, difficult job, especially if they are raising children without support from their family, friends or the community or they are dealing with relationship problems or financial difficulties. Caring for a child with a disability, special needs, or difficult behaviours is also a challenge. It is important for parents to get the support they need, so that they are emotionally and physically able to support their child.

Child abuse hotline

To get help or report child abuse, call:
Childhelp National Child Abuse Hotline: 1-800-4-A-CHILD (1-800-422-4453).

To get help or report child sexual abuse, call:
Stop It Now: 1-888-PREVENT (1-888-773-8368)
Rape, Abuse & Incest National Network (RAINN): 1-800-656-HOPE Network (RAINN)

What to do if you suspect child abuse

In terms of the Children's Amendment Act 38 of 2005, the healthcare professional is obliged to report reasonable grounds of suspicion of abuse to a social worker or the police. In case of a suspected/alleged sexual offence, the Criminal Law (Sexual Offences and Related Matters) Amendment Act 32 of 2007 demands that any abuse be reported to the police. It is an offence punishable with a prison sentence of five years and/or a fine if a person does not report abuse. No legal proceedings can be instituted against nurses who act in good faith and report the abuse or neglect to the designated officer (McQuoid-Mason et al, 2011).

When a child presents at a healthcare facility, usually accompanied by a parent or caregiver, the presenting problem should be attended to first. If, during the course of your examination, you detect anything suspicious such as injuries, behavioural cues or verbal disclosure of abuse, then it is a criminal offence if further investigations are not done.

A word of caution: where the nurse suspects that the parents may be involved, the nurse should persuade the parents to allow the child to be admitted for tests without accusing the parents of abuse or neglect. You can, however, explain to the child that sometimes parenting is difficult and that you would like to admit the child to help the family to deal better with stress or the presenting complaint.

Your institution will have a specific policy to deal with cases of abuse, but the following steps are a good indication of what is required (Pretorius et al, 2012):

- First assess the injuries and pain and manage them.
- A general consultation or forensic interview may follow.
- Document your observations and findings.

- Debrief the child immediately after the traumatic event.
- Report the child abuse on Form 22. Keep a copy in the patient file and a copy in the healthcare setting. Be particularly careful with your recordkeeping.
- Support the family and, if possible, introduce them to the policeman or policewoman or social worker who will assist them. The purpose of the intervention is to achieve the national norms and standards for child protection, which are:
  - to help the child and the parent to form a positive self-image
  - to establish and/or restore appropriate trust in other people
  - to acknowledge emotions – personal emotions and those of other people
  - to allow the child to vent aggression and to receive support in dealing with his or her anger
  - to help the child to experience positive adult and peer interaction
  - to help the child and the parent to communicate their needs and feelings verbally
  - to help the parent and the child to develop alternative and more acceptable modes of coping behaviour.

Intimate partner violence and rape

It is a sad reality that you will come into contact with some form of domestic violence during your career. South Africa has a very high incidence of intimate partner violence (IPV), particularly against women. In fact, South Africa has the highest reported incidence of intimate femicide (the killing of an intimate female partner) in the world. There is no doubt that you need to be prepared to handle such cases.

In the same way that there are many forms of child abuse, domestic or IPV can take many forms, such as emotional abuse, violence or even rape. Another similarity with child abuse is that the survivor of IPV is often too afraid or embarrassed to discuss the abuse with the healthcare professional.

The survivor may present at the healthcare facility with an unrelated complaint. According to national standards, a question about IPV must be included when taking a history from a patient presenting with depression, headaches or stomach pains, or who has a known abusive partner. For the busy nurse, a simple question such as either of the following may be helpful:

- Are you unhappy in your relationship?
- Are you in danger? Is someone hurting you?

Statistics concerning intimate partner violence

The lifetime prevalence of experiencing IPV is estimated to be between 15 per cent and 71 per cent among women worldwide (Garcia-Moreno et al, 2005).

In South Africa, which has among the highest rates of IPV in the world, violence has an extremely negative effect on women's health.

A nationally representative study found a 19 per cent lifetime prevalence of victimisation among female respondents, and a study on physical violence among South African men found that 27,5 per cent reported perpetration in their current or most recent partnership. Earlier studies report similar estimates. IPV is a leading cause of morbidity and mortality for South African women. Over half of female homicide victims are killed by their intimate partners. Women with violent partners are at increased risk of HIV infection and health-risk behaviours such as alcohol consumption (Gass et al, 2010).

What to do in cases of intimate partner violence and rape

This is a complex issue to consider. As with child abuse, your unit will have a standard policy to deal with IPV and you would be well advised to make sure that you know these procedures.

Some advice for the rape survivor on reporting to the police

- It is the survivor's choice to report the incident or not.
- If the survivor chooses not to report the incident, the case will not be investigated or prosecuted.
- If the rape survivor is under 14, there is no choice in the matter – incidents must be reported to the police or social worker.
- If the case is reported, the police may not refuse to investigate it. However, if there is too little evidence after an investigation, a prosecutor may decide not to prosecute the case.
- There is no time limit for reporting a rape case.

The flow chart in Figure 13.1 offers some guidance on the medico–legal– phychoshocial management of intimate partner violence.

Cues to identify IPV

- Vague non-specific symptoms
- History of mental illness, medication or psychological symptoms
- Fatigue, sleep problems, unexplained somatic complaints
- Symptoms of depression
- Feeling anxious/dizzy/thinking too much
- Chronic pain syndromes, headaches
- Repeated sexually transmitted infections
- Assault or trauma
- Suspected alcohol or substance abuse
- Antiretroviral use (HIV-positive)

Ask, 'Are you unhappy in your relationship?'

Yes

Clinical
1. Check for sexually transmitted infections/HIV
2. Document and care for injuries (use J88)
3. Check for pregnancy, offer contraception, termination, sterilisation

Legal
1. Refer to any or all of the following:
   a. Family court for a protection order
   b. Victim empowerment unit at police station for support
   c. NFO sector for legal aid

Psychological
1. Listen attentively to patient's story
2. Do mental problems checklist and consider anxiety disorder, depression, substance abuse, post-traumatic stress disorder
3. Follow-up counselling, support

Social
1. Assess current social support and explore future possibilities
2. Assess safety: risk assessment and feedback, make safety plans
3. Help with maintenance for children
4. Refer to relevant organisations

The therapeutic group process with 'Lifestyle intervention empowerment programme', chronic care model

Support group

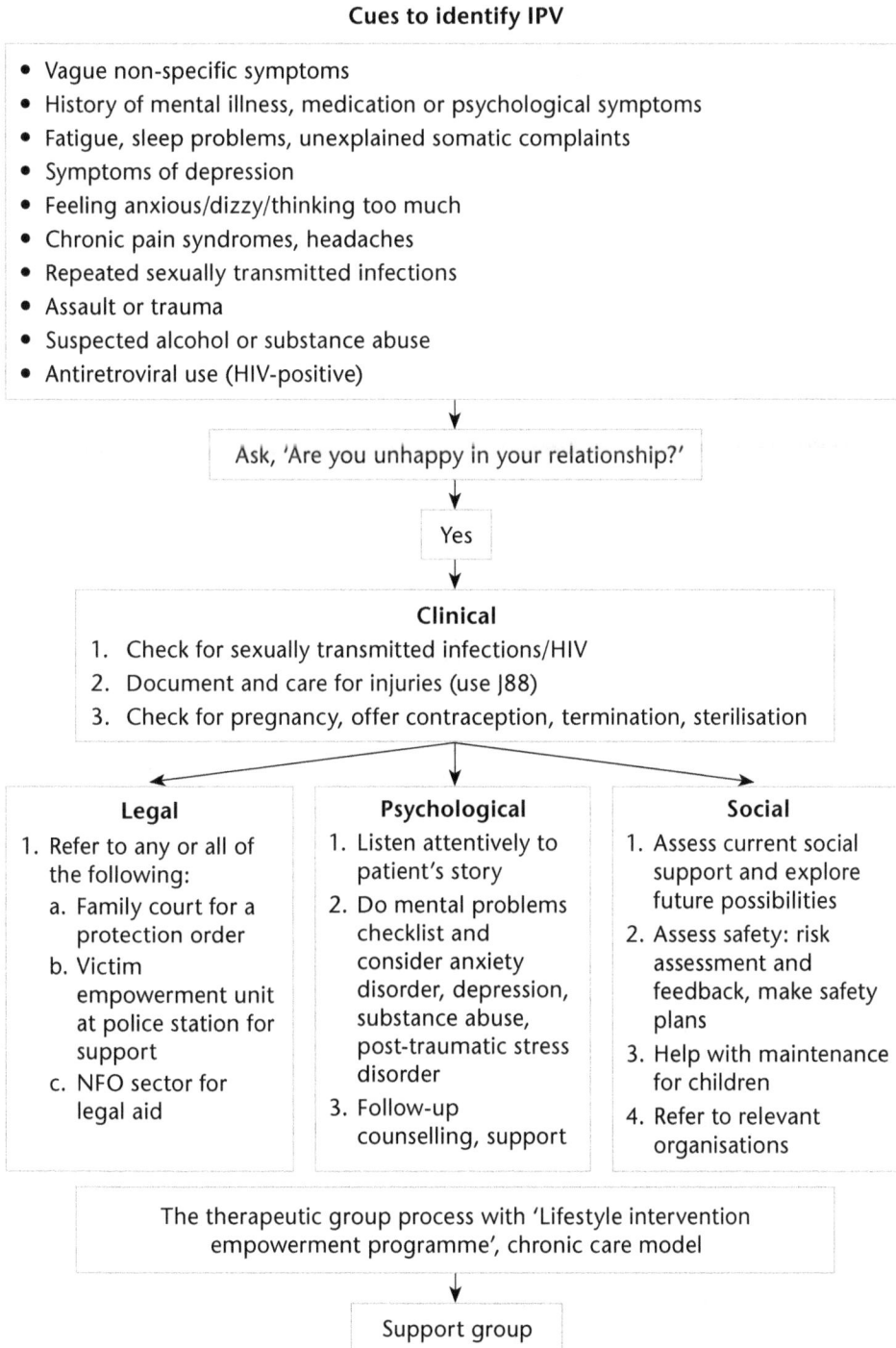

Figure 13.1 Flow chart for medico–legal–psychosocial management of intimate partner violence

Source: Joyner (2010)

Drug addiction

Drug addiction is a chronic, often relapsing brain disease that causes compulsive drug seeking and use despite harmful consequences to the individual. Drug addiction is a brain disease because the abuse of drugs leads to changes in the structure and function of the brain. Although it is true that for most people the initial decision to take drugs is voluntary, over time the changes in the brain caused by repeated drug abuse can affect a person's self-control and ability to make sound decisions, and at the same time send intense impulses to take drugs. These changes in the brain make it extremely difficult for an addict to stop abusing drugs.

Fortunately, there are treatments that help people to counteract addiction's powerful disruptive effects and regain control. Research shows that combining addiction treatment medications, if available, with behavioural therapy is the best way to ensure success for most patients.

Similar to other chronic, relapsing diseases, drug addiction can be managed successfully. As with other chronic diseases, it is not uncommon for a person to relapse and begin abusing drugs again. Relapse, however, does not signal failure; rather, it indicates that treatment should be reinstated and adjusted or that alternative treatment is needed to help the individual regain control and recover.

The effects of drugs on the brain

Drugs are chemicals that tap into the brain's communication system and disrupt the way that nerve cells normally send, receive and process information. There are at least two ways that drugs are able to do this:
- by imitating the brain's natural chemical messengers
- by overstimulating the 'reward circuit' of the brain.

Nearly all drugs, directly or indirectly, target the brain's reward system by flooding the circuit with dopamine – a neurotransmitter that controls movement, emotion, motivation and feelings of pleasure. The over-stimulation of this system, which normally responds to natural behaviours linked to survival (eating, spending time with loved ones, etc), produces euphoric effects in response to the drugs. This reaction sets in motion a pattern that 'teaches' people to repeat the behaviour of abusing drugs.

Mental health

The concept 'mental health' is complex and not easy to define. Whether or not an individual is considered 'normal' depends largely on the cultural norms and expectations of his or her society. What is considered to be normal behaviour in one society may not be considered so in another.

The WHO (2014) defines mental health as 'a state of well-being in which every individual realizes his or her own potential, can cope with the normal stresses of life, can work productively and fruitfully, and is able to make a contribution to her or his community'.

Many health workers have described the mentally healthy or mature individual as having the following characteristics:

- at least average intelligence
- effective contact with reality
- the ability to satisfy normal bodily desires without suffering from excessive feelings of guilt
- the ability to experience emotions freely and to express these emotions in a manner that is acceptable
- the capacity to form satisfactory and lasting interpersonal relationships
- a true assessment of his or her own abilities and the capacity to set realistic goals for himself or herself
- acceptance of failure or loss without reacting in an exaggerated manner
- adequate independence from the group while nevertheless still being able to satisfy the group's expectations of him or her
- moderately favourable levels of self-esteem.

The causes of mental conditions

There are many causes of mental conditions. In some it is possible to demonstrate a single cause, for example in AIDS dementia, or in Down syndrome where the cause is a chromosomal abnormality. In others, the condition is the result of an interaction between genetic endowment and socio-cultural and environmental factors, and in many mental illnesses the cause is uncertain.

Throughout the world and in South Africa too, the incidence of mental illness is highest at the lowest socio-economic levels. It appears therefore that socio-economic factors and a deprived or hostile environment play as important a part in the aetiology of mental illness as they do in physical illness.

Classification of mental conditions

Mental conditions are classified as disorders of the intellect, organic mental states, chronic mental states, psychoses, neuroses, personality disorders, psychosomatic illnesses and dementia due to HIV infection. Read more about each of these conditions below.

Disorders of the intellect

Mental sub-normality (mental retardation, mental deficiency) may be defined as a state of arrested development of the mind existing from birth or from an early age. It may be slight, moderate or severe.

The causes are many and include genetic abnormalities, chromosomal defects, infections of the mother during pregnancy (such as rubella), cerebral anoxia or brain damage during delivery, infections, or head injuries during infancy.

Organic mental states

These conditions arise as the result of some demonstrable pathology in the brain, such as a tumour or brain injury, or some underlying metabolic or toxic condition, such as acute delirium. This is an acute organic mental state that may be due to systemic infections, for example pneumonia, infections of the brain (meningitis), cerebral anoxia (in severe anaemia, or the use of hypotensive drugs), and the withdrawal of certain drugs (alcohol and drugs such as the barbiturates or bromide). Treatment of acute delirium is primarily treatment of the cause.

Chronic mental states

These may be defined as loss of mental capacity due to an organic condition of the brain. The term we use in connection with these chronic mental states is dementia. Dementia is characterised by loss of memory, emotional instability, poor judgement and difficulty in comprehension. Important causes of dementia include injury to the brain, chronic alcoholism, cerebral syphilis, pellagra and cerebral atherosclerosis.

Psychoses

- **Schizophrenia**: This is a severe mental illness, which is accompanied by severe disorders of emotion, perception and thought, as well as behavioural disturbances and a withdrawal from the social and physical environment. There are different types of schizophrenia, for example simple, hebephrenic, paranoid and catatonic. If you wish to know more about these conditions consult a psychiatric textbook.

- **Affective psychoses**: These are severe psychiatric illnesses that affect an individual's mood. Persons suffering from these illnesses may alternate between episodes of severe depression and mania or they may suffer from depression or mania only. When depressed, they feel unhappy and worthless, their behaviour and their thinking are slow and retarded, they experience sleep disturbances and loss of appetite and they lose weight. During bouts of mania they are excessively active, laughing and talking continuously and rushing from one task to another. Frequently they do not sleep or eat. They can become very aggressive.

Neuroses

The underlying cause of all neurotic behaviour is anxiety, and the particular behaviour represents an attempt by the person to deal with this anxiety. To use a simple example, in conversion hysteria the person 'converts' his or her anxiety into a bodily symptom such as hysterical paralysis or blindness. In this way the person tries to escape from the anxiety-producing situation. Such a reaction has secondary gains as well, as the person gains sympathy and attention.

Personality disorders

These are simply exaggerations of normal personality characteristics, for example we all get depressed from time to time but the person who is a depressive personality is more depressed more frequently than the average person.

Psychosomatic illnesses

These are physical illnesses where aetiological and psychological factors play a major part. It is important to bear in mind that these patients are suffering from a physical illness in which pathology or tissue damage can be demonstrated. In other words, they do not 'imagine' that they are ill, nor do they 'pretend' to be ill.

Dementia due to HIV infection

Decline in mental processes is a common complication of HIV infection (and many other conditions). Although the specific symptoms vary from person to person, they may be part of a single disorder known as AIDS dementia complex, or ADC. Common symptoms include a decline in cognitive functions, such as memory, reasoning, judgement, concentration and problem-solving. Other common symptoms are changes in personality and behaviour, speech problems and motor (movement) problems such as clumsiness and poor balance.

When these symptoms are severe enough to interfere with everyday activity, a diagnosis of dementia may be warranted.

Community mental health programmes

Community mental health programmes include primary, secondary and tertiary prevention. These are described below.

Primary prevention of mental illness

In this subsection we discuss the measures to be taken in health promotion and in specific protection.

Health promotion: All possible measures should be taken to improve the general health, both physical and psychological, of individuals and communities. These measures should be aimed at:

- improving the socioeconomic circumstances of deprived communities
- ensuring adequate nutrition, particularly of children and women of child-bearing age
- promoting a safe and psychologically healthy environment by providing suitable housing, adequate recreational facilities, sufficient schools, hospitals and clinics, suitable shelter and care for homeless and abandoned children, special facilities for the aged and the handicapped, and efficient means of communication to ensure that counselling and guidance services are available, for example child guidance and vocational guidance services; members of the community should be encouraged to make use of such services
- taking all possible steps to prevent family break-up and to promote a stable family life
- providing a physically safe and psychologically healthy work environment and taking all reasonable steps to remove occupational hazards.

Health education plays an important part in the achievement of the objectives listed above.

Specific protection: This includes the following measures:

- providing effective prenatal care to detect any conditions in the mother that could affect the health of the foetus (such as syphilis) or that could result in a difficult labour and possible damage to the infant
- directing all efforts towards the prevention of brain damage and asphyxia during the delivery
- encouraging the complete immunisation of all children to prevent diseases from occurring
- encouraging constant vigilance to prevent accidents during infancy and childhood, especially those that are likely to result in brain damage, such as motor-vehicle accidents and falls
- protecting the brain by encouraging the use of protective helmets when riding motorbikes or bicycles, horse riding, rock climbing or roller skating
- providing genetic counselling and prenatal diagnostic facilities, particularly for those couples who are 'at risk'; that is, where there is a family history of congenital defect or where a previous offspring has such a defect
- educating all people involved in caring for children, such as parents, nurses, teachers and workers in children's homes, in healthy child-rearing practices
- giving emotional support and reassurance during times of crisis such as bereavement, loss, illness and retirement, as this can do much to prevent psychological conditions such as anxiety, depression and even suicide.

Secondary prevention

The aim of secondary prevention is to reduce the number of cases of mental illness in a community. This may be done by means of early detection, accurate diagnosis and effective treatment.

- All possible measures should be taken to facilitate earlier detection. This will not only prevent the ill effects of long-term mental illness but will also reduce harmful effects on the family, friends and colleagues of the patient.

- While accurate diagnosis is an essential part of secondary prevention it is notoriously difficult. Medical practitioners, nurses and other healthcare workers require training directed specifically at improving their diagnostic skills in this field.

- Effective treatment requires, in the first instance, that there should be adequate facilities in the community that are freely available to all.

Tertiary prevention

The aim of tertiary prevention is to return the individual to the community with as little reduction in his or her social and occupational functioning as possible. In order to do this, it is necessary to avoid long-term hospitalisation of patients, for the longer a person has been in an institution the more difficult it is to rehabilitate him or her. When admission to an institution is unavoidable, all possible steps should be taken to ensure that the individual's social contacts are maintained. This can be done by encouraging frequent visits from family and friends. Facilities such as day and night centres, half-way houses and centres for sheltered employment, as well as the services of psychiatric social workers and community health nurses, are necessary if the patient is to be adequately rehabilitated.

Treatment

Treatment of mental illness may involve one or more of the following techniques:

Physical means

Physical means of treatment consists of the following:

- **Drugs:** Psychotropic drugs are drugs that have a powerful influence on the functioning of the higher centres of the central nervous system. These drugs have revolutionised the treatment of psychiatric illnesses and greatly reduced the need for hospitalisation. The most important drugs are hypnotics, sedatives, tranquillisers and anti-depressants.

- **Electro-convulsive therapy (shock treatment):** This was first used in the treatment of schizophrenia and severe depression. It has now to some extent been replaced by the use of drugs.

- **Psycho-surgery**: This surgical technique was once used commonly and was known as a leucotomy. It was used in cases of uncontrollable aggression. Once again, advances in drug treatment have replaced leucotomy as a treatment in psychiatric conditions.

Psychological means

The following are various psychological methods of treatment:

- **Psychoanalysis**: This type of treatment is based on the work of Freud, an Austrian psychiatrist who devised this method for the treatment of the neuroses. It is a time-consuming, expensive and intensive method.

- **Supportive psychotherapy**: This method relies heavily on communication between the therapist and the client. The clinical psychologist uses reassurance, suggestion, persuasion and emotional support in an attempt to help the client to adjust to his or her circumstances. This type of psychotherapy may be used to treat individuals, small groups or families.

- **Behaviour therapy**: This treatment applies the principles of learning and conditioning to the treatment of neurotic symptoms.

- **Hypnotherapy**: Hypnosis may appear to be similar to sleep but physiologically there are important differences between them. Hypnosis is an artificially induced state of suggestibility. While the patient is under the influence of hypnosis, the therapist makes certain suggestions hoping that they will be acted upon after termination of the hypnotic state.

- **Muscular relaxation**: This treatment is based on the theory that it is impossible to feel anxiety or fear while one is in a state of complete relaxation because the two responses, namely tension and relaxation, are physiologically incompatible. Complete muscular relaxation is not easy to attain and requires considerable practice.

- **Manipulation of the environment**: This is usually, but not always, the task of the social worker. There are occasions when unfavourable environmental conditions, such as an unsuitable occupation, poverty, a chronically ill person in the home, inadequate housing or conflict within a family, may be the cause of psychological problems. It is sometimes possible to reduce such stress by arranging for help in the home, advising on a change of employment or simply giving sound financial or other advice, or referring the client to the appropriate agency.

Conclusion

This chapter has outlined ways to manage one's health with regular exercise, correct eating habits, moderation in alcohol consumption, and by seeking ways to reduce stress levels. The community nurse should be able to offer guidance on these preventative measures.

Self-assessment

1. Describe the health education you would provide to a group of adolescents on the prevention of tobacco smoking.

2. A young male client is visiting your clinic and explains that he may have a problem with alcohol consumption. Describe the advice you would provide and the possible referrals you could make for this client.

3. Explain the factors associated with obesity and the preventative measures that may be instituted.

4. Discuss how you would deal with a case of suspected child abuse.

5. Discuss the prevention of mental illness using the following headings:
   - Primary prevention
   - Secondary prevention
   - Tertiary prevention.

Bibliography

Cancer Association of South Africa (CANSA). 2016. Fact sheet on a health profile of South Africa and related information. Available: https://www.cansa.org.za/files/2016/08/Fact-Sheet-Health-Profile-of-SA-Related-Info-web-Aug-2016.pdf (Accessed 4 October).

Coulson, N., Goldstein, S. & Ntuli, A. 1998. *Promoting Health in South Africa: An Action Manual.* Sandton: Heinemann.

Department of Transport. 2020. Road safety: Arrive Alive. Available: https://www.gov.za/about-government/government-programmes/road-safety-arrive-alive-0 (Accessed 8 October 2020).

Garcia-Moreno, C., Jansen, H.A.F.M., Ellsberg, M., Heise, L. & Watts, C. 2005. WHO multi-country study on women's health and domestic violence against women: Initial results on prevalence, health outcomes, and women's responses. Available: https://www.who.int/reproductivehealth/publications/violence/24159358X/en/ (Accessed 5 October 2020).

Gass, J.D., Stein, D.J., Williams, D.R. & Seedat, S. 2010. Intimate partner violence, health behaviours, and chronic physical illness among South African women. *South African Medical Journal*, 100(89):582–585.

Gilbert, L., Selikow, T.A. & Walker, L. 1996. *Health & Disease: An Introductory Reader for Health Professionals.* Randburg: Ravan Press.

Health Systems Trust. 2000. *South African Health Review.* Durban: The Press Gang.

Help Guide. 2019. Child abuse and neglect. Available: https://www.helpguide.org/articles/abuse/child-abuse-and-neglect.htm (Accessed 4 October 2020).

Joyner, K. 2010. *Aspects of Forensic Medicine: An Introduction for Healthcare Professionals.* Cape Town: Juta.

Mathews, S., Abrahams, N., Jewkes, R., Martin, L.J., Lombard, C. & Vetten, L. 2004. Intimate femicide-suicide in South Africa: a cross-sectional study. Available: semanticscholar.org (Accessed 4 October 2020).

McQuoid-Mason, D., Dada, M. & Geyer, N. 2011. *A-Z of Nursing Law*. Second edition. Cape Town: Juta.

Pretorius, D., Mbokazi, A.J., Hlaise, K.K. & Jacklin, L. 2012. *Child Abuse: Guidelines and Applications for Primary Healthcare Practitioners*. Cape Town: Juta.

South African Medical Research Council (SAMRC). 2014. South African women show high levels of obesity and overweight. Available: http://196.21.144.194/Media/2014/14press2014.htm (Accessed 5 October 2020).

Stanhope, M. & Lancaster, J. 2000. *Community Health Nursing: Process and practice of promoting health*. St. Louis, VA: Mosby.

World Health Organization (WHO). 2014. Mental health: A state of well-being. Available: http://tdr.who.int/features/factfiles/mental_health/en/ (Accessed 6 October 2020).

World Health Organization (WHO). 2015. Obesity and overweight fact sheet. Available: https://www.who.int/gho/ncd/risk_factors/overweight/en/ (Accessed 6 October 2020).

World Health Organization (WHO). 2018. Alcohol. Available : https://www.who.int/newsroom/fact-sheets/detail/alcohol (Accessed 6 October 2020).

Sustainable development

14 CHAPTER

Sindi Mthembu

Learning outcomes

After studying this chapter, you should be able to:

- Define the terms development, sustainable development and empowerment.
- Explain how poverty impacts on health.
- Describe the 17 sustainable development goals (SDGs).
- Discuss how sustainable development is necessary to improve the health status of communities.
- Describe health and development in southern Africa and the organisations involved.
- Explain what is understood by the intersectoral approach to development.
- Describe what is meant by community development.

Key terms

Community participation: A process whereby the residents of a community are given a voice and a choice to participate in issues affecting their lives. In this way the members of the community might, if the process is managed well, take ownership of the projects that are implemented by the government.

Economic development: A process whereby an economy's real national income as well as per capita income increase over a long period of time. It is measured in an increase in living standards, improvement in self-esteem, needs and freedom from oppression as well as greater choice. The most accurate method of measuring development is the Human Development Index (HDI), which takes into account the literacy rates and life expectancy that affect productivity and could lead to economic growth.

Economic growth: An increase in a country's real level of national output that can be caused by an increase in the quality of resources (education, etc), increase in the quantity of resources, improvements in technology, or in other ways an increase in the value of goods and services produced by every sector of the economy. Economic growth can be measured by an increase in a country's gross domestic product.

Intersectoral action: Actions affecting health outcomes undertaken by sectors outside the health sector, possibly, but not necessarily, in collaboration with the health sector.

Poverty alleviation: Strategies and programmes that are aimed at increasing people's access to goods, services and opportunities; increasing people's ability to withstand the socioeconomic shocks entailed in job loss, crop failure and illness; and expanding the horizon of opportunities to improve quality of life of the poor.

Sustainable development: Refers to development that meets the needs of communities without compromising the ability of future generations to meet their own needs. It means integration of social, economic and environmental factors into planning, implementation and decision-making to ensure that development serves present and future generations.

Introduction

Sustainable development can be defined as the efforts to meet the basic needs of people today without ruining the chances of future generations to do the same. It is easy for development to occur when economies are strong and can provide for all the people in a country. In South Africa, where so many people are presently living in poverty, economic growth is needed before the country's economy will be able to provide sufficient resources to overcome poverty. Sustainable development is a worldwide aim and on the agenda of many countries, especially those that are developing and least developed, such as most countries in Africa.

Seventeen municipalities in South Africa and four organisations, including three universities, are members of the International Council for Local Environmental Initiatives (ICLEI). ICLEI is a global network committed to sustainable urban development, by influencing sustainability policy and driving local action for low emission, nature-based, equitable, resilient and circular development. The emphasis for ICLEI is on environmental, social and economic concerns as three distinct, but interrelated, components of sustainable development. ICLEI's general mandate is to build an active and committed municipal membership of local spheres of government (local and regional governments and authorities) as well as international, regional, national and sub-national local government associations (ICLEI, nd).

The core objective of sustainable development is optimising human welfare. Welfare includes income and material consumption, along with education, health, equality of opportunity and human rights.

All these social welfare factors are needed for people's survival and the country's economic growth. The country's economy has to grow to be able to embrace the increasing number of people and cater for the welfare of those people. If social and welfare needs are well catered for, less poverty and fewer poverty-related challenges will emerge.

Traditionally, poverty has been defined on the basis of a household's income. If people earn below a certain amount per month, they are regarded as living 'below the bread line' or unable to meet the basic needs of the household members.

Lately, definitions are moving beyond this single dimension to be multi-dimensional, including utility and capability-based concepts.

Poverty is also about health, education, security, political voice, discrimination and equality (in a country, region or household) and the total environment that influences how a person lives. Not all of these measures are necessarily at work in every context, but generally each one is needed to capture something missing in the others.

It can be said that poverty is therefore the result of people's lack of a sustainable livelihood or good health, as well as their vulnerability to the environment in which they live.

Many of the people living in poverty are disempowered because they lack the ability to make decisions, or to influence those in their community who have the authority to make the right decisions that will help them.

It is very difficult for people to break out of the poverty cycle or trap that they find themselves in. Only the government's commitment and appropriate policies that can be implemented at community level, with the participation and involvement of the people, can help solve the problem.

Communities must be given the tools and all the help they need to develop the necessary practical skills to be able to earn money and make their own decisions to improve their environment and their community in a way that will make them poverty-free. Through this process, people are said to be empowered. Empowerment will enable communities to earn money.

However, people can only make use of their skills if they live in a secure country or community and are given the opportunities they need to lift themselves out of the poverty trap.

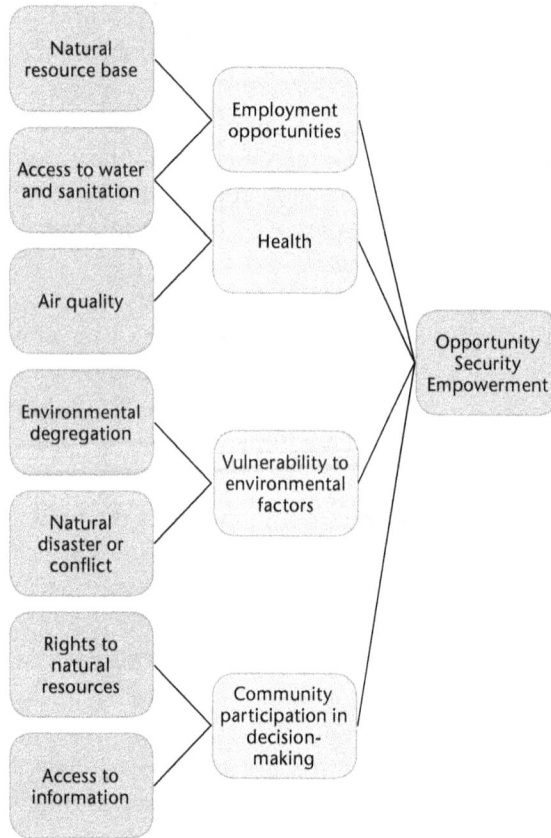

Figure 14.1 Environmental links to poverty

The sustainable development goals (SDGs)

The SDGs are a planned set of objectives aimed at ending extreme poverty in all its forms. Replacing the millennium development goals (MDGs) in 2015, the SDGs were first formally discussed at the United Nations Rio+20 conference on sustainable development held in Rio de Janeiro in June 2012, and are set to be achieved by 2030. SDGs are universal and apply to national and local governments, businesses and civil societies in all countries. The conference outcomes reaffirmed the commitment of all nations in the world to freeing humanity from poverty and hunger as a matter of urgency. There are 17 goals with 169 targets covering a broad range of sustainable development designed to be a blueprint to achieve a better and more sustainable future for all. SDGs were adopted by all United Nations (UN) member states in 2015 as a universal call to achieve a better and more sustainable future for all by 2030 as per UN Resolution 70/1 of the 2030 Agenda.

The 17 SDGs are broad based, interconnected and interdependent, and each has a list of targets which are measured with indicators. In an effort to make the SDGs successful. They address the global challenges we face, including those related to poverty, inequality, climate change, environmental degradation, peace and justice and ensure that all people enjoy peace and prosperity.

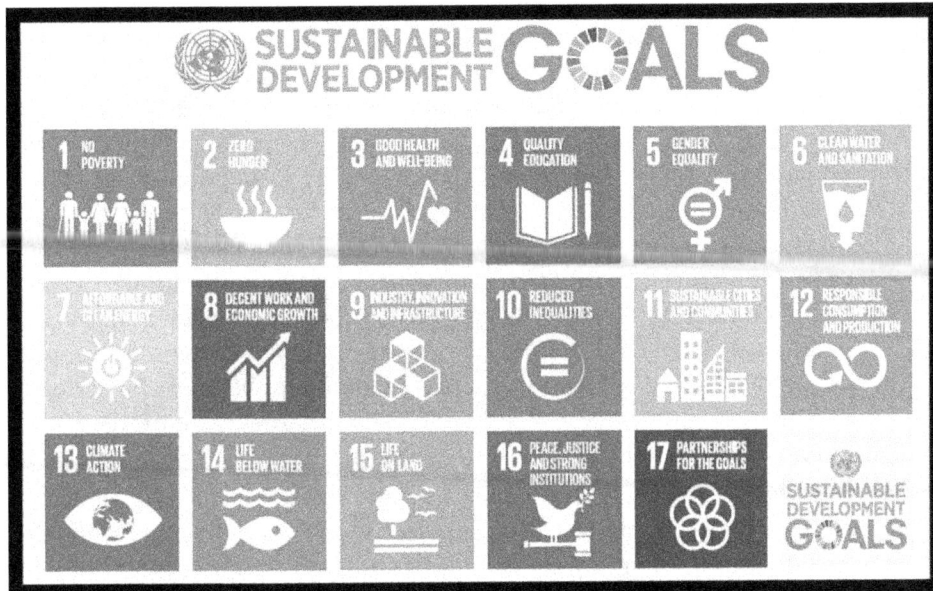

Figure 14.2 A diagrammatic representation of the 17 SDGs
Source: Adapted from United Nations (2015)

The 17 SDGs can be summarised as follows:

1. **No poverty**: End poverty in all its forms everywhere so that by 2030, extreme poverty for all people everywhere is eradicated. This goal aims to eliminate all forms of poverty everywhere, highlights the disproportionate effects of climate change on impoverished and marginalised communities, and calls for a sound policy framework to support accelerated poverty eradication actions. It addresses equality by requiring all nations to ensure both men and women have equal access to economic resources, basic services, ownership of property and inheritance, natural resources, new and appropriate technologies (especially in information and communication) and financial services, including microfinance.

2. **Zero hunger**: End hunger, achieve food security and improved nutrition and promote sustainable agriculture. This would be accomplished by doubling agricultural productivity and incomes of small-scale food producers (especially women and indigenous peoples), by ensuring sustainable food production systems, and by progressively improving land and soil quality. Emphasis is on maintaining genetic diversity

of seeds, increasing access to land, preventing trade restriction and distortions in world agricultural markets to limit extreme food price volatility, eliminating waste with help from the International Food Waste Coalition, and ending malnutrition and undernutrition of children.

3. **Good health and well-being**: Ensure healthy lives and promote well-being for all at all ages. This goal is directly linked to health and aims to reducing maternal mortality to less than 70 deaths per 100 000 live births and to reduce under-five mortality to at least as low as 25 per 1 000 live births. Key strategies for meeting this goal are to reduce adolescent pregnancy (which is strongly linked to gender equality), provide better data for all women and girls and achieve universal coverage of skilled birth attendants. Furthermore, this goal aims to achieve universal health coverage, including access to essential medicines and vaccines. It proposes to end the preventable death of newborns and children under five and to end epidemics such as HIV and AIDS, tuberculosis (TB), malaria, and water-borne diseases. Attention to health and well-being also includes targets related to the prevention and treatment of substance abuse, deaths and injuries from traffic accidents and from hazardous chemicals and air, water and soil pollution and contamination.

4. **Quality education**: Ensure inclusive and equitable quality education and promote lifelong learning opportunities for all. The target for this goal is to ensure that, by 2030, all girls and boys complete free, equitable and quality primary and secondary education.

5. **Gender equality**: Achieve gender equality and empower all women and girls. The targets for this goal are to end gender discrimination and to empower women and girls through technology. Providing women and girls with equal access to education, healthcare, decent work and representation in political and economic decision-making processes will nurture sustainable economies and benefit societies and humanity at large.

6. **Clean water and sanitation**: Ensure availability and sustainable management of water and sanitation for all. This gaol is mainly for the provision of clean drinking water supply and sanitation. Attending school and work without disruption is critical to successful education and successful employment. Therefore, toilets in schools and workplaces are specifically mentioned as a target to measure.

7. **Affordable and clean energy**: Ensure access to affordable, reliable, sustainable and modern energy for all. Targets for 2030 for this goal include access to affordable and reliable energy while increasing the share of renewable energy in the global energy mix. This would involve improving energy efficiency and enhancing international cooperation to facilitate more open access to clean energy technology and more investment in clean energy infrastructure.

8. **Decent work and economic growth**: Promote sustained, inclusive and sustainable economic growth, full and productive employment and decent work for all. The targets for this goal are to reduce youth unemployment and operationalise a global strategy for youth employment. Implementation of the Global Jobs Pact of the International Labour Organization is also mentioned.

9. **Industry, innovation and infrastructure**: Build resilient infrastructure, promote inclusive and sustainable industrialisation and foster innovation. Manufacturing is a major source of employment and this goal encourages the manufacturing of high products in industrialised economies in the least developed countries as well.

10. **Reducing inequality**: Reduce inequality within and among countries. This goal, known as 'shared prosperity', complements SDG 1, the eradication of extreme poverty, and it is relevant for all countries in the world. The main aim is to reduce the transaction costs for migrant remittances to below 3 per cent.

11. **Sustainable cities and communities**: Make cities and human settlements inclusive, safe, resilient and sustainable. The target for 2030 is to ensure access to safe and affordable housing. The indicator named to measure progress toward this target is the proportion of urban population living in slums or informal settlements.

12. **Responsible consumption and production**: Ensure sustainable consumption and production patterns. The targets of this goal include using eco-friendly production methods and reducing the amount of waste. By 2030, national recycling rates should increase, as measured in tons of material recycled. Further, companies should adopt sustainable practices and publish sustainability reports.

13. **Climate action**: Take urgent action to combat climate change and its impacts. The UN encourages the public sector to take initiative in this effort to minimise negative impacts on the environment.

14. **Life below water**: Conserve and sustainably use the oceans, seas and marine resources for sustainable development. This goal aims to prevent and reduce marine pollution and acidification, protecting marine and coastal ecosystems, and regulating fishing as well as the call for an increase in scientific knowledge of the oceans.

15. **Life on land**: Protect, restore and promote sustainable use of terrestrial ecosystems, sustainably manage forests, combat desertification, and halt and reverse land degradation and halt biodiversity loss. This goal articulates targets for preserving biodiversity of forest, desert, and mountain eco-systems, as a percentage of total land mass. It calls for more attention to preventing invasion of introduced species and more protection of endangered species.

16. **Peace, justice and strong institutions**: Promote peaceful and inclusive societies for sustainable development, provide access to justice for all and build effective, accountable and inclusive institutions at all levels. The target is to see the end to sex trafficking, forced labour and all forms of violence against and torture of children. It also targets universal legal identity and birth registration, ensuring the right to a name and nationality, civil rights, recognition before the law, and access to justice and social services.

17. **Partnerships for the goals**: Strengthen the means of implementation and revitalise the global partnership for sustainable development in terms of finance, technology, capacity building, trade and systemic issues. This goal promotes the development of multi-stakeholder partnerships to share knowledge, expertise, technology and financial support. The goal aims to improve North–South and South–South cooperation, and public-private partnerships involving civil societies. (North and South refer to social, economic and political differences between developed countries (North) and developing countries (South).)

- *South–South cooperation* refers to the technical cooperation among developing countries in the global South. It is a tool used by states, international organisations, academics, civil society and the private sector to collaborate and share knowledge, skills and successful initiatives in specific areas such as agricultural development, human rights, urbanisation, health, climate change, etc.

- *North–South cooperation* occurs when a developed country supports a developing country, such as with financial aid during a natural disaster or humanitarian crisis. This has been highly observed during the COVID-19 pandemic.

- *Triangular cooperation* involves three countries, two from the South and one from the North. The one from the North can also be an international organisation, which will provide financial resources to countries from the South in exchange of technical assistance on specific agreed upon topics.

Health and sustainable development in southern Africa

The African continent has some of the poorest countries in the world. It is a concern that, instead of gaining equity within the African region, inequity has increased among and within countries. As inequity in development has widened, so has the health gap. To add to the situation in sub-Saharan Africa, it was identified as the region that carries the greatest burden of disease in the world. Communicable diseases that are a public health problem in the region include HIV and AIDS, tuberculosis, malaria, measles, hepatitis B, cholera and bilharzia. The worst of these is the HIV and AIDS epidemic that, by virtue of its magnitude, has affected societies and inflicted irreparable damage on families and communities. The epidemic has affected all people in the region without distinction, but it is the women, children and youth who have suffered the most. It has influenced both social and economic development.

Southern Africa is also challenged by an increased incidence of non-communicable diseases such as diabetes and hypertension, and cardiovascular and circulatory diseases. All these examples are lifestyle diseases. This means that they are associated with rapid urbanisation, industrialisation and changing lifestyles. These diseases are thought to account for more than 40 per cent of all deaths in developing countries.

Food production has declined in the region due to droughts, lack of skilled farmers and political instability. As a result of food shortages, both mother and child malnutrition are on the increase. Access to safe water is still a major problem in the southern parts of the African continent.

In the past 25 years, the South African government has implemented successful development programmes to increase access to safe water to many within the country. However, there are still millions of people who do not have access to safe water or adequate sanitation and even more who do not have access to electricity. The lack of basic resources needed for development challenges the process.

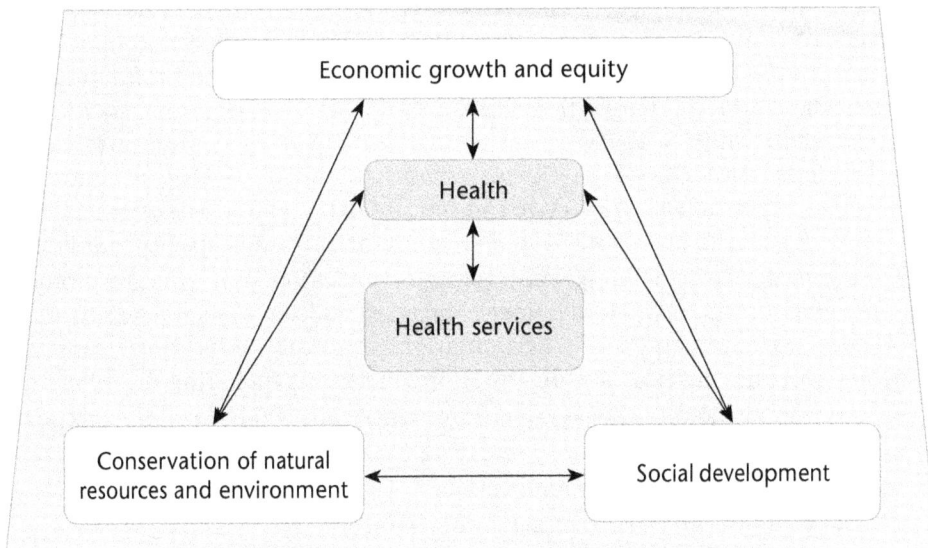

Figure 14.3 The triad of health and sustainable development

Organisations involved in sustainable development in Africa

The **Southern African Development Community (SADC)** was established in 1992 to encourage closer cooperation among the people and governments of the region and to rationalise their policies and strategies for sustainable development. The 14 countries in the southern part of Africa together address the needs of more than 200 million people living in the region whose level of development is generally low. Improved strategies have been put in place with the assistance of the WHO for development, but control of communicable diseases is important before strides can be made in development programmes.

The **New Partnership for Africa's Development (NEPAD)** was conceptualised in 1999 to create an environment for economic growth and development on the continent. It is an organisation whose membership consists of heads of state and other senior officials from most of the countries in Africa. The continent has a poor record in implementing development strategies in the past and this organisation aims to disprove this notion.

The aims of the partnership include poverty alleviation and broad-based improvement in incomes and quality of life. It has plans for countries in Africa to work together to implement development programmes mobilising their own resources, with the richer and more developed countries helping those that are poorer and less developed. Only once they are making a difference do they plan to seek help from outside Africa in the form of funding and/or specialised expertise. The ultimate outcome of NEPAD is to turn around the negative view people have of the continent and make it more attractive to investors.

Africare is one of the most experienced and largest African–American led non-profit international development organisations, and leaders in development assistance to Africa. Since its founding in 1970, Africare has delivered more than $1 billion in assistance to tens of millions of men, women and children across the African continent. Through Africare projects, it has been able to nurture valuable relationships with key local figures ranging from community leaders and traditional authorities to presidents and prime ministers. Africare centres its development approach around active community participation and partners with local organisations to ensure institutional strengthening and capacity building.

Conserve Africa is a non-governmental organisation that aims to promote and implement sustainable development practices, policies and strategies through knowledge management and dissemination, training, education, research, advocacy and campaigning. The organisation's objectives including the following:

- Promote sustainable development in Africa for the benefit of the public by preserving, conserving and protecting the environment.
- Relief of poverty and the environment of the conditions of life in socially and economically disadvantaged communities.
- Promote sustainable means of achieving economic growth and regeneration.
- Advance the education of the public in subjects related to sustainable development and the protection, enhancement and rehabilitation of the environment and to promote study and research in such subjects.
- Increase the knowledge base within the public and local civil society organisations about environment and sustainable development issues.
- Influence regional and international response to the environment and poverty linkages and to the root causes of the current state of the environment in Africa.

The **African Sustainable Development Association (A-SDA)** is a South African based organisation that drives an active public–private partnership (PPP) ecosystem, implementing collaborative projects towards sustainable and inclusive development in South Africa and beyond. A-SDA aims to equip South African and African corporate businesses to partner with local small and medium enterprises (SMEs) to be globally competitive and enhance their value chain performance.

To date, a number of projects have been initiated but few results have materialised. Leaders in Africa will have to show their commitment to development programmes by supporting them not only in word but by committing resources to the programmes as well.

Intersectoral collaboration in sustainable development

As implied by the term 'intersectoral', we will see in this section how the full range of social, governmental and organisational sectors needs to be mobilised and brought together in striving for the goal of sustainable development. The emphasis is on community participation.

The need for an intersectoral approach

Poverty is the root of much of the unreasonably high level of burden of disease. It increases the vulnerability of people to ill-health. It also leads to ill-health through economic underdevelopment, unemployment and low incomes, environmental degradation, poor agricultural production, inequitable land reform, lack of education, poor infrastructure and the oppression of women. To meet these problems, there is a need for broad intersectoral interventions.

Countries face health-related problems associated with poverty and lack of access to basic services and resources on the one hand, and with industrialisation, technical development and rapid urbanisation on the other hand. This complicates the management of health problems and therefore requires a multidisciplinary response. The sectors responsible for water, sanitation, the environment, housing, education and energy are all indirectly involved with health as they all aim to improve the way people live, either directly or indirectly.

Global problems have been identified but each country, region or community will have its own unique challenges. To resolve these challenges, it is necessary to look at each problem within the context of the community and its specific customs and values and the resources it has, as well as the multidisciplinary team tasked to resolve these problems.

Community participation

The concept of community participation has developed over the years and has been interpreted in many different ways. The objective is to get community members involved in implementing development strategies to ensure that community members accept and buy into the programme. Community members should be involved in one of the following ways:

- **Contribution**: Community members assist employees or health professionals to implement a development project in the community.
- **Compliance**: Participation is the result of health-promotion programmes where people are informed and encouraged to accept the programme based on the knowledge they have acquired from the employees or health professionals involved in the project.
- **Control**: Community members are assisted to develop the necessary skills to implement and manage a project and then allocated the task. They report back to the authorities from time to time.
- **Collaboration**: Community assistance is requested from the beginning and at each stage of the project. The members of the community become part of the project team.

The success of community participation is dependent on the members of the community giving their time, labour and other resources. In undeveloped areas this is difficult when people are unemployed and hungry. In South Africa, volunteers are encouraged to participate in projects and in return a stipend is paid for people's travel and food. This way the unemployed are engaged to good purpose and are taught skills, and their expenses are paid. This is a form of empowerment that gives people experience, which makes them more employable, while at the same time initiating programmes that will improve the environment or well-being of the whole community. To manage local and national health concerns it is necessary to:

- identify and assess health hazards associated with the environment and development
- develop an environmental health policy incorporation principles and strategies for all sectors responsible for development
- communicate this policy to all levels of the community
- use a participatory approach, engaging all sectors and community members to implement health and environmental programmes.

Development allows for the simultaneous achievement of a number of goals. For example, addressing environmental issues will help to achieve health goals, and achieving these goals will help to ensure environmental sustainability. The outcomes of the process provide hope for developing countries.

Conclusion

Sustainable development covers different aspects of social development, environmental protection and economic growth. The main benefits from this process is the maintenance of health and the bio-capacity of the environment. Through sustainability, the well-being of individuals and communities is supported, the economy is promoted for enhancement of liveability, where there is little waste and pollution, fewer emissions, more jobs and a better distribution of wealth. This will ensure that all human beings can enjoy prosperous and fulfilling lives and that economic, social and technological progress occurs in harmony with nature.

Self-assessment

1. What are the challenges in achieving sustainable development and how can they be overcome?

2. Sustainable Development Goal No. 3 (SDG 3) is linked to health and promotion of health. Explain the main objectives and targets for this goal and give practical examples for your response.

3. Which of the following best describes sustainable development? (Choose the most correct response.)

    a) Development that provides for economic and social viability even if that results in environmental degradation for the future.

    b) Development that provides environmental sustainability even if that results in economic and social degradation for future generations.

    c) Development that meets the needs of the present without compromising the ability of future generations to meet their own needs.

    d) Development that meets the needs of the future generations even if that means the needs of present societies go unmet.

4. For sustainable development to be successful, which key systems must work together? (Choose the most correct response.)

    a) Economic, social, environmental

    b) Economic, environmental, executive

    c) Economic, legislative, environmental

    d) Economic, social, legislative, environmental

5. Which of the following terms describes the point beyond which the environment exceeds its ability to provide essential resources? (Choose the most correct response.)

    a) Sustainable development

    b) Sustainable consumption

    c) Environmental development

    d) Environmental limits

6. Explain four ways in which community members can be involved in implementing development strategies in their own areas.

Bibliography

International Council for Local Environmental Initiatives (ICLEI). nd. About ICLEI: Mission and mandate. Available: http://iclei.org/index.php?id=744 (Accessed 11 September 2020).

Unicef. 2014. Levels and trends in child mortality. Available: https://data.unicef.org/resources/levels-trends-child-mortality-report-2014/# (Accessed 11 September 2020).

United Nations (UN). 2012. The history of sustainable development in the United Nations. Rio+20 UN conference on sustainable development. 20-22 June 2012.

United Nations (UN). 2015a. Sustainable development goals. Available: https://www.un.org/sustainabledevelopment/sustainable-development-goals/ (Accessed 11 September 2020).

United Nations (UN). 2015b. Transforming our world: The 2030 agenda for sustainable development. United Nations sustainable development knowledge platform. Available: https//sdgs.un.org/2030agenda (Accessed 21 September).

United Nations (UN) Official. 2015c. The sustainable development document. Available: www.un.org (Accessed 1 April 2020).

World Health Organization (WHO). 2015. World health statistics. Available: https://www.who.int/gho/publications/world_health_statistics/2015/en/ (Accessed 11 September 2020).

Environmental sustainability

Roelien Els

Learning outcomes

After studying this chapter, you should be able to:

- Identify the basic elements that have an impact on environmental sustainability.
- Discuss the adverse effects that air pollution and inadequate ventilation have on health.
- Describe the requirements to ensure optimal domestic lighting.
- Differentiate between natural and artificial heating.
- Explain the association between overcrowding and health.
- Describe the impact of global warming on the health of the community.
- Discuss the community nurse's role and responsibilities to reduce the environmental impact on healthcare.

Key terms

Airborne transmission: The transmission of diseases caused by the spread of droplet nuclei that remains infectious when suspended in air over long distances and time. The evaporated droplets enter the upper and lower respiratory tract to cause certain diseases.

Droplet transmission: Droplet transmission occurs when a person is in close contact (within 1 metre) with someone who has respiratory symptoms (eg coughing or sneezing) and is therefore at risk of having his or her mucosae (mouth and nose) or conjunctiva (eyes) exposed to potentially infective respiratory droplets. Transmission may also occur through fomites in the immediate environment around the infected person.

➡

Biomass fuels: Fuels that come from natural resources, such as firewood, charcoal, crop residue and animal dung; methane from waste; and alcohol made from sugar or starch.

Sustainability: The principle of adapting our exploitation and consumption of natural resources, and controlling our waste products, to prevent further damage to the earth and its environment.

Environmental sustainability: The capability to improve the quality of human life according to the carrying capacity of the earth's supporting ecosystems. Sustainability aims to stabilise the existing disruptive relationship between the human culture and the living world to prevent further damage to the environment.

Recycling: Reducing the use of natural resources by re-using products and materials for domestic, commercial and industrial purposes.

Introduction

In this chapter we are going to take a closer look at one aspect of sustainable development that was introduced in Chapter 14 – environmental sustainability and, in particular, the importance of clean air and adequate ventilation, requirements for safe housing and environmental cleanliness.

As a reminder, when we speak of environmental sustainability, we are concerned with caring and maintaining the world and its natural resources so that current and future generations will be able to enjoy the basics of life. These 'basics of life' are things such as:

- clean water
- clean air
- a clean environment (including safe housing, electricity and sanitation)
- food security
- non-economic variables such as education and health.

The Constitution of the Republic of South Africa (1996) provides the overarching legislative foundation for environmental management in South Africa. The care of the environment is entrenched in the Constitution, which stipulates that:

- every person has the right to an environment that is not harmful to his or her health or well-being
- the environment must be protected through reasonable legislative measures to prevent pollution and ecological degradation
- environmental conservation must be promoted
- sustainable ecological development must be secured by careful use of natural resources, while promoting justifiable economic and social development.

The community nurse can play a vital role in educating the community about the importance of caring for the environment and the positive impact that good environmental practices can have on preventing illness.

Sustainable Development Goals

The Sustainable Development Goals (SDGs) were introduced in Chapter 14. The United Nations developed a set of action-oriented SDGs to address the three dimensions of sustainable development, namely economic, social and environmental development. The overarching challenge underpinned in all environmental goals is to ensure environmental sustainability. Sustainable energy is one of the 17 global goals that make up the 2030 agenda for sustainable development. Efficient management of our natural resources may impact all other environmental goals positively.

The South African government has developed the National Development Plan (NDP) 2030 as an overarching policy to address the most urgent challenges, such as ensuring access to sustainable energy and climate change. The NDP links directly to SDG 7 and addresses specific targets for 2030, such as:

- providing access to affordable electricity and other clean forms of energy to at least 90 per cent of South Africans according to a targeted pro-poor electricity tariff system to qualifying electricity customers
- increased utilisation of renewable energy
- a 15 per cent energy efficiency improvement in the mining and mineral processing sector
- hybrid and electric vehicles to be widely used.

This chapter supports the local SDG initiatives, which are aimed at the promotion of healthy lives and well-being for everyone.

Air quality is linked to several SDGs, which are aimed at reducing exposure to climate-related extreme events, and social and environmental shocks and disasters. The following section on air quality and ventilation introduces you to the factors that cause air pollution and the health conditions associated with poor air quality.

Air quality

Air is essential to life. All cells require a constant supply of oxygen for the metabolic processes and will die if deprived of it. Standard dry air is composed of mainly three gasses: nitrogen, oxygen and argon. Standard dry air also contains water vapour and carbon dioxide. There could also be small traces of neon, helium, krypton and xenon but this will depend on local conditions. Table 15.1 gives a breakdown of the main elements of air.

Table 15.1 The main elements of air

Component	Inspired air	Expired air
Nitrogen	78.08%	78.08%
Oxygen	20.94%	16.94%

Component	Inspired air	Expired air
Water vapour	Variable	Saturated
Argon	0.93%	0.93%
Carbon dioxide	0.03%	4.03%

The main elements that constitute air are described below:

- **Nitrogen** is a colourless, odourless, tasteless gas that makes up 80 per cent of our atmosphere and serves to dilute oxygen. We are dependent upon green plants and microbes to convert nitrogen into a usable form for human absorption. Nitrogen helps in protein synthesis, amino acids that influence growth, assists brain function and plays a role in the immune system.

- **Oxygen** maintains life because it supports combustion and enables the process of metabolism. It acts as a purifier because it combines with organic substances. In some cases, it destroys bacteria. This process is known as oxidation.

- **Water vapour**: The amount of moisture present in the air is known as the *humidity* of the air. The humidity level is influenced by air temperature, as warm air can hold more moisture than cold air. We say that air is *saturated* with water when it cannot take up any more moisture at a given temperature.

- **Argon** is element 18 on the Periodic Table and is colourless, odourless, non-flammable and non-toxic as a solid, liquid or gas. It is classified as a non-reactive gas and although it does not contain biologically active characters, research continues to explore its medical uses in the treatment of brain injury.

- **Carbon dioxide** is a waste product of respiration and all metabolic processes. It is being added to the air continually, yet the amount remains fairly constant because the carbon is utilised by green plants for photosynthesis. Photosynthesis is the process whereby plants use the sun's energy in order to synthesise, or manufacture, carbohydrates.

Air pollution

Air pollution is a combination of natural and man-made substances in the air we breathe. The *quality* of the air is of importance because air pollution affects our health, productivity levels and eventually our economic sustainability. There are two types of air pollution: indoor pollution caused by cooking fumes from fireplaces and wooden stoves, and outdoor (ambient) pollution caused by emissions from industries and road transport. Air pollution consists of chemicals such as particulate matter, invisible gasses such as nitrogen dioxide, sulphur dioxide and carbon monoxide, and semi-volatile liquids such as methane and benzene. Particulate matter is a highly lethal pollutant and consists of tiny particles and liquid droplets suspended in the air.

South Africa's Air Quality Act of 2004 enabled the formulation of national norms, standards and measures for the prevention of pollution. The Act permits the minister to label certain substances such as carbon dioxide (CO_2), methane (CH_4), nitrous oxide (N_2O) as priority air pollutants and to require that coal mines, cement production industries as well as electricity production facilities have to submit pollution prevention plans for approval. Examples of the measures entrenched in standards and norms to prevent and manage air pollution are the following:

- National Framework for Air Quality Management, 2012
- Regulations Regarding the Phasing-out and Management of Ozone-Depleting Substances
- National Atmospheric Reporting Regulations, 2015
- National Greenhouse Gas Emissions Reporting Regulations, 2016.

South Africa has a 97 per cent reliance on coal for energy, which in turn worsens outdoor pollution. A recent study done by the International Growth Centre indicates that 7,4 per cent of all deaths in South Africa in 2012 were related to chronic exposure of fine particulate matter (Altieri & Keen, 2016). Examples of air pollution are:

- domestic fires
- vehicle emissions
- industrial emissions
- acid rain.

Domestic fires

Air pollution levels are frequently high in informal settlements, where electricity is not readily accessible, and the community cannot afford electricity. Smoke, soot, sulphur oxides and particles of matter, such as ash, are added to the air by domestic fires. Fires used for cooking and heating are still considered one of the most serious sources of atmospheric pollution. Pollution levels are especially high in under-serviced settlements.

Vehicle emissions

In the urban industrial areas of the world motor vehicles are probably the major source of atmospheric pollution. Exhaust fumes add carbon monoxide, hydrocarbons (a chemical compound of hydrogen and carbon), lead (which is added to petrol) and the oxides of nitrogen and sulphur to the air.

Industrial emissions

Over half of the global population is reliant on solid biomass fuels such as wood, coal, crop residues and animal dung for their domestic energy requirements. When burned indoors in open fires or rudimentary appliances, the incomplete combustion of solid biomass fuels releases high concentrations of toxic pollutants such as particulate matter, carbon monoxide, oxides of nitrogen, sulphur dioxide and volatile organic compounds into the living environment.

Industry adds the products of combustion to the air such as toxic chemicals, which may escape into the atmosphere and cause not only disease, but also death. Metals such as cadmium and arsenic, and fluorides and asbestos are known carcinogens that may pollute the air as a result of industrial processes. All of these substances are detrimental to health. From time to time accidents occur and these are responsible for acute local episodes of pollution. A series of studies conducted in Mpumalanga has reported a connection between the pollution in the area and the people's health challenges.

In addition, some chemicals used by industry are life-threatening on contact, and some persist in the environment, accumulate in the food chain, travel long distances from where they are released and are harmful to human health in small amounts. Human exposure can occur at different stages of the life cycle of a chemical, including through occupational exposure during manufacture, use and disposal, consumer exposure, exposure to contaminated products or environmental exposure to toxic waste.

> Exposure to air pollutants has been associated with diseases affecting various body systems, as discussed in Table 15.2. Acute lower respiratory infection (ALRI) such as pneumonia is considered one of the leading causes of death among children under five worldwide.

Acid rain

The main sources of sulphur dioxide in South Africa are coal-fired power stations and metal working industries. Acid rain is caused by the release of sulphur dioxide and nitrous oxides. When sulphur and nitrogen dioxides combine with atmospheric moisture, a highly acidic rain, hail or fog is produced. Acid rain changes the acidity of soil, water and shallow groundwater and removes essential nutrients such as calcium from the soil. Acid rain may also activate the release of aluminium, which makes it hard for trees and other plants to absorb water.

Exposure to pollutants

Exposure can occur via various direct or indirect pathways, such as:

- inhalation of contaminated air and dust (eg nitrogen oxide found in tobacco smoke)

- ingestion of contaminated water and food (eg through exposure to household aerosols, contaminated vegetation and soil contaminants)
- dermal exposure to chemical or contaminated products such as lipid-soluble chemicals in soil
- indirect foetal exposure during pregnancy (eg there is a possible association between air pollutants and autism spectrum disorder (ASD)).

Health effects of air pollution and inadequate ventilation

When solid biomass materials are burned indoors using open fires, high concentrations of toxic pollutants such as particulate matter, carbon monoxide, sulphur dioxide and nitrogen oxides are released. In 2013 the International Agency for Research on Cancer has classified outdoor pollution, and specifically particulate matter (PM), a major component of outdoor air pollution, as carcinogenic to humans (WHO, 2013).

The World Health Organization (WHO) (2020a) indicates that an estimated 4.2 million premature deaths globally are linked to air pollution, mainly from heart disease, stroke, lung cancer, chronic obstructive pulmonary disease and acute respiratory infections in children. The effects of air pollution on health is more serious in vulnerable populations such as people with pre-existing health conditions and those from a lower socioeconomic status.

Children may be more vulnerable to the effects of air pollutants than adults, because their:

- pulmonary epithelial linings are more permeable and can therefore absorb toxic substances more readily
- immune systems are not fully developed, limiting the body's defence against infection
- respiration rate is higher
- lung surface per kilogram of body weight is larger than that of an adult, resulting in them inhaling 50 per cent more polluted air than adults.

Table 15.2 details some of the conditions caused by air pollution. However, you should bear in mind that it is very difficult to separate the effects of such pollution from other environmental factors that may be associated with a particular disease. NASA uses air quality forecasters and satellites such as Aqua, Terra and Suomi-NPP to orbit the earth to monitor air pollution.

It is generally accepted that the ill effects detailed in Table 15.2 result from air pollution.

Table 15.2 The systemic results of air pollution and inadequate ventilation

Affected system	Health effects
General effects on the human body	• Stuffiness and discomfort, lassitude and loss of energy, and decreased mental efficiency occur due to poor ventilation. • Cancer, neurotoxicity and birth defects may be caused by pesticide poisoning. • Long-term arsenic exposure causes bladder, kidney and lung cancer, peripheral neuropathy, enlarged liver, bone marrow depression, diabetes and adverse reproductive effects.
Cardiovascular health	• Association in women between air pollution and ischaemia. • Increased incidence and mortality from coronary artery disease. • Development of a stroke due to vascular changes. • Hypertension associated with high lead levels in the air.
Respiratory health	• Decreased lung function due to air pollution. • Chronic obstructive pulmonary disease, including chronic bronchitis and emphysema, due to exposure to cotton, grain and wood dusts. • Increased risk of developing asthma from exposure to traffic-related air pollution. • Streptococcal throat infections. • Tuberculosis. • Exposure to asbestos, arsenic and cadmium causes lung cancer, mesothelioma and asbestosis (fibrosis of the lungs). • Nasopharyngeal cancer.
Possible links with cancer	• High nitrogen oxide concentrations and other air pollutants are associated with several forms of cancer, including cervical cancer and brain cancer.
Haematopoietic system	• Prolonged exposure to volatile organic compounds, benzene, ionising radiation, ethylene oxide and formaldehyde is associated with the development of leukaemia. • Inadequate ventilation exacerbates the risk of diseases that are spread through airborne transmission, eg meningitis.
Integumentary system	• Irritation of the skin and mucous membranes, including the conjunctiva of the eyes. • Arsenic in drinking water causes skin cancer.
Immune system	• Allergies, eg hayfever and allergic rhinitis.
Effects on children	• Exposure to air pollutants may cause asthma, pneumonia and lower respiratory diseases as well as low birth weight. • Lead exposure leads to reduced intellectual functioning.

Ventilation

Ventilation is the intentional introduction of outdoor air into a space such as inside a building. As people breathe, the oxygen content of expired air is decreased, the carbon-dioxide content is increased, the air becomes saturated with water vapour and the temperature of the air is raised. Airborne transmitted diseases such as pulmonary tuberculosis, influenza and meningitis are spread when pathogens are expired in air.

Natural ventilation

Natural ventilation is the use of natural forces such as wind pressure and pressure generated by the density differences between indoor and outdoor air. The purpose of ventilation is to replenish oxygen by both diluting and removing pollutants originating in the building. Ventilation also helps regulate internal temperatures and reduce the accumulation of moisture, odours, bacteria, smoke and carbon dioxide by creating air movement. There are two basic types of natural ventilation:

- **Thermal buoyancy-driven ventilation**: Wind ventilation supplies air from a positive pressure through openings on the windward side of a building and exhausts air to a negative pressure on the leeward side. Cooler air enters the building at low level, is heated by equipment, occupants and heating systems and becomes less dense. This increase in buoyancy makes the air to rise through the building for ventilation to the outside at the top.
- **Wind-driven cross ventilation**: In summer, the indoor–outdoor temperature difference is not high enough to drive buoyancy ventilation, and wind is used to supply as much fresh air as possible. Pressure differences between the one side of the building and the other draw air in on the high-pressure side and out on the low-pressure side of the building.

The success of using natural ventilation depends on climate, building design and human behaviour. Natural methods of ventilation of houses include:
- windows and doors
- airbricks, solar chimneys and wind towers
- trickle ventilators.

Windows

Various legal requirements have to be complied with in urban areas, for example windows have to be at least one-tenth of the floor area and they must be situated in an outside wall. It must be possible to open the windows. There are many types of windows on the market today and all are effective if correctly placed. Louvred panes in a window improve the ventilating properties and have the added advantage that they can be adjusted in order to eliminate draughts. Using windows to facilitate natural ventilation depends on outside conditions relative

271

to the indoor environment. It can be difficult to generate airflow (ie wind and temperature difference) because natural ventilation only works when natural forces are available. Climate, security and cultural criteria may dictate that windows and vents remain closed, resulting in lowered ventilation rates.

Airbricks

These are perforated bricks, which are placed in walls just below the ceiling. Warm air that rises leaves the room through the perforations in the bricks, thus using thermal buoyancy as a mechanism to promote ventilation. They are also placed in the foundation of houses for sub-floor ventilation. Their use in buildings is compulsory.

While the number, size and placement of ventilating openings is most important in ensuring adequate ventilation, these alone are not sufficient; unless the rooms are large enough for the number of people who will occupy them, ventilation will be poor irrespective of how many windows, doors and airbricks there are in a room.

Natural ventilation forces are unable to come into play in enclosed spaces. It is therefore essential to have adequate ventilation to ensure a free flow of air, which helps disperse certain pathogens, such as *Mycobacterium tuberculosis*, which causes pulmonary tuberculosis.

External ventilation

In order to achieve good indoor ventilation, external ventilation has to be good. Narrow streets, houses within a few metres of one another, back-to-back dwellings and an absence of grass or trees, all stop the free circulation of air and thus hamper indoor ventilation.

Mechanical ventilation

In securing efficient ventilation, natural forces are used as far as possible, but where circumstances make this impossible, artificial means, using electricity to power the mechanism, have to be used. All artificial ventilation systems other than regular air conditioners must be authorised by the local authority according to specified standards. In large urban areas more and more public buildings, including hospitals and schools, as well as large department stores, places of entertainment and factories, rely entirely on mechanical ventilation, which is driven by fans. Mechanical ventilation systems are designed to deliver a specific ventilation flow rate of air, regardless of the impacts of wind and outdoor temperature. In hospitals (eg isolation rooms and contained areas such as the laboratory) the airflow direction is designed to flow from clean to dirty zones. Filtration systems can be installed to remove microorganisms, particulates, gasses and odours. Ventilation in the operating theatre requires many air-quality requirements such as positive pressure and directional airflow to maintain the sterile environment. There are a number of mechanical methods, such as:

- **Air conditioning**: This process controls the temperature and moisture content of the air before it is introduced into a building.
- **Fans**: Fresh air may be forced into a building by means of large fans – this is known as the plenum system – or extraction fans can be used to draw air out of a building.

Housing

Safe housing is addressed in SDG 11, which emphasises the promotion of access for all to adequate, safe and affordable housing and basic services. Section 24 of the Bill of Rights states that everybody has a right to 'an environment that is not harmful to their health or well-being'. Between 1994 and December 2018, the South African government built over 3.2 million homes funded from the Human Settlement Development Grant (HSDG). The General Household Survey of 2018 (StatsSA, 2018) showed that about 81 per cent of South African households reside in formal dwellings, 31 per cent in informal dwellings and 5 per cent in traditional dwellings. The large-scale subsidised housing programme enabled families to receive a government subsidy at an increased rate of 5.6 per cent in 2002 to 13.6 per cent in 2018. Of the households living in formal dwellings, 25 per cent were renting, 62 per cent owned their homes and 12 per cent resided rent free. The Department of Human Settlements aims to transform the country's residential areas and build communities with closer access to work and social amenities, including sport and recreational facilities.

The requirements of good housing

Building regulations and functional guidelines are contained in South Africa's National Building Regulations (SABC, 2018) to ensure safety when building houses. The physical aspects of housing such as structural design, foundations and floors, walls and roofs, lighting and ventilation and sanitary disposal are important to ensure that the main features of good housing are adhered to. Poorly constructed dwellings with inadequate lighting, ventilation, energy usage and sanitary disposal are essentially unconstitutional and pose adverse health effects on the occupants. When a house is to be erected, drawings and plans must be submitted to the local authority before you are allowed to build any sort of structure. The plans must include:

- a site plan and layout drawings
- a fire installation drawing
- a drainage installation drawing.

The site

The nature of the soil on which the house is built is important. For example, if a house is constructed on soil that is predominantly clay it may be cold and damp because clay retains moisture. These houses are also more likely to crack than houses built on lighter soils. Areas where the subsoil water lies close to the surface are also not suitable for the erection of dwellings as this may lead to dampness in the house. Made soil – that is, areas that have been filled in by the controlled tipping of refuse – may not be used for building purposes for at least three years.

Ideally, residential sites should be located in the healthiest part of the town and approved by the local authority. In most cities only one residence may be erected on each stand unless permission has been granted to build another cottage or dwelling. This will depend on the municipal by-laws and the size of the site.

Planning and building

In urban areas the erection of buildings is strictly controlled and must comply with the municipal by-laws. Plans must be approved by the local authority. Building inspectors and health inspectors keep a close watch on each house during the construction period.

Minimum standards, especially those concerning the floor space, size of the windows, materials that may be used, drainage and many other aspects, are laid down and have to be complied with. A local authority has the power to order the demolition of a building if the plans have not been submitted for approval or the building does not meet with certain requirements.

Maintenance of buildings

It is always the responsibility of the occupant to ensure that his or her home/premises and surroundings are kept clean and tidy. Local authorities are empowered to enforce this. Health inspectors visit buildings in their area regularly to ensure the following:

- Premises must be in a sanitary condition, with no situation likely to endanger health.
- Factories and shops are inspected and particular attention is paid to rodent proofing.
- Refuse storage on premises is strictly supervised to ensure that no danger or nuisance exists.

Health inspectors are empowered to point out conditions that need attention; should their instructions be ignored they can be enforced by law.

Sub-economic housing

In South Africa, people who have the financial means to build or buy their own homes usually do so with the assistance of a loan from a bank or other financial institution. It is the responsibility of the government and/or the local authority to provide low-cost housing for people of limited means.

National housing subsidy scheme

The Department of Human Settlements has updated the RDP housing plan and now calls it 'Breaking New Ground' (BNG). The local authority, who are not allowed to profit from the plan, rents out or sells the houses to approved people. Only people who do not already own property are eligible for this type of housing. Homeowners must live in their house for a minimum of eight years before they are legally able to sell or rent it out.

Characteristics of poor-quality housing can include poor structural integrity, ventilation and temperature regulation and the presence of condensation, which in turn may lead to health risks, creating a favourable breading environment for pathogens, moulds and animal infestation. Overcrowding is particularly severe in developing countries and when combined with the process of urbanisation, it is expected to increase and intensify in the future. Many households need to accommodate extended families and family visits to deal with illness, mourn a death in the family, or sometimes for cultural reasons. Research conducted between 2002 and 2014 showed that more than one-quarter of formal low-cost dwellings in South Africa are overcrowded.

Association between overcrowding and health

The United Nations Human Settlements Programme, UN-Habitat, defines dwellings as moderately overcrowded if occupied by more than two but fewer than five people per room, whereas extreme overcrowding is defined as a dwelling with more than six people per room (Nkosi et al, 2019).

A range of controlled studies have shown significant associations between overcrowded housing and ill health. These are some of the risk factors associated with overcrowded housing:

- Diseases transmitted by airborne droplets, such as respiratory diseases (eg streptococcal throat infections, pneumococcal infections and pulmonary tuberculosis) as well as meningococcal disease.

- Infections of the gastrointestinal tract, such as diarrhoea and vomiting, because inadequate or absent sanitation coupled with limited water supply increase the risk of oral–faecal contamination due to bacteria such as E. Coli.

- Skin infections (eg scabies), eye-infections (trachoma), and chronic ear infections (eg otitis media).

- An increase in the incidence of the diseases that can be transmitted from animals to humans especially where domestic animals live in close association with the family. Diseases such as *brucellosis, anthrax, tetanus* and *salmonella* infections may be transmitted to the family by direct contact or indirectly through contaminated soil and dust.

- Diseases spread by rodents and insects such as fleas, lice and flies.

- Infectious disease outbreaks such as measles, cholera, SARS, COVID-19 with severe adverse epidemic and even pandemic consequences.
- An absence of the basic necessities and an increased frequency of home accidents due to a lack of separate facilities for cooking, sleeping and playing because dwellings are often structurally unsafe or functionally in a state of disrepair with broken stairs, floors and windows.
- Negative impact on mental health of adults and children exacerbated by a lack of privacy contributing to depression, anxiety, stress and self-harm with adverse outcomes such as suicide among adults and children.
- Family violence, child maltreatment, including sexual abuse, and increased violence in the community.

When looking at the ill-effects of poor housing one must remember that it is difficult to pinpoint how much the actual dwelling contributes to the problem because there are many other factors at play in such situations, and poor housing is often also associated with inadequate education, unemployment and poorly paid jobs, illness and social discrimination. The community nurse can contribute to the country's National Development Plan and goals for a healthy South Africa in educating the community.

Lighting and heating

The General Household Survey Report (GHSR) of 2016 indicates that 60 per cent of South African rural households have no access to electricity and more than 5 per cent of South Africa's 16.6 million households use candles as a main source of lighting (StatsSA, 2016). Government continues to invest in renewable energy products across the country, especially in rural areas. The Free Basic Alternative Energy Policy instructs local municipalities to select and assist with the provision of suitable off-grid energy sources for indigent households. The policy lists paraffin (kerosene), liquid petroleum gas, bio-ethanol gel (or fire gel), coal and solar energy as options to assist with energy for cooking, heating, lighting and electricity. With quality light, a family can continue to be productive – cooking, studying and earning money for the family. A statement made in line with South Africa's goal to provide some form of energy to the entire country states that 'South Africa aims to ensure that by 2030 at least 90 per cent of people have access to grid electricity' (Naidoo, 2014).

Natural light

Natural light is emitted from the sun and may be direct or indirect. Indirect light is light that is reflected from various surfaces. During the day and under normal circumstances natural light is usually sufficient for most purposes, but the amount of light entering a building depends on a number of factors:

- **The position and size of the windows**: The more windows there are in a building, and the larger they are, the greater the amount of light that will enter the rooms. Although sunlight entering a room makes it look bright and cheerful, and warms it as well as lighting it, it is not the best type of light in which to work because it is of high intensity and it causes a glare. In classrooms, for example, it is advisable to have windows on the south side of the room in order to prevent such a glare.
- **The presence of tall buildings, walls or trees that will throw a shadow on the windows**: In areas of high population density tall blocks of flats are built close to one another and very little natural light may enter some parts of the building.
- **The clearness of the atmosphere**: The presence of smoke or smog will darken the atmosphere and therefore the room.

Artificial light

This light is made available by the release of stored energy. It is used when there is insufficient natural light available or when a building is designed in such a way that the use of natural light is not possible.

The characteristics of good artificial lighting

Good artificial lighting should be sufficient for the activity that is normally carried out in the room or building. There should be no glare or flicker, and the light should not cast harsh shadows. Ideally, the method used should not pollute the air or raise the temperature. Artificial light may be produced by:

- combustion
- electricity.

Factors such as seasonality, the availability and price of fuels as well as cultural aspects all influence residents' fuel choices and the quantity consumed. During the warmer months, un-electrified households use paraffin and liquid petroleum gas for cooking and lighting. During winter, low-income households favour solid fuels such as wood and coal.

Fuel types using *combustion lighting* include the following:

- **Candles**: These are used extensively for lighting in areas where electricity is not available, and in many parts of the country no other method of lighting is possible; however, their use has many disadvantages, for example:
  - the amount of light given off is not sufficient for most visual tasks
  - the light flickers
  - the products of combustion are added to the air
  - there is always the danger of fire.

- **Oil lamps:** Paraffin (kerosene) oil is the fuel most commonly used in these lamps. Depending on the size and design, a lamp should provide adequate light. However, the paraffin fumes generate air pollutants, such as carbon monoxide, nitrogen dioxide and a host of hydrocarbons and volatile organic compounds, and raise the room temperature. Paraffin lamps are a health hazard as they can be knocked over, leading to domestic fires and extensive burn wounds, especially in young children and the elderly.

- **Gas lamps:** Various kinds of gas such as coal gas, petrol gas or acetylene gas may be burnt to obtain light. Gas lamps provide adequate light but have the same disadvantages as oil lamps as the gases may emit toxic fumes. There is also the danger of explosion if the mechanism becomes defective.

- **Electric lighting:** This is the best kind of artificial lighting available. It does not pollute indoor air quality, nor does it warm the environment noticeably, it is relatively cheap, and it is possible to direct the light exactly where it is needed. South Africa is experiencing an ongoing energy crisis where 'rolling blackouts' or 'load shedding' has been implemented countrywide since 2007 to reduce the load on the national power system to curb imbalances between the demand for and availability of electricity. To avoid this situation, South Africans should keep striving to use electricity more efficiently.

Harnessing the sun's energy

The sun is the natural source of all radiant energy. Without sunlight, life on earth would not be possible because all life processes are dependent on this energy.

Scientists are working on ways to harness this energy and developing various types of renewable energy sources. One idea is a light called the Nokero ('No Kerosene') N200 LED light. These renewable solar lights have been manufactured in South Africa since 2010 and operate with a rechargeable AA-sized battery. The battery charges in the sun by day without the harmful effects of chemicals, paraffin, gas or other toxic materials.

Another solar solution is solar heating, which is a method of heating water that makes use of the sun's rays. There are a number of different types of solar heating systems on the market but essentially they consist of a glass panel or 'collector' that focuses the rays of the sun onto a plate containing metal tubes filled with water. The water flowing through the tubes is heated by the sun's rays and this hot water is then conducted to storage tanks. From the tanks the water is carried to the hot-water taps. Although solar heating systems are relatively expensive, solar heating has a number of advantages:

- It can be used in areas where electricity is not available.
- Once the system has been installed, the energy is free.
- It does not pollute the atmosphere.
- It is fuel-saving.

Artificial heating

During the winter months it is necessary to provide sufficient heat so that people remain comfortable in their workplace and at home.

Heat is transmitted in a room by means of convection, conduction and radiation.

- **Convection**: When air is heated it expands, becomes lighter and rises, and cold air flows in to take its place. This in turn is heated and rises up, and so currents of air, known as convection currents, are set up in a room.
- **Conduction**: A warm object in contact with a cooler object will lose heat to the cool object, the heat being passed from molecule to molecule by conduction. A poker placed in a fire is heated this way – the heat is conducted from the tip of the poker, which is in contact with the fire.
- **Radiation**: This is the transfer of heat from a source to an object without the intervening air being heated.

When a room is warmed by an open fire, for example, all three forces come into play. People and objects in front of the fire are warmed by radiation, and they, in turn, warm the surrounding air by conduction. This warm air will expand and rise and cool air will move in to take its place, causing convection currents.

Climate change

In addition to reducing South Africa's carbon footprint, the NDP also recommends steps to prepare South Africa for the effects of climate change. A strong emphasis on adaptation to climate change includes having an effective climate change mitigation and adaptation response, which is closely aligned with SDG 13. Climate change, or global warming, is defined as an ongoing series of changes in the earth's general weather conditions as a result of a rise in the temperature of the earth's surface. This, in turn, increases the temperature of the earth's atmosphere and oceans.

Between 2030 and 2050, climate change is expected to cause approximately 250 000 additional deaths per year related to malnutrition, malaria, diarrhoea and heat stress (WHO, 2018). The rise in the global temperature points to an increase in gas concentrations, known as greenhouse gases (GHGs). Gases are emitted into the atmosphere directly or indirectly as products of electricity generation. Carbon dioxide, a by-product of burning fossil fuels, is called a greenhouse gas because it contributes to global warming. GHGs form an insulating layer in the atmosphere, called the 'greenhouse effect', reducing the amount of the sun's heat that radiates back into space. The trapped radiation causes an increase in the temperature on earth.

Over the last 50 years, human activities, particularly the burning of fossil fuels, have released large quantities of carbon dioxide and other greenhouse gases to trap additional heat in the lower atmosphere, affecting the global climate. In the last 130 years, the world has warmed by approximately 0.85 °C.

Since 1850 each of the last three decades has been successively warmer than any preceding decade. Sea levels are rising, glaciers are melting and precipitation patterns are changing. Extreme weather events are becoming more intense and frequent (WHO, 2018). There is strong evidence to suggest that climate change will increasingly affect the world's agriculture and water supplies in years to come. There is also evidence that changes in land use through agriculture and deforestation has contributed to climate change.

Substantial changes in South Africa's climate are likely to be caused by variables such as rising temperatures, unusually heavy rainfall events and droughts. These changes in climate have a direct and/or indirect impact on the environment and put pressure on the natural resources necessary for survival.

Going green

Because of global warming, more and more people are becoming aware of their personal impact on the earth and environment. The term 'going green' has become synonymous with certain behaviours and includes a number of different practices designed to reduce waste, conserve energy and resources, promote sustainable living and encourage the use of environmentally friendly products. Examples of going green include:

- reducing waste and recycling reusable items
- reducing energy consumption and water usage
- buying local green products to reduce packaging and transporting
- growing a garden or composting kitchen waste
- buying sustainable building materials such as bamboo and recycled steel to conserve natural resources
- using public transport to reduce vehicle emissions
- using alternative energy sources, such as wind or solar energy.

The South African government supports green economy programmes and has implemented a number of projects that are geared towards a resource efficient, low carbon and pro-employment growth path. Natural resources are national economic assets and our economy depends on energy and mineral resources, biodiversity, agriculture, forestry, fishing and tourism. Every citizen has a fundamental responsibility to develop a green economy.

Household recycling – something we can all do

The underlying principle of recycling is to reduce the utilisation of natural resources and to re-use products before these are finally discarded and placed in landfills. When products such as plastic cold-drink containers are recycled, they are broken down into their constituent parts. These constituents are then re-used in the production of new products, for example pillow and duvet stuffing. Each of us can help by recycling:

➡

- metal (eg cold-drink and beer cans, food tins and aluminium cans)
- glass (eg beer bottles, jam jars and mayonnaise bottles)
- paper (eg newspapers, magazines, white office paper and cardboard boxes)
- plastic (eg milk and cold-drink bottles).

Much of the recycling in South Africa is collected by informal recyclers (bin pickers) who recover much of the waste material from dustbins and landfill sites. This situation is not ideal because of the potential health hazards, for example infection and toxification due to skin breakage, as well as cross contamination where recyclable material is contaminated with other waste. However, certain municipalities now provide a separate bin for recyclables.

Impact of climate change on environmental sustainability

Climate change affects the social and environmental determinants of health – clean air, safe drinking water, sufficient food and secure shelter. In this section we will examine some of the effects of climate change on the environment and society; these include threats to water security, agriculture and the built environment, as well as the social and health aspects of increased migration and change in rainfall patterns.

Water security

As South Africa's climate is characterised by dry, warm conditions, the country suffers periodic water shortages. Water shortages are made more severe by overpopulation, migration of people from other African countries to South Africa and continued urbanisation. All these factors increase the problem of access to water and adequate sanitation. Cholera outbreaks can be related to climate-induced circumstances such as seasonal changes brought on by wetter, warmer climatic conditions. As water is a vital natural resource for agriculture and fisheries, there could be severe implications for food security. Climate change is likely to lead to more intensely variable weather conditions, for example sudden high volumes of rainfall leading to flooding, in addition to severe droughts in other areas. Increased variability in rainfall patterns will result in less reliable stream flows, which will consequently lead to an increase in the unit cost of water from dams and thus an increase in consumer tariffs.

Agriculture

The increase of water scarcity and drought severely affects national water resources, which impacts on food production. Maize production falls in summer-rainfall areas, and fruit and cereal production fall in winter-rainfall areas. Droughts increase the frequency of wildfires brought about by the increasing number of hot days.

The built environment

Droughts and floods are capable of causing structural damage to roads and buildings, preventing the normal delivery of healthcare services and schooling. Sea levels rise, and storm surges may damage the built environment in coastal regions. Extreme wet and dry rainfall cycles cause greater soil movement, resulting in water and sewage pipes being more prone to cracking. This increases the financial burden of repairing and replacing drainage infrastructure.

Migration

Climate is believed to be a driver of migration out of the central areas of South Africa, where conditions are very dry and less hospitable. Lack of facilities and economic opportunities in remote rural areas has resulted in increased migration to the urban areas. Where population growth is highest, there tend to be more people living in poverty because of the detrimental impacts of overcrowding and competition for resources. As South Africa is a country where refugees and asylum seekers have freedom of movement and the right to work, the impact of climate change is likely to intensify the demand for scarce or depleted resources.

The impact of climate change on health

The WHO assessment concluded that climate change is expected to cause approximately 250 000 additional deaths per year between 2030 and 2050; 38 000 due to heat exposure in elderly people, 48 000 due to diarrhoea, 60 000 due to malaria, and 95 000 due to childhood undernutrition (WHO, 2018).

The influence of changes in the climate on the lives and health of people has huge implications:

- Extreme high air temperatures contribute directly to deaths from cardio-vascular and respiratory disease, particularly among elderly people. Rising temperatures and variable precipitation are likely to decrease the production of staple foods in many of the poorest regions. This will increase the prevalence of malnutrition and undernutrition.
- High temperatures also raise the levels of ozone and other pollutants in the air that worsen cardiovascular and respiratory disease. Pollen and other aeroallergen levels are higher in extreme heat and trigger asthma attacks, which affect around 300 million people worldwide.
- More than half of the world's population lives within 60 km of the sea. Rising sea levels and extreme weather may cause flood damage to homes, disrupt supplies of medical and health services and result in physical injuries and drownings.
- By the late 21st century, climate change is likely to increase the frequency and intensity of drought at global scale. A lack of safe water compromises hygiene and community diseases especially gastrointestinal conditions.

- Changes in climate are likely to lengthen the transmission seasons of important vector-borne diseases and to alter their geographic range. Climatic conditions strongly affect water-borne diseases and diseases transmitted through insects, snails or other cold-blooded animals.
- The prevalence of waterborne, airborne and vector-borne diseases such as diarrhoea, cholera and bilharzia may increase, especially where this coincides with inadequate access to sanitation.
- Malaria is strongly influenced by climate. Transmitted by Anopheles mosquitoes, malaria kills over 400 000 people every year – mainly children under five years old in certain African countries. The Aedes mosquito vector of dengue fever is also highly sensitive to climate conditions, and studies suggest that climate change is likely to continue to increase exposure to dengue.
- Where rainfall levels are projected to decrease (notably in the west of the country), issues of land degradation, soil erosion and lowered agricultural food production arise, resulting in food shortages, which in turn may lead to malnutrition.

Conclusion

It is clear that environmental sustainability is an important contributor to achieving health and alleviating poverty in South Africa. It is also clear that environmental health is not just the responsibility of government but also the responsibility of each of us living in South Africa; each of us should be aware of the impact of our actions on the environment.

Self-assessment

1. What is the composition of air?
2. Discuss causes of air pollution with applicable examples of each.
3. Discuss how you as a nurse can contribute in the community to sustain the environment.
4. Develop a mind map to depict the association between overcrowding and health.
5. Describe the impact of climate change on health.

Bibliography

Africa Check. 2019. Historical delivery of housing opportunities funded from the HSDG. DMNGT 2019/01/17. Available: https://africacheck.org/wp-content/uploads/2019/02/Housing-delivery-1994-to-2018.pdf (Accessed 14 September 2020).

Altieri, K. & Keen, S. 2016. The cost of air pollution in South Africa. International Growth Centre. Available: https://www.theigc.org/blog/the-cost-of-air-pollution-in-south-africa/ (Accessed 15 September 2020).

Barnes, B., Mathee, A., Thomas, E. & Bruce, N. 2009. Household energy, indoor air pollution and child respiratory health in South Africa. *Journal of Energy in Southern Africa*, 20(1). February 2009.

Bertollini, R., Haefliger, P., Prüss-Ustün, A. & Vickers, C. 2011. Knowns and unknowns on burden of disease due to chemicals: A systematic review. Available: http://www. biomedcentral. com/content/pdf/1476-069X-10-9.pdf (Accessed 14 September 2020).

Business Dictionary. nd. Available: http://www.businessdictionary.com/definition/ environmental-sustainability.html#ixzz1y8c7IMFv (Accessed 14 September 2020).

Cant, R.L., O'Donnell, M., Sims, S. & Harries, M. 2019. Overcrowded housing: One of a constellation of vulnerabilities for child sexual abuse. ScienceDirect. *Child Abuse & Neglect*, 93: 239-248. Available: https://www.sciencedirect.com/science/article/abs/pii/ S0145213419301796 (Accessed 14 September 2020).

Centre for Alternative Housing Finance (CAHF) in Africa. nd. South Africa. Macroeconomic overview 2019. Available: http://housingfinanceafrica.org/countries/south-africa/ (Accessed 14 September 2020)

Chutel, L. 2018. This picturesque corner of South Africa has the world's deadliest air pollution. Available: https://qz.com/africa/1441504/highest-concentration-of-deadly-air-pollution-found-in-south-africa/ (Accessed 14 September 2020).

Designing Buildings Ltd. 2020. Natural ventilation of buildings. Available: https:// www.designingbuildings.co.uk/wiki/Natural_ventilation_of_buildings (Accessed 14 September 2020).

Dreamstime. nd. Environmental pollution problems. Available: https://www.dreamstime. com/environmental-pollution-problems-set-pollution-air-water-deforestation-warning-signs-vector-illustrations-image123898630] (Accessed 15 September 2020).

ESKOM. nd. Load shedding – Frequently asked questions. Available: http://www. google.com/url?sa=t&rct=j&q=&esrc=s&source=web&cd=&ved=2ahUKEwjv1 oTQo-vrAhWSasAKHWzjDkQQFjABegQICxAD&url=http%3A%2F%2Fwww. eskom.co.za%2Fdocuments%2FLoadSheddingFAQ.pdf&usg=AOvVaw1oSu-wwtMX9FgRwnqWs3fd (Accessed 15 September 2020).

European Environment Agency. 2020. Health impacts of air pollution. Available: https:// www.eea.europa.eu/themes/air/health-impacts-of-air-pollution/health-impacts-of-air-pollution (Accessed 14 September 2020).

Frost, S. 2019. Definition of going green. Available: https://www.hunker.com/12000238/ definition-of-going-green (Accessed 15 September 2020).

Goyal, S. 2017. Is nitrogen important for human body? Available: https://www.jagranjosh. com/general-knowledge/is-nitrogen-important-for-human-body-1509531787-1 (Accessed 14 September).

Hamilton, C. & Bastianoni, S. 2019. Environmental protection and ecology. Available: https://www.sciencedirect.com/topics/earth-and-planetary-sciences/environmental-protection (Accessed 14 September 2020).

Heart and Stroke Foundation South Africa. nd. Air Pollution. Available: http://www. heartfoundation.co.za/pollution/ (Accessed 14 September 2020).

Helmenstine, A. 2019. The Chemical composition of air. Available: https://www.thoughtco. com/chemical-composition-of-air-604288 (Accessed 14 September 2020).

Impact Amplifier. 2018. South Africa's energy schizophrenia: Why hasn't the country achieved affordable power for the poor? 2018. Available at: https://www. impactamplifier.co.za/news/south-africas-energy-schizophrenia-hasnt-country-achieved-affordable-power-poor/ (Accessed 14 September 2020).

Langhof, O. & Tuele, R. 2011. The face of climate change in South Africa. Greenpeace Africa. Available: http://www.greenpeace.org/africa/en/News/Blog/the-face-of-climate-change-in-africa/blog/38164/ (Accessed 14 September 2020).

Naidoo, S. & Piketh, S. 2014. Domestic fuel combustion in un-electrified low-income settlements in South Africa. Available: https://www3.epa.gov/ttn/chief/conference/ei21/session2/naidoo.pdf (Accessed 14 September 2020).

NASA Climate Kids. nd. Available: https://climatekids.nasa.gov/air-pollution/ (Accessed 14 September 2020).

National Institute of Environmental Health Sciences. nd. Air pollution and your health. Available: https://www.niehs.nih.gov/health/topics/agents/air-pollution/index.cfm (Accessed 14 September 2020).

Nkosi, V., Haman, T., Naicker, N. & Mathee, A. 2019. Overcrowding and health in two impoverished suburbs in Johannesburg, South Africa. *BMC Public Health*. Available: https://bmcpublichealth.biomedcentral.com/articles/10.1186/s12889-019-7665-5 (Accessed 14 September 2020).

Novrangi, D.S., Tang, J. & Zhang, J.H. 2014. Argon gas: A potential neuroprotectant and promising medical therapy. Available: https://medicalgasresearch.biomedcentral.com/articles/10.1186/2045-9912-4-3 (Accessed 14 September 2020).

Pagalan, L., Bickford, C., Weikum, W., Brauer, M., Lanphear, N., Hanley, G.E., Oberlander, T.F. & Winters, M. 2019. Association of Prenatal Exposure to Air pollution with autism spectrum disorder. *JAMA Pediatrics*.2018.3101.doi 10.1001.

Republic of South Africa. 1996. Green paper on an environmental policy for South Africa (October). Available at: http://www.info.gov.za/greenpapers/1996/environmental. htm. (Accessed 14 September 2020).

Republic of South Africa. 1997. Housing Act 107 of 1997, as amended. Pretoria: SA Government.

Republic of South Africa. 2004. Library of Congress (LOC). Regulation on air pollution. Available: https://www.loc.gov/law/help/air-pollution/southafrica.php (Accessed 14 September 2020).

Republic of South Africa. 2015. Housing. Available: https://www.gov.za/links/housing-0?gclid=EAIaIQobChMIk9-jzb7r6wIVz9_tCh2nuA2iEAAYASAAEgIo9PD_BwE (Accessed 15 September 2020).

Republic of South Africa. 2018. Department of Statistics. General household survey 2018. Available: http://www.statssa.gov.za/?p=12180 (Accessed 15 September 2020).

Republic of South Africa. 2019. Department of Environment, Forestry and Fisheries. About green economy. Available: https://www.environment.gov.za/projectsprogrammes/greeneconomy/about (Accessed 15 September 2020).

Rhodes University. 2020. Environmental legislation and policies 2020. Available: https://www.ru.ac.za/environmentalsustainability/resources/envirolegislation/ (Accessed 14 September 2020).

Schilder, P. 2018. Trends in SA health care HVAC design. Available: https://www. refrigerationandaircon.co.za/index.php/features/air-conditioning/344-trends-in-sa-health-care-hvac-design (Accessed 14 September 2020).

South African Alternative Energy Association (SAAEA). nd. Available: http://saaea.org (Accessed 14 September 2020).

South African Bureau of Standards (SABS). nd. South African National Standards (SANS): National Building Regulations. Available: https://www.sans10400.co.za/ (Accessed 14 September 2020).

South African Bureau of Standards (SABS). nd. South African National Standards (SANS): Good lighting and ventilation is vital for healthy living. Available: https://www.sans10400. co.za/lighting-and-ventilation/comment-page-2/ (Accessed 14 September 2020).

Statistics South Africa (StatsSA). 2016. General household survey report (GHSR). Available: http://www.statssa.gov.za/?p=9922&gclid=EAIaIQobChMI3-qIq83q6wIVWODtCh0u eQDlEAAYASAAEgKDMvD_BwE (Accessed 15 September 2020).

Statistics South Africa (StatsSA). 2018. Energy and the poor: A municipal breakdown. 2018. Available: http://www.statssa.gov.za/?p=11181 (Accessed 14 September 2020).

Sustainable Businesses. 2019. What is environmental sustainability? Available: https://www. thebalancesmb.com/what-is-sustainability-3157876 (Accessed 14 September 2020).

United Nations (UN). 2015. Sustainable Development Goals. Knowledge Platform. Transforming our world: The 2030 agenda for sustainable development. Available: https://sustainabledevelopment.un.org/post2015/transformingourworld (Accessed 15 September 2020).

Wikipedia. nd. Air pollution. Available: http://en.wikipedia.org/wiki/Air_pollution (Accessed 14 September 2020).

Wikipedia. nd. Rolling blackout. Available: wikipedia.org/wiki/Rolling_blackout (Accessed 14 September 2020).

World Health Organization (WHO). 2005. Air quality guidelines for particulate matter, ozone, nitrogen dioxide and sulfur dioxide. Global update: Summary of risk assessment. Available: https://www.who.int/airpollution/publications/aqg2005/en/. (Accessed 15 September 2020).

World Health Organization (WHO). 2013. Outdoor air pollution a leading environmental cause of cancer deaths. Available: https://www.iarc.fr/wp-content/uploads/2018/07/ pr221_E.pdf (Accessed 15 September 2020).

World Health Organization (WHO). 2014. 7 million premature deaths annually linked to air pollution. Available: https://www.who.int/mediacentre/news/releases/2014/air-pollution/en/ (Accessed 15 September 2020).

World Health Organization (WHO). 2018. Climate change and health. Available: https:// www.who.int/news-room/fact-sheets/detail/climate-change-and-health (Accessed 14 September 2020).

World Health Organization (WHO). 2020a. Ambient air pollution. Available: http://www. who.int/airpollution/ambient/health-impacts/en/ (Accessed 14 September 2020).

World Health Organization (WHO). 2020b. Modes of transmission of virus causing COVID-19: implications for IPC precaution recommendations. Available: https://www. who.int/news-room/commentaries/detail/modes-of-transmission-of-virus-causing-covid-19-implications-for-ipc-precaution-recommendations (Accessed 14 September 2020).

Safe water and sanitation

Roelien Els

16

Learning outcomes

After studying this chapter, you should be able to:

- Discuss different sources of water.
- Define the terms 'water service' and 'basic water supply'.
- Outline the management of water resources in South Africa.
- Describe the most important water-related diseases.
- Explain the term 'basic sanitation service'.
- Outline the management of refuse disposal.
- Discuss the general diseases associated with inadequate sanitation.
- Make suggestions about the responsibility of the nursing profession towards the realisation of Sustainable Development Goal (SDG) 6.

Key terms

Aquifer: A geological formation which has structures or textures that hold water or permit water movement through them.

Borehole: A well, excavation or any artificially constructed or improved underground cavity which can be used for the purpose of intercepting, collecting or storing water in or removing water from an aquifer.

Catchment: The area from which any rainfall will drain into the watercourse through surface flow to a common point.

Conservation: The efficient use and saving of water by using measures such as water saving devices, water-efficient processes, water demand management and water rationing.

Pollution: The presence in or introduction into the environment of a substance that has harmful poisonous effects.

Purification: A process of removing undesirable chemicals, biological contaminants, suspended solids and gases from water with the goal of producing water fit for a specific purpose.

Waste: Any solid material that is suspended, dissolved or transported in water (including sediment) that is spilled or deposited on land or into a water resource that it is likely to cause pollution of the water resource.

Watercourse: A river or spring, a natural channel in which water flows regularly or intermittently, a wetland or dam into which or from which water flows and any collection of water that the Minister declares to be a watercourse.

Introduction

At the World Summit on Sustainable Development in 2002, former President Nelson Mandela said: 'Among the many things that I learned as president was the centrality of water for social, political and economic affairs of the country, the continent and the world' (RSA, 2002).

It is estimated that demand for water will exceed supply by 2025 if nothing is done to supplement current water resources. The World Health Organization (WHO) estimates that half of the world's population will be living in water-stressed areas by 2025 (WHO, 2019). South Africa's status as a water-scarce country is reflected in the formulation of our legislative framework. According to the Constitution, actual delivery of water is the responsibility of local government. Meeting this universal service obligation requires that each South African has access to at least a basic water supply. The National Water Act 36 of 1998 and Water Services Act 108 of 1997 specifically address water resource and catchment management strategies to meet our future water needs. In 2013, the Department of Water and Environmental Affairs (now the Department of Water and Sanitation, or DWS) published the National Water Resource Strategy (NWRS2) to secure and protect our current water resources in South Africa. Some of the achievements made on national level by the DWS are extracted from this report (DWS, 2015):

- Installation of water meters in priority catchment areas to monitor water use
- Installation of additional water pipelines and pump stations, raising dam walls and completion of dam constructions
- Allocation and provision of water to households and resource poor farmers
- Implementation of measures to optimise water plant capacity
- Generating hydropower
- Compulsory licensing of Catchment Management Areas

- Assess wastewater treatment collector systems for compliance with effluent standards (Green Drop progress report)
- Assess water supply systems for compliance to drinking water standards (Blue Drop report).

In the sections that follow, we will look more closely at water sources, the protection thereof, goals for water provision and general principles of water use. As a nurse working in the community setting, you need to know about impurities present in water and apply this knowledge to promote the general health of the community, and more specifically, educate the public to prevent waterborne diseases.

Water

Water is derived from the moisture that evaporates from the surface of the oceans, dams and rivers and that later falls as rain. When rain falls, about one-third of water runs off, one-third percolates into the soil, and one-third evaporates. The two main natural catchment sources of water derive from surface water and ground water.

Surface water

Surface water refers to water bodies on the surface of the earth, such as rivers, streams and wetlands. It is further divided into upland and lowland surface water, as described below.

Upland surface water

This is water that has its source above the level of human or animal habitation, usually in high mountainous areas. It is therefore free from impurities and pathogens. The water drains down the mountainside into the valleys where it may form streams, dams, or rivers. Dams may also be constructed by engineers to dam up water in a valley.

Rivers that flow through densely populated areas are particularly heavily polluted. Where a town obtains its water from such a source, it must undergo intensive purification before it can be distributed to consumers.

Lowland surface water

In this case the source of the water lies below the level of human and animal habitation, and as the water is likely to be polluted it is an unsafe source of supply for human consumption.

Groundwater

The nature of groundwater depends on the geological formation of the earth. The earth's crust is formed by the soil, which consists of powdered rock and organic matter, including bacteria. The subsoil consists of powdered rock only and there is no organic matter present in it.

Below the subsoil is a rock layer, known as the first impervious (non-porous) layer. Water cannot pass through this rock unless it finds a fissure or crack in the rock.

A second layer of rock, which lies below the first, is known as the second impervious layer. A layer of subsoil may be found between these two rock strata. None of these layers lies straight and level, and they can be pictured rising and falling much as the surface of the earth rises and falls when it forms mountains, hills and valleys.

When it rains, the water that seeps into the soil comes to rest above the rock at different levels.

- *Subsoil water* is water that has come to rest above the first impervious layer. It is also known as shallow water.

- *Deep water* is water that has seeped through a fissure or crack in the rock and lies above the second impervious layer.

Springs

If underground water is under pressure it may be forced to the surface and form a spring, which will flow out of an opening called the eye of the spring. An artesian well is one from which the water gushes to the surface and does not have to be pumped out.

The quality of underground water depends on whether it lies above or below the first impervious layer. Water from below the first impervious layer is generally free from bacterial contamination because impurities are removed as the water percolates through the soil, which acts as a filter; but water from above this layer may contain pathogenic organisms.

All underground water has a high mineral salt content because it dissolves out of the soil. It is known as hard water.

Wells

To obtain water from an underground source, a well or a borehole has to be constructed. It is important that these are effectively constructed and maintained to prevent contamination of the water. Pollution of a well takes place in two ways:

- Impurities are washed into the mouth of the well from the surface.
- There may be seepage into the well through the sides.

The division of water according to its natural source is greatly influenced by the following:

- *The nature of the soil:* water seeps more readily into sandy soils than into clay.
- *The nature of the countryside*: if it is hilly, then more of the rain will run off into the streams and rivers.
- *The temperature of the atmosphere*: the higher the temperature, the more water will evaporate.

Protection of water sources

The protection of water resources is closely linked to its uses, conservation, management and control. If a local authority obtains water from a catchment area, the rights to the catchment area is also acquired to prevent humans and animals from gaining access to it, ie the right to fence the area in. Water in transit will be conducted in pipes and not open channels from the source of the reservoirs to prevent contamination.

Water pollution occurs as a result of activities on land. When people litter on land, it collects in rivers and ultimately washes down to the ocean. Industries such as oil refineries, paper mills and chemical, electronics and automobile manufacturers pump toxic effluent into nearby water sources, which end up in dams and oceans. Ocean pollution has become a problem of epic proportions. Untreated sewage, including household and medical chemicals and industrial pollutants are pumped into the ocean where marine outfall pipes extend deep into the ocean with long-term consequences on water quality and serious threats to marine systems. Examples of pollutants that affect water ecosystems include:

- human sewage
- microplastics (small plastic beads) found in toothpaste, facial cleaners and kitchen rubs
- agricultural fertilisers and pesticides
- industrial sulphur, heavy metals and cyanide
- coal mining processes that contaminate groundwater, rivers and the ocean with heavy metals, coal ash and mercury from acid-mine drainage, causing acid rain and thermal pollution.

The person who owns, controls, occupies or uses the land is responsible for taking measures to prevent pollution of water resources. If appropriate measures to prevent pollution are not followed, the catchment management agency may intervene and recover the costs incurred from the person responsible for the pollution.

The following measures must be taken to prevent and remedy the effects of water pollution:

- Stop, adjust operations and control any act or process that causes the pollution.
- Contain and prevent further spread of pollutants.

- Eliminate all sources of pollution.
- Comply with prescribed waste standards.
- Remedy the effects of the pollution, such as the bed and banks of a water-course.

Catchment management

A catchment management strategy is a legislative requirement in South Africa and supports the national water resource strategy. The norms and standards for levels of water services align with the principles of universal access, human dignity, user participation, service standards, redress, and value for money. The principles of sustainability, affordability, effectiveness, efficiency and appropriateness should be maintained in supplying safe water to the community. The National Water Act 36 of 1998 (RSA, 1998) differentiates between the basic human needs reserve and the ecological reserve. Basic human needs reserve includes water for drinking and food preparation and for personal hygiene. A *basic water supply* is defined as a minimum volume of potable water to a formal connection at the boundary of a stand or site of public institutions such as schools, clinics and hospitals (DWS, 2017). The ecological reserve relates to the water required to protect the aquatic ecosystems of the water resource.

Conventional water-treatment processes remove organic substances from raw water up to the stage of chemical treatment to ensure a safe drinking-water supply to the community. This causes changes in the physical and chemical composition of water. Local municipalities are responsible for monitoring changes and preventing a decline in water quality through quality surveys. Water services refer to water supply and sanitation services and include:

- regional water schemes
- local water schemes
- on-site sanitation
- collection and treatment of wastewater.

Water provision goals

The National Water Act 36 of 1998 (RSA, 1998) defines 'water use' as activities which reduce stream flow, waste discharges and disposals, controlled activities which impact detrimentally on a water resource, altering a watercourse, removing water found underground for certain purposes, taking and storing of water, and water used for recreation. The goal of water provision to households and public facilities links to specific goals for water services. These goals are discussed below:

- *Water quality* – Goal: people have access to potable water that is fit for human use and comply with the national water quality standards. The SANS 241 guideline (2015) specifies the quality of acceptable drinking water in terms of microbiological, physical, aesthetic and chemical characteristics (SABS, 2015).

- *Pressure in water reticulation systems* – Goal: people have access to potable water for human use at a constant pressure. Potable water shall be made available at a water point at a minimum of 10 liters per minute, to the minimum of quantity potable water of 25L/c/d to consumers, at a typical water pressure in the water inlet between 40 and 45 psi (290 kPa) to a household.
- *Water metering* – Goal: all water use is measured and metered to ensure sustainable and effective use of water. All users shall be educated that water is an economic good which needs regulation by metering.
- *Water tariffing* – Goal: all water use will be charged for to enable effective and productive water use. The DWS will review water tariffs along the water provisioning cycle, including water management charges, raw water, water board and municipal tariffs.
- *Water re-use and recycling* – Goal: water re-use and recycling must be investigated and advocated to promote water conservation.
- *Asset management* – Goal: implementing effective asset management practices to ensure sustainable and reliable water services in the protection of public health and the environment.

The community nurse supports government's water services goals by cultivating an awareness and motivating the community to conserve water where possible.

Water re-use and recycling

The 'National Strategy for Water Re-use' support safe and efficient strategies of water recycling (DWA, 2013). Treated water can be supplied directly to households (direct re-use) or be discharged back to the freshwater resource where it is blended with other water and subsequently treated and distributed for indirect re-use. The overall demand for fresh water should be reduced through water-wise landscaping, rainwater harvesting, and water-efficient appliances and manufacturing processes with lower water needs than conventional methods. Previously used water (wastewater and effluent) can be treated to a standard fit for domestic use (drinking purposes).

Re-using greywater

Greywater from kitchen sinks, dishwashers and washing machines can be re-used as a biologically active topsoil layer to provide nutrients for plants because soil bacteria quickly break down the organic solids. The value of soil bacteria as biological water purifier contributes to the protection of ground and surface water quality. Greywater systems for the safe re-use of greywater from baths, showers and hand basins are available and easy to install. Greywater re-use systems can also be economically installed for:

- gardening and irrigation
- flushing toilets, washing yards, cars, pavements and driveways
- agriculture and aquaculture
- industrial cooling
- fire fighting.

Rainwater conservation

Unpredictable changes to our climate, such as erratic rainfall patterns, droughts and heatwaves that affect natural water supplies, have made it necessary to develop certain self-help plans to conserve water in an economical way. Rainwater harvesting is part of this plan and has been implemented as a technique to collect, concentrate and store rainwater that runs off a natural or constructed catchment surface. Rainwater from roofs and ground surfaces can be collected in above-ground or underground storage tanks. (See Chapter 15 for a full discussion on climate change.)

Access to water using this method will enable poor households to grow fresh food at home, and surplus growth can generate income.

The disadvantages of relying on rain as a source of water include the following:

- It is an uncertain source of supply and there are very few parts of South Africa where rain will meet a community's needs for water.
- It is not as palatable as other water because of its lack of mineral salts.
- It can be polluted during collection and storage.

Common water contaminants

As a result of water pollution, water is loaded with impurities. Each impurity in water carries its own biological or chemical risk and poses serious health problems and even death. Appearance and taste are not indicative of the purity of water, and water may be grossly contaminated without its clarity or taste being affected. Contaminated water contains different elements known as total dissolved solids (TDS). Impurities in the water may be suspended or dissolved.

- *Suspended impurities* consist of substances that are insoluble in water. They may be inorganic, for example silt, dust, rust, clay and sand, or organic, for example biological contaminants such as bacteria, viruses and the ova and larvae of parasites. Chemical contaminants cannot be removed by simple filtration processes.
- *Dissolved impurities* are mainly inorganic and consist of mineral salts and metals such as calcium, magnesium, lead, nitrate, mercury, fluoride and arsenic, which are present in the waste dumped by industries.

The purity and chemical composition of water may be examined by taking samples of the water for chemical and bacteriological examination. Clean

Winchester bottles may be used for collecting water for chemical analysis, but if bacteriological examination is required, laboratory-certified, sterile sample containers must be used. Water samples must be kept below 0 °C to maintain the cold chain for analysis purposes.

Inadequate waterborne sanitation systems, malfunctioning pumps, inefficient treatment plants, poor plant designs, and poor operating and maintenance also lead to deposits of the following impure components in wastewater:

- overdose in chlorine residue in the final effluent, which affects the aquatic ecosystem's ability to support aquatic life
- unbalanced levels of biological oxygen, dissolved oxygen and total nitrogen and phosphate
- high concentrations of potassium and nitrogen in groundwater
- high levels of *Escherichia coli* – these spills cause massive fish kills, with health and economic implications.

Water-related diseases

Waterborne diseases are any illness caused by drinking water contaminated by human or animal faeces, as it contains pathogenic microorganisms. In developing countries four-fifths of all illnesses are caused by waterborne diseases, with diarrhoea being one of the leading causes of childhood death.

Contamination is likely to occur where public and private drinking water systems obtain water from surface waters (rain, creeks, rivers, dams), which can be contaminated by infected animals or people. Runoff from landfills, septic fields, sewer pipes, and residential or industrial developments can also contaminate surface water. Waterborne diseases can have dramatic outbreaks of faecal–oral diseases such as cholera and typhoid.

Water sanitation and hygiene have an important impact on both health and disease. Diseases and infections may be due to the presence of pathogenic organisms or the ova and/or larvae of parasites in the water, or indirectly because certain insect vectors require water for part of their life cycle. Chemicals such as mercury and lead, insecticides, radioactive wastes and many other substances may cause serious toxic conditions. Examples of water-related diseases include:

- those due to microorganisms in drinking water causing diarrhoea, hepatitis A and E, salmonellosis, dysentery, cholera, typhoid and para-typhoid fever
- arsenicosis, fluorosis and lead poisoning caused by chemicals in drinking water
- diseases like schistosomiasis and giardiasis, malaria and dengue fever, where the vectors spend part of their life cycle in water
- breathing in mists from water sources such as air conditioning, cooling systems and spas, which could be contaminated by Legionella bacteria
- bathing or drinking water contaminated with blue-green algae.

A lack of water leads to poor personal hygiene and conditions such as pediculosis, scabies, trachoma, leprosy and ringworm (tinea).

Activity: Using water to transform poverty

Rural households in South Africa continue to face hunger, malnutrition and lack of income. Former state president Thabo Mbeki once demonstrated the individual responsibility of every citizen of South Africa to conserve water by asking the residents from a rural village how they are using their water to be economically active (The Mvula Trust, nd).

To facilitate interactive group discussion, review literature resources with related topics on the internet. An appropriate website to browse is http://www.mvula.co.za/.

Brainstorm the effects of inadequate water supply on a rural community. Make suggestions on practical, sustainable methods to educate people on the conservation of water in different kinds of communities.

Explain the application of the terms 'multiple use system' (MUS) and 'securing water to enhance local livelihoods' (SWELL) as tools to improve a community's economic viability.

Purification of drinking water

When rain falls on the earth's surface, it mixes with substances such as silt, minerals and even bacteria from the land. By the time the water reaches dams and rivers, it contains various hazardous substances and must be purified to make it fit for human consumption. The purification process starts when this 'raw water' is piped to a treatment plant where it passes through wire screens that trap solid objects such as water plants, animal carcasses, sand, silt, clay particles, sticks, leaves and litter. The raw water also contains bacteria, viruses and hazardous minerals such as iron, aluminum and manganese.

The water then enters a spiral flocculator where slaked lime is added. The water moves around very quickly to ensure good contact with the slaked lime to attract the sand, silt and clay particles. A chemical coagulant is used to enable microscopic dirt particles to coagulate into larger flocks, which then sink to the bottom of the sedimentation tank. The sedimentation at the bottom of the tank is called sludge and is sucked out to a sludge deposit site. The surface water in the tank is now much cleaner and flows over the side of the sedimentation tank into the carbonation tank.

The lime that is added in the purification process during flocculation changes the water's pH to about 10.5, making it taste and feel soapy. Carbon dioxide is added to make the water less alkaline (ie a pH of between 8.0 and 8.4). The water is maintained at this pH because it tastes and feels better and causes calcium carbonate deposits to form a protective layer inside the pipes.

From here the water flows into a filter house, then slowly through big sand filter beds to remove small water plants and animals. It then enters underground pipes, where chlorine gas is released into the water to remove pathogens such as bacteria.

The clean water is then pumped through underground pipes to booster pumping stations. Chlorine is effective for six to eight hours and therefore chloramine (chlorine and ammonia) is added to kill any remaining pathogens. From the booster pumping station water is pumped into reservoirs and then sold to municipalities to supply to homes and factories.

Purification of water on a small scale

Small-scale methods of water purification are boiling, distillation, filtration and disinfection. Each of these methods is described below.

Boiling

Boiling water for 10 minutes will destroy most pathogens but will not kill spores. If the water is required for domestic purposes only, this is of no consequence to health. When completely sterile water is required, it must be distilled, as even boiling for 20 minutes will not destroy spores. Boiling makes water less palatable because it removes the dissolved gases from it, but this can be remedied by pouring the water from one container to another, the two containers being held some distance from each other. This process will aerate the water.

Distillation

This is done by bringing water to the boil and then leading the steam to another container where it condenses and forms water again. Distilled water is pure, but distillation is not used to produce drinking water because it lacks dissolved minerals such as magnesium and calcium.

Filtration

Various kinds of domestic filters are available for the filtration of relatively small amounts of drinking water, but filters may become colonised by pathogenic bacteria that will enter the water as it passes through the filter. Filters must therefore be cleaned thoroughly and boiled from time to time to prevent contamination of water.

A fairly reliable filter for small-scale use in rural areas can be constructed by filling a steel drum with layers of small stones, gravel and sand, and allowing the water to run through. This method is illustrated in Figure 16.1.

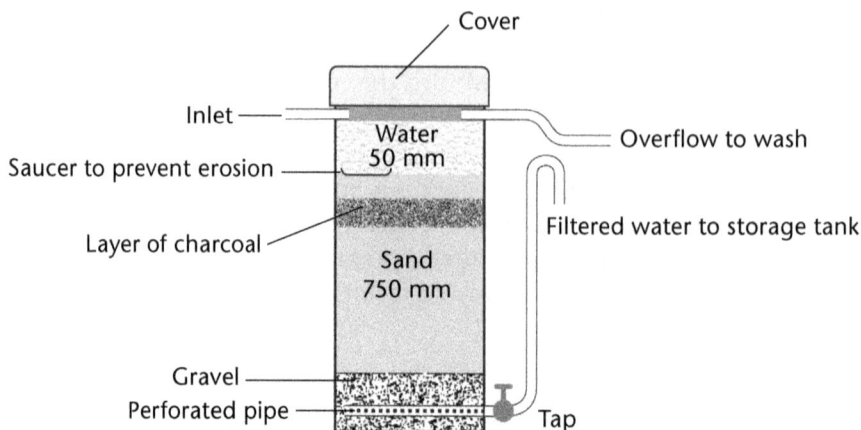

Figure 16.1 Water filter suitable for rural areas

Disinfection

On a small scale, disinfection of water may be achieved by the addition of small quantities of chemicals such as chlorine or bleach. Mix 8 drops (0.75 millilitres) of bleach to 4 litres (16 cups) of water. If the water is cloudy, mix 16 drops (ie 1,5 millilitres or 1/4 teaspoon) of bleach to 4 litres (16 cups) of water. The water needs to stand for 30 minutes or more before it is safe to drink. Many commercial preparations are available for the sterilisation of water and these should be used according to the directions on the label. They are useful when travelling or camping in areas where water supplies are likely to be contaminated.

The water services authorities (WSA) in South Africa (NBI, 2019) also regulate sanitation services in order to promote hygiene for all citizens in our country. This chapter deals with important aspects of sanitation to enable the nurse to serve the community in the promotion of health and prevention of sanitation-related diseases.

Environmental hygiene

Healthy populations are essential for the advancement of human development, well-being and economic growth. The 2030 Agenda for Sustainable Development (UN, 2015) underpins the importance of hygiene in goalsetting to 'achieve access to adequate and equitable sanitation and hygiene for all and end open defecation, paying special attention to the needs of women and girls and those in vulnerable situations' by 2030.

South Africa's 826 landfill sites take in 98 million tons of waste each year. Just less than 39 per cent of general waste is recycled and more than 61 per cent treated or landfilled, while just 6 per cent of hazardous waste is re-used or recycled and 94 per cent treated or landfilled. Human communities produce many kinds of waste.

The amount and type of household refuse depends on the characteristics of the community and usually includes the following types of waste:

- Household refuse, which consists of liquid waste from sinks, baths and basins, as well as dry refuse such as bottles, tins, paper, containers and wrappings of all kinds, and food waste
- Human excreta in the form of sewage.
- Industrial waste.

Household refuse: Dry or solid refuse

If refuse is not stored properly, removed regularly and disposed of adequately, it will pollute the environment, attract rodents, and provide breeding areas for flies and mosquitoes.

Household refuse must be stored in bins with tight-fitting lids, which should always be kept sealed. These containers may be made of galvanised iron or a hard-composition material. Many local authorities require the householder to line the bin with a large plastic bag. The use of plastic bags is hygienic and reduces the risk of littering as it keeps the litter contained once it is removed from the bin. In urban areas, the refuse is removed once or twice a week and the vehicles used for refuse collection are specially designed to prevent garbage from spilling out onto the streets.

In rural areas, where refuse is not collected on a regular basis, domestic refuse must be dealt with regularly and not be allowed to accumulate. It should be kept in suitable containers with tight-fitting lids. Organic material can be composted and used as fertiliser, while food waste and plant material can be used to feed animals. Refuse that is not suitable for these purposes may be buried or burned.

Industrial disposal of household refuse

Once the local authority has collected the waste, it may be disposed of in several ways:

- **Incineration**: The refuse is burned in large incinerators and the ash and clinker that remain are used for road works. More recently, building blocks for the construction of dwellings have been made from the clinker. The heat from these incinerators may be used for industrial purposes. Incineration is not the ideal method of disposal as it is expensive, it pollutes the atmosphere and it is wasteful as it destroys material that could have been recycled.
- **Controlled tipping**: The local authority has to select a suitable site, usually well away from residential areas. Refuse is deposited in layers of about 2 metres in depth. Each layer is covered with 220 millimetres of soil or ash at the end of the day's tipping. This is done to prevent flies and rodents

from gaining access to the refuse. Controlled tipping is often used to fill in and reclaim land for later use as parks, sports fields and, in some cases, for buildings. However, it does have some disadvantages, for example:

- in urbanised, industrialised areas, land close to towns and cities is expensive; on the other hand, if the site is too far from the town the cost of transporting the refuse to the site becomes prohibitive
- slow combustion occurs within the dump and this causes certain substances to ignite. Once this happens the dump may burn for some time. This pollutes the atmosphere and creates a health hazard.

- **Pulverisation**: Where this method is used the refuse is ground down to a fine powder in large machines and then either tipped, as in controlled tipping, or packed into bags and sold as fertiliser. This method of refuse disposal is common in many Western European countries.

- **Recycling**: Because the removal and disposal of refuse is a costly operation, it is desirable to reduce the volume of the waste. The best way of doing this is to remove anything that may be recycled. Paper, cardboard, glass, tins and plastic can all be salvaged and reprocessed. This serves not only to reduce the volume of the refuse, and therefore the cost of the operation, but also helps to preserve the world's rapidly dwindling resources. The topic of recycling is dealt with in more detail in Chapter 15.

Government policy underpins pollution risk management. Safe human excreta and sludge-effluent management, in return, prevent water contamination and contribute ultimately to the protection of our water resources.

Human excreta: Treatment of wastewater in the sewerage system

Raw sewage is screened to remove large objects and then passed on to primary settling tanks, where sludge particles sink to the bottom. The overflow from primary settling tanks then gravitates into the balancing tanks and from there into an activated sludge reactor. The by-now clear effluent goes through an anaerobic zone, where it is deprived of oxygen, and from there it is transferred to the secondary settling tanks. Chlorine is added at this stage to kill harmful human bacteria and viruses. The water then remains in a maturation river for about 12 hours before being discharged into a natural river.

Sanitation

South Africa has placed an on-going focus on the reduction of the sanitation backlog with regular sanitation policy reviews and legislative amendments. The National Sanitation Policy 2016 (RSA, 2016) addresses the following minimum criteria for basic sanitation:

,opriate health and hygiene awareness and behaviour

.ne lowest cost for an appropriate system of disposing of human excreta, household wastewater and grey water without having a detrimental impact on the environment

- Adequate toilet and handwashing facilities to ensure clean living environments at household and community level
- Consideration of defecation practices of small children and people with disabilities and special needs.

Many different types of sanitation technology are currently used in South Africa, including buckets (priority has been given to eradicating this system), pit latrines (with or without ventilation), chemical toilets (also to be replaced with more appropriate technology types such as dry sanitation toilets), flush toilets with on-site septic tanks and disposal, and flush toilets with waterborne and central treatment works.

An efficient method of disposal will prevent the contamination of water supplies and pastures, reduce the possibility of insect infestation (eg flies and mosquitoes), and prevent the occurrence of insect-related disease transmission.

Disposal of human excreta

Safe disposal of human excreta is a major priority for the health of all beings. The National Norms and Standards for Domestic Water and Sanitation Services (DWS, 2017) has as one of its goals, an environment free from human faeces. The following standards (DWS, 2017) address the safe disposal of excreta:

- Excreta disposal and/or containment measures shall protect surface water, groundwater and groundwater sources from faecal contamination. Therefore:
  - All excreta containment measures, ie trench latrines, ventilated improved privy (VIP) toilets and soakaway pits, shall be at least 50 metres away from groundwater sources. This distance needs to be increased for fissured rocks and limestone.
  - The bottom of any toilet or soak-away pit shall be at least 1.5 metres above the water table. This distance needs to be increased for fissured rocks and limestone. Sanitation facilities shall not contaminate freshwater resources or create health risks for people or the environment.
- The necessary measures and training shall be put in place and enforced to raise awareness and change practices to ensure the appropriate disposal of human faeces.

Human excreta may be dealt with in one of two ways:
- the conservancy method
- the sewerage or water-carriage system.

The conservancy method

- **The VIP toilet:** The ventilated improved privy (VIP) toilet is the minimum acceptable level of basic sanitation in South Africa (Still et al, nd). VIP toilets provide effective sanitation to the majority of rural and peri-urban households. Since 2003, all new VIPs funded by the government have been made from concrete blocks and panels. The concrete slab has two holes over the pit. In places where the soil is unstable, the pit of the VIP toilet needs to be lined to prevent it from collapsing. Later initiatives led to a design where the pit was lined by putting wedge-shaped blocks in place, backfilling and compacting the soil, which resulted in a shorter construction time of the pit and a cost-effective lining that boosted local economic development. Most VIPs are constructed for a 10-year life span, leading to sanitary problems when the VIP pits are full. Possible solutions were trialed around the world, one of which included digging a new pit close to the existing toilet, using a portable petrol-driven suction pump to transfer the contents to the new pit, and then closing the old pit over with soil. VIP toilets cannot be built in landscapes with shallow rocks or high water tables. Many alternatives have been explored and a combination of a urine diversion toilet and external compost heap has been found to be the most effective solution. A special toilet seat is applied to separate urine from faeces. The faeces drop into a small chamber beneath the seat. Soil is added each time the toilet is used to help dry out the faeces. The waste is removed monthly and transferred to a compost heap. The heat in the compost heap destroys pathogens, and the waste breaks down into compost that is safe to use.

- **Borehole latrines:** These are made by drilling a hole, about 400 mm in diameter and as deep as possible, into the earth. The latrine is then constructed in a similar way to a pit privy and the same precautions are taken to prevent the transmission of pathogens.

- **Dry-earth closets:** A pail is used to receive the excreta and a small amount of dry earth is deposited on the excreta when a handle is released. Bacteria present in the soil act on the faeces, rendering them harmless. The pail must be removed, emptied and cleansed.

- **Chemical closets:** These closets also contain a pail that receives the excreta. A chemical that breaks down the excreta and deodorises it is poured over the contents of the pail. The pails must be removed, emptied and cleaned. The contents of the pails can be buried.

- **Bucket system:** The local authority is responsible for the removal of the pails from the householders' premises at regular intervals. One pail is in use while a second pail is removed for cleaning and disinfection. The used pails are exchanged at regular intervals for clean ones. It is advisable to use pails that are fitted with lids that can be clamped tightly over the top of the pail. The lid can then be clamped onto the pail and the pail removed together with its contents. This means that the pail does not have to be emptied into a tank wagon in the street, and so spilling of the contents and the release of offensive odours are prevented. Government is committed to replacing this system, which is currently the most used system.

- **The sewerage or water-carriage system**: Although this method of disposal eliminates the danger of the transmission of pathogens such as salmonella, it is an expensive method of disposal and very wasteful of water.

Human excreta and liquid wastes are transported from the building by means of water. Soil pipes and waste pipes carry the wastes from the building to large underground sewers. These sewers transport the wastes to the sewage disposal works where they are safely and effectively dealt with.

A sewerage system comprises:

- water closets or toilets to receive the excreta
- basins, baths and sinks
- waste pipes that lead from toilets to sewers
- waste pipes that lead from basins, baths and sinks to sewers
- sewers
- sewage disposal works (sewage treatment plants).

Industrial waste disposal

The local government sector is mandated to provide waste management services. There are special problems associated with the disposal of industrial waste, because it is produced in vast quantities and often contains toxic chemicals. Landfills in Gauteng and the Western Cape are almost at capacity and these cities are constantly in search of more landfill facilities. Factories are obligated by law to ensure that the waste they produce is rendered harmless before it is disposed of into rivers or the sea. Non-toxic effluent may be disposed of into sewers.

Conclusion

South Africa faces many challenges in managing its water resources and stopping the illegal dumping of pollutants. Though progress has been made in providing access to clean water and an acceptable sewerage system for all, much still needs to be done in this area. It should be remembered though that South Africa has limited resources when it comes to water, and it is each person's responsibility to manage his or her own water usage.

Self-assessment

1. List the legislation related to national water management.
2. Discuss the two sources from which water is derived.
3. Describe how water is supplied to urban areas.
4. Discuss the management of water quality in urban areas.
5. Discuss the two ways in which human excreta are disposed of.
6. List diseases related to inadequate sanitation management.

Bibliography

Agri News. 2019. The deadly effects of water pollution in South Africa. 2019. Available: http://www.farmingportal.co.za/index.php/agri-index/76-water-and-irrigation/1676-the-deadly-effects-of-water-pollution-south-africa (Accessed 15 September 2020).

Definitions.net. nd. Water purification. Available: https://www.definitions.net (Accessed 15 September 2020).

Department of Water and Environmental Affairs. 2013. Release of the National Water Resource Strategy (NWRS2). Available: https://www.gov.za/release-national-water-resource-strategy-nwrs2. (Accessed online 16 September 2020).

Department of Water Affairs (DWA). 2013. National water resources strategy. Available: http://www.dwa.gov.za/documents/Other/Strategic%20Plan/NWRS2-Final-email-version.pdf. (Accessed 16 September 2020).

Department of Water and Sanitation (DWS). 2015. Reporting on implementation of the 2nd national water resources strategy (NWRS2). Detailed implementation progress report: June 2013 to July 2015. Available: http://biodiversityadvisor.sanbi.org/wp-content/uploads/2016/08/NWRS2-Detailed-Implementation-Progress-Report-Jun-2013-Jul-2015.pdf (Accessed 16 September 2020).

Department of Water and Sanitation (DWS). 2016. National sanitation policy 2016. Available: https://www.fsmtoolbox.com/assets/pdf/194_-_17005SC_POLICY_National_Sanitation_Policy_2016_FINAL310117.pdf (Accessed 16 September 2020).

Department of Water and Sanitation (DWS). 2017. National norms and standards for domestic water and sanitation services. 2017. Available: https://cer.org.za/wp-content/uploads/1997/12/National-norms-and-standards-for-domenstic-water-and-sanitation-services.pdf (Accessed 14 September 2020).

Helmenstine, AM. 2020. ThoughtCo. Is it ever safe to drink bleach? Available: https://www.thoughtco.com/is-it-safe-to-drink-bleach-606151 (Accessed 16 September 2020).

Kent TO Systems. 2019. Harmful impurities found in drinking water. Available: https://www.kent.co.in/blog/harmful-impurities-found-in-drinking-water/ (Accessed 15 September 2020).

Kneale, L. 2019. The solid waste management industry. Available: https://www.whoownswhom.co.za/store/info/4718 (Accessed 15 September 2020).

Lawyers for Human Rights. 2009. Water supply and sanitation in South Africa: Environmental rights and municipal accountability. LHR publication series, 1/2009. Available: http:// cer.org.za/wp-content/uploads/2011/11/LHR-DBSA_Water_Report. pdf (Accessed 15 September 2020).

Lenntech Water Treatment Solutions. nd. Waterborne diseases. Available: http:// www. lenntech.com/library/diseases/diseases/waterborne-diseases.htm (Accessed 15 September 2020).

Mema, V. 2010. Impact of poorly maintained wastewater and sewage treatment plants: Lessons from South Africa. Water Institution of South Africa (WISA). Paper presented at WISA 2010 Biennial Conference & Exhibition, Durban. Available: https://www. semanticscholar.org/paper/IMPACT-OF-POORLY-MAINTAINED-WASTEWATER-AND-SEWAGE-%3A-Mema/afa6d6ff3a25061a5c9b8f2194680f1b5c682fbc?p2df (Accessed 16 September 2020).

National Business Initiative. 2019. Strengthening South Africa's water services authorities report (02/2019). Available: https://www.nbi.org.za/wp-content/uploads/2019/05/ NBI_KYM-Report-2_Strengthening-WSAs.pdf (Accessed 16 September 2020).

National Institute of Environmental Health Sciences. 2017. Waterborne diseases. Available: https://www.niehs.nih.gov/research/programs/geh/climatechange/health_impacts/ waterborne_diseases/index.cfm (Accessed 15 September 2020).

Rand Water. nd. How is tap water cleaned? Available: http://www.waterwise.co.za/site/ water/purification/story-tap-water.html (Accessed 16 September 2020).

Republic of South Africa (RSA). 1997. The Water Services Act No 108 of 1997. Available: http://www.info.gov.za/gazette/acts/1997/108-97.pdf (Accessed 14 September 2020).

Republic of South Africa (RSA). 1998. National Water Act No 36 of 1998, as amended). Pretoria: Government Printer. Available: http://www.energy.gov.za/files/policies/act_ nationalwater36of1998.pdf. (Accessed 16 September 2020).

Republic of South Africa (RSA). 2002. Address by Nelson Mandela at opening of the Waterdome during the world summit on sustainable development, 2002. Available: http://www.mandela.gov.za/mandela_speeches/2002/020828_waterdome.htm (Accessed 16 September 2020).

Roberts, J. 2010. SA water demand will exceed supply by 2025. *Mail & Guardian*, 4 February 2010. Available: https://mg.co.za/article/2010-02-04-sa-water-demand-will-exceed-supply-by-2025/ (Accessed 16 September 2020).

South African Bureau of Standards (SABS). 2015. South African National Standard (SANS) 241-1:2015. Edition 2. Drinking water. Available: https://store.sabs.co.za/pdfpreview. php?hash=d3d0b4e624a31e2a7a68cf1a3f4fb181b864dcdf&preview=yes (Accessed 16 September 2020).

South African Human Rights Commission. 2014. Report on the right to access sufficient water and decent sanitation in South Africa. Available: www.sahrc.org (Accessed 15 September 2020).

South African Instrumentation and Control. 2000. Water quality monitoring. Available: http://www.instrumentation.co.za/news.aspx?pklnewsid=5810 (Accessed 15 September 2020).

Still, D.A., Salisbury, R.H., Foxon, K.M., Buckley, C.A. & Bhagwan, J.N. 2018. The challenges of dealing with full VIP latrines. Available: https://wisa.org.za/wp-content/uploads/2018/12/WISA2010-P148.pdf (Accessed 16 September 2020).

Technology Networks. 2018. Eight common water contaminants and how to prevent them. Available: https://www.technologynetworks.com/tn/lists/8-common-water-contaminants-and-how-to-prevent-them-296339 (Accessed 15 September 2020).

The MVULA Trust. nd. How to use water for poverty alleviation. Available: (http://www.themvulatrust.org.za/how-to-use-water-for-poverty-alleviation/ (Accessed 15 September 2020).

United Nations (UN). 2013. International Day of Peace. Secretary General's message for 2013. Available: https://www.un.org/en/events/peaceday/2013/sgmessage.shtml (Accessed 16 September 2020).

United Nations (UN). 2015. UN Water Target 6.2 – Sanitation and hygiene. Available: https://www.sdg6monitoring.org/indicators/target-6-2/ (Accessed 6 September 2020).

United Nations Development Programme (UNDP). 2015. Sustainable development goals 2015. Available: http://www.undp.org/content/undp/en/home/sdgoverview/post-2015-development-agenda.html (Accessed 14 September 2020).

Van Niekerk, AM. & Schneider, B. 2013. Implementation plan for direct and indirect water re-use for domestic purposes – Sector Discussion Document. Available: https://www.green-cape.co.za/assets/Sector-files/water/Reclamation-and-reuse/WRC-Implementation-plan-for-direct-and-indirect-water-re-use-for-domestic-purposes-sector-discussion-document-2013.pdf (Accessed on 16 September 2020).

World Health Organization (WHO). 2019. Drinking-water. Available: https://www.who.int/news-room/fact-sheets/detail/drinking-water (Accessed 16 September 2020).

World Health Organization (WHO). nd, Water. Available: https://www.afro.who.int/health-topics/water (Accessed 15 September 2020).

Nutrition and food safety

Roelien Els

Learning outcomes

After studying this chapter, you should be able to:

- Describe the various food groups and their functions.
- Discuss the factors that influence food choices.
- Outline the food groups, functions of nutrients and diseases associated with them.
- Discuss the factors that cause contamination of food.
- Describe the regulation of food safety in South Africa.
- Describe strategies to promote food hygiene at home.
- Describe the types of food preservation.
- Explain the processes involved in the preservation of milk.
- Outline the food security challenges in South Africa. Discuss the community nurse's role and responsibility in assisting with food security.

Key terms

Mechanical transmission: The transfer of pathogens from an infected host or a contaminated substrate to a susceptible host, without a biological association between the pathogen and the vector.

Obesity: The condition of excessive accumulation and storage of fat in the body occurs when more calories are consumed than are expended in the form of energy and is evidenced when body weight is greater than 20 per cent of the expected weight for males and 25 per cent for females.

➡

> **Pasteurisation**: A process whereby non-spore-bearing pathogenic organisms in fluid (especially milk) are killed by heat without affecting the food properties or flavour of the fluid.
>
> **RDA**: Recommended dietary/daily allowance. Refers to the recommended daily amounts of specific nutrients and/or vitamins and minerals required to maintain health.

Introduction

Nutrition is the scientific study of food and nourishment, including food consumption, dietary guidelines and the role that nutrients play to maintain physiological health processes in the human body. We know that food is needed to fulfil the following functions:

- provide the body with heat and energy (eg maintaining activities of daily living and body processes such as digestion and metabolism)
- supply chemical elements necessary for tissue building and repair (eg wound healing)
- supply the substances needed for the regulation of body processes (eg gastrointestinal motility)
- maintain health and protect the body against infection (eg mineral elements maintain cardiac function and vitamin deficiencies compromise the body's immune system).

Globally 88 per cent of countries face a serious burden of malnutrition. Malnutrition refers to deficiencies related to excesses or imbalances in a person's energy intake. The WHO (2020b) proposes that malnutrition addresses three broad groups of conditions:

1. Undernutrition, including wasting (low weight-for-height), stunting (low height-for-age) and underweight (low weight-for-age). Around 45 per cent of deaths among children under five years of age are associated with undernutrition. At the same time, rates of childhood overweight and obesity are rising in these same countries.

2. Micronutrient-related malnutrition where there is a lack of dietary vitamins and minerals or they are taken in excess in the diet.

3. Overweight, obesity and diet-related non-communicable diseases are linked to heart disease, diabetes and some cancers, such as colorectal cancer, which is associated with a high saturated fat intake.

The way people make food choices and prepare food is not solely based on economical, psychological or nutritional needs. The community nurse needs to understand the challenges underlying food choices and meal preparation in the specific community that he or she serves. Some of the factors that influence food choice and food consumption include the following:

- **Biological determinants**, such as hunger, appetite and taste. Taste preferences are often regarded as a primary motivator of the individual's food choices. Food preferences may be influenced by early exposure. For example, several studies done on taste preferences propose that foods eaten by a woman during pregnancy and lactation may influence the infant's early taste preferences. Food deprivation and irregular availability of food during childhood have been found to explain poor eating behaviours.

- **Economic determinants**, such as cost, income and availability. A household needs sufficient money and time to prepare healthy meals. As financial resources and food security decline, low-income populations focus more on price and quantity than on food preference and quality.

- **Physical determinants**, such as physical health, cooking skills, availability of kitchen equipment, attitude and knowledge about food. The person that prepares the food must have the physical ability and necessary knowledge to preserve nutrients during the cooking process. Food choices are influenced by knowledge of food preparation and the availability of kitchen equipment to refrigerate, prepare and cook food. The inability to preserve food at refrigerated temperatures, limits purchasing of fresh produce such as fruit, vegetables, meat and milk.

- **Social determinants**, such as culture, family, peers and meal patterns. Family structure and the role of each family member in food choices influence the ability to be food secure and have access to a healthy diet. For example, women who work full-time or are the single head of the household have limited time to prepare healthy, balanced meals.

- **Psychological determinants**, such as mood, stress and energy levels. Having multiple jobs, working long and inflexible hours, working night shifts and using public transport all have an impact on the time and energy available to purchase and prepare food. These households are more likely to revert to skipping meals, eating take-away meals, or eating away from home, resulting in limited time to meet the family's nutritional needs. When work–life stress increases, the motivation to sustain a nutritious diet decreases and the tendency to consume more fast-foods and sugar-sweetened beverages increases.

No individual food or food group contains all the nutrients to support life. The information that follows is intended to provide some foundational knowledge on diet, nutrition and food safety. We will also provide guidance on the correct way to store, preserve and handle food to promote nutritional health and when to refer incidents of foodborne disease timeously to prevent large-scale community outbreaks.

Food groups and classifications

Dietary guidance should be based on the principles of moderation and variety to sustain growth, development, reproduction and longevity. Table 17.1 splits food into four groups – a simplified way of explaining nutritional needs when working in the community.

Table 17.1 Four major food groups

Food groups	Example of food types	Chemical value	Recommended daily allowance (RDA)
GROUP 1 Body building foods Milk and milk products	Milk, cheese yoghurt and cream. Skimmed milk reduces the amount of saturated fatty acids, but is unsuitable for infants.	Source of high-quality protein, fat and vitamins A, B and D, mineral salts and calcium.	Adults 400 ml milk. Pregnant/ lactating women 700 ml milk. Children 500 to 700 ml milk. Reduce amount of milk if cheese is served.
GROUP 2 Body and tissue-building foods Animal products and legumes	Red meat including animal organs, poultry, fish, eggs. Beans, seeds and nuts.	Supply protein of high biological value. Contain fats, fat-soluble vitamins A and D and B-group vitamins, mineral salts and iron.	One or two servings per day.
GROUP 3 Protective foods Fruit and vegetables	**Fruit:** apples, strawberries, bananas, limes and pineapple, grapes and fruit juice. **Vegetables:** *Dark green vegetables:* spinach, broccoli. *Starchy vegetables:* potato, sweet potato, corn, green peas. *Orange vegetables:* squash and carrots. *Dried beans and peas:* black beans, pinto beans. *Additional vegetables:* cauliflower and artichoke.	Supply the body with carbohydrates eg starch in potatoes and sugar in grapes. Contain mineral salts and vitamins, especially vitamin C.	One starchy serving, one green vegetable, plus one other vegetable. One serving of fruit juice per day.
GROUP 4 Energy producing foods Grains	**Refined grains:** White flour, white rice, white bread, pasta and oats. **Whole grains:** Brown rice, oatmeal, whole-wheat flour and whole-grain pasta.	Rich in carbohydrates to meet body's energy requirements. Unrefined cereals contain protein, vitamins and mineral salts.	Two to three servings per day, depending on the individual's energy requirements.

The classification of food into groups according to their nutritional value, enables a person to plan a balanced diet that contains all the different nutrients. Dietary diversity promotes a balanced diet and should aim to contain nutrients in the correct proportions.

The food groups are divided according to their nutritional properties. Nutrients can also be classified into macronutrients needed in large quantities and micronutrients that are required in small amounts. For the purpose of developing foundational knowledge, nutrients are divided into six major classes:

- carbohydrates, including cellulose
- proteins
- fats
- vitamins
- mineral salts
- water (this is not strictly a nutrient, but as it is required in the diet in sufficient amounts it is included here).

Carbohydrates

The most useful classification scheme divides carbohydrates into groups according to the number of individual simple sugar units. Carbohydrate molecules are made up of carbon, oxygen and hydrogen atoms. Monosaccharides contain a single sugar unit; disaccharides contain two sugar units; and polysaccharides are long chains of monosaccharides linked by glycosidic bonds.

Carbohydrates are compounds that contain starches and sugars. They are derived almost entirely from plants. Carbohydrates are readily available, relatively inexpensive and can have a longer shelf life than other foods, which is why carbohydrate deficiencies are not as common as some of the other nutritional deficiencies, except in times of starvation and famine. About 55 per cent (or more) of one's daily energy requirements (kilojoules) should come from carbohydrates, particularly starches, and not more than 10 per cent from sugars.

There are a variety of interrelated classification schemes, as demonstrated in Table 17.2.

Table 17.2 Classification of carbohydrates

Common carbohydrates	
Name	Derivation of name and source
Monosaccharides (simple sugars)	
Glucose	From the Greek word for sugar or sweet 'glucos'. Found in cane sugar, honey, fruit and vegetables. High in ripe bananas, watermelon and raisins and vegetables, such as green peas and carrots and boiled potatoes.
Fructose	Latin word for fruit 'fructus'. Found in fruits and honey.
Galactose	Greek word for milk 'galact'. Found as a component of lactose in milk.

➡

Common carbohydrates	
Name	**Derivation of name and source**
Disaccharides (contain two monosaccharides)	
Sucrose	French word for sugar 'sucre', a disaccharide containing **glucose and fructose**, found in sugar cane, honey, jams, sweets, mayonnaise, salad dressings and processed meat products such as sausages, ham and patés.
Maltose	From the word 'malt', a disaccharide containing two **units of glucose**, found in germinating grains, used to make beer. Formed during the digestion of starch.
Lactose	Latin word for milk 'lact', a disaccharide found in milk of mammals containing **glucose and galactose.** Lactose (found in dairy products) and glycogen (stored in the liver and muscle of animals) are the only animal-derived source of carbohydrate.
Common carbohydrates	
Name	**Derivation of name and source**
Oligosaccharides (compound sugars, containing 2–10 sugar molecules)	
Raffinose	Foods naturally high in raffinose are beans, asparagus, sugar beet molasses, cabbage, broccoli, sweet potatoes and whole grains. It is a trisaccharide containing glucose, galactose, and fructose units. They pass unchanged to the colon where the normal intestinal bacteria ferment them to gasses such as methane and hydrogen.
Stachyose	Stachyose is composed of four sugar molecules: two galactoses, glucose and fructose. It is mainly found in beans and peas.

Sources: Aryal (2020); Nutrients Review.com (2016)

Daily requirements of carbohydrates

The optimal daily carbohydrate intake for a man who weighs 79 kg and needs about 12 000 kJ a day is 412 g. The corresponding figure for a woman who weighs 63 kg and needs 9 000 kJ, is 309 g.

Functions of carbohydrates

- Carbohydrates are the body's most important source of heat and energy.
- They are necessary for the complete metabolism of fat: 'Fat burns in the flame of carbohydrate.'
- They are 'protein sparers' because protein will not be used for heat and energy if carbohydrates are available.
- They play a part in the detoxification of certain metabolites and drugs.
- Lactose (milk sugar) plays a role in the synthesis of B-complex vitamins by promoting the growth of specific bacteria.

Sources of carbohydrates

- Cane sugar and all manufactured products containing cane sugar, such as sweets and jam
- Fruits and some vegetables, such as peas, which also contain sugars, as well as skins and peels of fruit and vegetables and leafy green vegetables
- Bread, cereal, rice, potatoes and pasta, which are rich in starchy carbohydrates
- Cellulose, which is found in the skins or peels, seeds and leaves of plants; it also forms the framework of plant cells
- The husks of grains and cereals.

Refined carbohydrates

These include bread containing white flour, many breakfast cereals, white rice, pastries, pasta and pizza, cakes, cookies and sweets.

Refined carbohydrates are whole grains that have been stripped of valuable nutrients, such as vitamins, minerals and fibre, during food processing. The excessive intake of refined carbohydrates is associated with increased fasting triglyceride levels and increased risk for type 2 diabetes and heart disease.

Cellulose

Dietary fibre is mainly made up of cellulose. This is a large carbohydrate polymer that cannot be digested by our body because we lack the necessary enzymes.

Functions of cellulose

Fibre promotes digestive health and adds bulk to the intestinal contents, while insoluble fibre promotes peristalsis and reduces the risk of colon cancer. Some serious conditions such as diverticulosis and carcinoma of the bowel are associated with constipation. Soluble fibre slows down the movement of food and reduces insulin spikes to assist with blood glucose control.

Sources of fibre

Only plant-based foods contain fibre, many of which also contain high amounts of protein. The following foods are good sources of fibre:

- Whole grain foods, such as barley, brown rice, oatmeal and wholewheat bread
- Fruits, such as bananas, mangoes, strawberries, prunes, plums and figs
- Vegetables, such as broccoli, spinach, beetroot and carrots.

Protein

Protein molecules are made up of nitrogen, carbon, oxygen and hydrogen atoms. Protein is the only nutrient that contains nitrogen and it cannot be replaced by any other substance in the diet. Protein also contains small amounts of sulphur, phosphorus and magnesium. These nitrogen monomers are essential amino acids needed by the body for metabolism. There are 20 different amino acids, nine of which are known as essential amino acids because they cannot be produced by the body and have to be obtained from the diet. Essential amino acids include isoleucine, leucine, phenylalanine, threonine, lysine, tryptophan, methionine, valine and histidine. Proteins may be classified according to their essential amino acid content:

- **Complete (or first-class) proteins** contain an adequate amount of all the essential amino acids needed to build new proteins. These proteins are derived mainly from animal sources and include meat, fish, poultry, cheese, eggs and yoghurt. Complete proteins do not need to be combined with other food to provide adequate protein.
- **Incomplete (second-class) proteins** are any proteins that lack one or more essential amino acid(s) in the correct proportions. Examples include grains, nuts, beans, seeds, peas and maize.

Daily requirements of protein

Adults require 0.8 g of protein per kilogram of body weight. The daily requirement of dietary protein is 63 g for men and 50 g for women. For children (1 to 10 years of age) the requirement ranges from 16 g to 28 g. Adolescent boys need about 59 g of protein a day, and girls 44 g daily. Pregnant or lactating women need an extra 30 g of protein a day. At least one-quarter of this protein should be derived from animal sources.

> One 250 ml cup of milk contains 8 g of protein
>
> One egg contains 6 g of protein
>
> 30 g of meat, fish or poultry contains about 7 g protein
>
> 125 ml cooked dried beans contain 8 g protein.

Functions of protein

- Protein is essential for the growth, maintenance and repair of body tissues.
- Proteins are the building blocks of all body tissues.
- Protein is required for the provision of energy when there are not enough carbohydrates in the diet and fat stores are depleted.
- Protein is required for endocrine gland secretion.

- The plasma proteins albumin, globulin and fibrinogen exert an osmotic pressure that retains fluid in the blood vessels.
- Protein is required for the synthesis of enzymes, plasma proteins, antibodies (immunoglobulins) and some hormones.
- Protein is essential for the formation of hemoglobin in the red blood cells.

Sources of protein

One of the main differences between plant and animal proteins is their amino acid content. Most animal products are complete sources of protein whereas plant proteins are incomplete because they lack some of the essential amino acids.

- **Animal protein**: fish, various types of eggs, dairy products such as cheese, milk and whey, red meat and poultry. These proteins are considered a better-quality protein as they contain all the amino acids needed.
- **Plant protein**: legumes (eg peas, beans and lentils), nuts, wholewheat and unrefined cereals (eg maize and rice) and fruit like guava, avocado, kiwifruit and dried apricots. The best-quality plant protein is found in soya beans.

Iron deficiency is one of the most common nutrient deficiencies in the world, affecting more than 25 per cent of people worldwide. It is important that vegetarians and vegans mix dietary protein sources to ensure that their diet contains all the essential amino acids. Quinoa and buckwheat are good examples of complete plant-based sources of protein.

Protein-energy malnutrition

Protein-energy malnutrition is a term that has replaced 'protein-calorie' malnutrition and refers to two the conditions kwashiorkor and marasmus.

- **Kwashiorkor**: This condition occurs most commonly in children between the ages of one and two years and is primarily due to a deficiency of high-quality protein, although it is accompanied by deficiencies of other nutrients, as well as an inadequate kilojoule intake. The condition is frequently precipitated by an infection, often a gastrointestinal infection. The child is apathetic, listless and irritable. The hair becomes reddish, sparse and straight, and there are skin changes. Oedema occurs and is due to the hypo-proteinaemia. The child suffers from diarrhoea and vomiting. Anaemia is present.
- **Marasmus**: This condition is associated with failure to thrive and the child usually weighs less than 60 per cent of his or her expected weight. It is the result of an insufficient intake of kilojoules. The child is small and wrinkled. There is muscular wasting and a marked lack of subcutaneous tissue. The infant is often found to be suffering from bacterial and parasitic infections.

Prevention and control of kwashiorkor and marasmus

- Encourage breastfeeding and avoid, at all costs, any circumstances that may lead to the separation of an infant from its mother.
- Postpone weaning until the infant is at least two years old, if possible.
- Provide parents and caregivers with health education on the importance of a balanced diet in the growth and development of their child.
- Provide at-risk babies, falling below the third percentile on the growth and development graph, with vitamin supplements and milk powders, where possible, at community health facilities.
- Promote improved hygienic practices, for example hand washing as well as environmental hygiene, to reduce the susceptibility to infection in immuno-compromised people.

Fats

Fats are compounds of carbon and hydrogen, with a small amount of oxygen. Fats are made up of the same kinds of atoms as carbohydrates. The fat in a normal diet is a neutral fat and consists of three fatty acid chains linked to one molecule of glycerol (a triglyceride). After food consumption, calories that are not immediately used by body tissues are converted into triglycerides and stored in the body's fat cells. When triglyceride levels become excessive, risk for hypertension, obesity and heart disease increase. It is recommended that people with high triglyceride levels make dietary lifestyle changes to avoid saturated and trans fats (trans fatty acids) in their diet and drastically reduce the intake of simple carbohydrates, sugars and alcohol because very high ranges of triglyceride levels increase the risk of developing other medical problems (Cleveland Clinic, 2019).

Saturated fats

These are found primarily in animal-derived foods such as beef, veal, lamb, pork, poultry fat, butter, cream, full cream milk, full cream ice cream, full cream cheeses and 2 per cent milk. Plant sources of saturated fat include cocoa butter, coconut oil, palm oil and palm kernel oil. Refined carbohydrate products, such as cake, cookies, pastries and doughnuts, also contain high amounts of saturated fat. According to the AHA, saturated fats are a primary source of triglycerides and high cholesterol levels in the body. A maximum of 7 per cent of total daily calories should come from saturated fat.

Trans fats

Trans fats are found in margarine, hydrogenated vegetable oils, deep-fried foods, baking mixes, pastries, instant soups, processed snack foods and in fast-foods (take-aways)s. Trans fats are made by adding hydrogen to vegetable oils to create a longer-lasting, solid-form fat. Trans fats contain triglycerides and probably increase cholesterol and triglyceride levels in the body. The AHA recommends that no more than 1 per cent of a person's daily calories stem from trans fats.

Dietary cholesterol

Most animal-derived saturated fat sources, such as red meat, poultry fat, processed meats, hard cheeses, full cream milk, cream, 2 per cent milk and commercially prepared pastries, cookies and snack foods, contain dietary cholesterol. The AHA suggests consuming no more than 300 mg of dietary cholesterol daily for most adults. People with heart disease, high cholesterol or high triglyceride levels should limit cholesterol intake to under 200 mg per day.

Daily requirements of fats

Not more than 25 to 30 per cent of the body's daily energy requirement should be obtained from fats. This means that an adult man weighting 79 kg who needs 12 000 kJ a day should eat no more than 97 g of fat. The corresponding figure for a woman who weighs 63 kg and who needs 9 000 kJ a day is 73 g.

Many South Africans are suffering from overnutrition, eating too many calories in a diet filled with convenience foods such as hamburgers, fried chicken, pizza and chips (French fries). Fried take-away foods contain high levels of saturated and trans fats that clog arteries, leading to ischaemic heart disease.

The high kilojoule and sugar contents lead to obesity. Obesity is a key risk factor for the development of type 2 diabetes and heart disease. Studies have shown that the overall prevalence of overweight and obesity in South Africa is high. More than 29 per cent of men and 56 per cent of women are classified as overweight or obese.

An average small serving of chips from a fast-food restaurant contains 11 g of fat.

Functions of fats

- Fats are a concentrated source of heat and energy; 1 g of fat yields 38 kJ (9 calories) when oxidised in the body.
- Fats provide the source of fat-soluble vitamins A, D, E and K as well as essential fatty acids.
- Fats delay the emptying of the stomach and therefore the onset of hunger.
- They have 'satiety value' and make food more palatable.
- Fats protect and support various organs such as the kidneys.
- Dietary fat supplies essential fatty acids – linoleic and linolenic acid – which cannot be formed in the body but are needed for synthesis of prostaglandins and are essential for growth and brain development.
- Omega-3 and omega-6 fatty acids promote cardiovascular health.

Sources of fat

Fats may be derived from animal, fish or plant sources.

- **Animal-derived sources**: meat, butter, cream, cheese, bacon and egg yolk – foodstuffs rich in saturated fatty acids
- **Fish-derived sources**: fish, such as herring, and fish-liver oils, such as cod-liver oil
- **Plant-derived sources**: olives, sunflower seeds, nuts and avocado pears.

Vitamins

Vitamins are organic compounds present in most nutrients and are essential for normal growth and development because they perform vital functions in body cells. A balanced diet, by definition, provides an adequate intake of all vitamins. Several studies have shown that vitamin supplementation must be taken with medical supervision as it may cause toxicity in large amounts, such as vitamin A. Table 17.3 introduces the classification, sources and functions of the various vitamins that we obtain when we eat a balanced diet. Vitamin deficiencies and the prevention of vitamin-related diseases are addressed under the different types of vitamin.

Table 17.3 Classification of vitamins

Vitamin	Sources	Functions	Deficiency diseases	Prevention
Vitamin A A fat-soluble vitamin. Synthesised by animals from the precursor carotene. Heat-stable, thus very little loss occurs during food preparation and cooking.	Milk and milk products, egg yolk, fish liver oils and animal liver, yellow and green leafy vegetables, eg spinach, carrots, yellow maize, pumpkin, sweet potatoes.	• Required for the health of epithelial tissues such as the skin and mucous membranes. • Necessary for normal vision, partly because it forms part of the retinal pigment and is needed for health of the cornea of the eye. • Necessary for normal growth.	• Stunted growth. • Lowered resistance to infections, especially infections of the respiratory tract. • Dry, scaly, rough skin ('toad's skin'). • Night blindness. • Xerophthalmia.	• Breastfeeding. • Infants and children should receive sufficient full-cream milk. • Supplement with dried milk powder and vitamins when necessary. Deficiency can be prevented by the intermittent administration of vitamin A as the vitamin is stored in the liver. • Education of parents and other adults in infant and child nutrition. • Vitamin A immunisation regimen.

➡

Vitamin	Sources	Functions	Deficiency diseases	Prevention
Vitamin D A fat-soluble vitamin. Heat-resistant and not readily destroyed during food preparation and cooking. Toxic when administered in large amounts.	Small amounts in plants. Mainly animal sources such as milk, cream, butter, cheese, liver, egg yolk and fish liver oils. Fortified milk and dairy products. Non-dietary source: the action of the sun's rays on certain steriods in the skin results in the formation of vitamin D.	• Necessary for the absorption and metabolism of calcium and phosphorus. • Needed for the development of healthy bones and teeth.	• *Rickets:* Primarily due to an inadequate dietary intake of vitamin D in children. It can occur because of failure to absorb the vitamin; this is the cause of the rickets that occurs in coeliac disease. • *Steatorrhoea.* • *Osteomalacia* in adults due to impaired absorption and use of calcium and phosphate. De-mineralisation of bone.	Fortification of milk and diary products. Moderate exposure to direct sunlight.
Vitamin E A fat-soluble antioxidant vitamin, not readily destroyed during food preparation and cooking.	Vegetable oils and margarine. Wheat germ and wheat germ oil, whole grains, legumes, nuts, egg yolk, leafy green vegetables. Papaya, mango.	• Protects body membrane lipids from being destroyed in oxidative reactions. • Protects against coronary heart disease.	• Deficiency is more often due to failure of absorption than to a dietary insufficiency, eg in premature babies and cystic fibrosis. The absence of bile in the intestine or the use of laxatives containing mineral oils hampers its absorption. A deficiency of the vitamin results in delayed clotting of blood and spontaneous haemorrhages.	• Create public awareness by giving health education to maintain and promote dietary health and prevent associated disease by preserving nutrients.

➡

Vitamin	Sources	Functions	Deficiency diseases	Prevention
Vitamin K A fat-soluble antioxidant vitamin. Heat-resistant and not readily destroyed during food preparation and cooking.	Liver, leafy green vegetables, eg spinach, vegetable oils, tomatoes, fat, pork, beef liver, cheese, egg yolk, cabbage, cauliflower.	Vitamin K is necessary for the formation of prothrombin, and factors essential for the clotting of blood.	Deficiency prevents normal blood coagulation. Occurs in adults where there is obstruction of flow in bile, severe liver damage, and in malabsorption, eg in coeliac disease. Newborn infants' intestines are sterilie and require several weeks to become colonised with vitamin K-producing bacteria.	*Adults*: dietary management. *New born infants*: Vitamin K injection as per diagnosis.
Vitamin C (ascorbic acid) A water-soluble vitamin that is readily destroyed by drying, storage and oxidation. Overcooking results in serious vitamin C loss. Toxic effects and formation of kidney stones and red blood cell destruction when taken in very high doses.	Fresh citrus fruit, guavas, berries, eg strawberries, kiwi fruit. Leafy green fresh vegetables, eg raw cabbage, broccoli, cauliflower, and tomatoes.	• It is necessary for the formation and health of the inter-cellular substance of the tissues. • It plays a part in the formation of red blood cells. • It is needed for the healing of wounds. • It increases resistance to infection. • It acts as an antioxidant to protect body molecules from damaging oxidative reactions. • It increases iron absorption.	A deficiency of this vitamin results in a weakening of the capillary walls and spontaneous haemorrhages. This condition is known as scurvy. Collagen production is affected, leading to fragility of blood vessels, delayed wound healing and poor bone repair. Gums become swollen and spongy and teeth loosen in their sockets.	A glass of fresh orange juice, or a fresh citrus fruit per day is sufficient to supply the body's needs for the vitamin. To preserve as much of the vitamin C in vegetables as possible they should be cooked for a short time in rapidly boiling water and eaten immediately after cooking. Frozen vegetables probably retain the largest amount of vitamin C. People should be encouraged to grow their own fruit and vegetables.

➡

Vitamin	Sources	Functions	Deficiency diseases	Prevention
Vitamin B₁ (Thiamine) A water-soluble vitamin that is relatively stable at high temperatures. Thiamine is lost when the cooking water for rice or meat is discarded.	Thiamine is found in small amounts in a wide variety of foods such as brewer's yeast and yeast extract, nuts, the outer husks of grains, wheat germ, legumes, liver, green vegetables, eggs and pork.	• Thiamine plays a part in tissue respiration. • It is a co-enzyme that is necessary for the release of energy from carbohydrate. • It is necessary for the normal functioning of the nervous system. • Plays an important role in carbohydrate, protein and fat metabolism.	A deficiency of this vitamin results in fatigue, loss of appetite, depression and irritability, and polyneuritis. *Beriberi:* Occurs in the eastern countries among people whose staple diet is polished rice, which is rice from which the outer husks have been removed. The condition is characterised by muscular weakness, peripheral neuritis, cardiac involvement and oedema. Neurological damage, eg irreversible memory loss, ataxia and visual disturbances in alcoholism.	Health education to create awareness of sources of Vitamin B₁, disease risks, factors affecting the loss of vitamin. Motivation and referral of alcoholics for appropriate dietary management. Vitamin preservation during food preparation and cooking.
Vitamin B₂ (Riboflavin) A water-soluble vitamin. Stable to heat but is destroyed by exposure to light and alkalis.	Diary products, eggs, cheese, liver, yeast, fish roe, leafy green vegetables, and meat.	• Necessary for normal growth and development. • Forms a part of the enzyme system that is responsible for the release of energy from carbohydrate. • Plays an important part in tissue respiration. • Necessary for the health of the eyes.	A deficiency of this vitamin is usually found in association with deficiencies in other B-group vitamins. It leads to cracks in the corners of the mouth (angular storatitis), roughening of the skin, eye strain. Inflammation of the tongue (glossitis), seborrhoeic dermatitis.	Create public awareness by giving health education to maintain and promote dietary health, and prevent disease by preserving nutrients. Adjustment in food preparation methods, eg avoid adding soduim bicarbonate during cooking process.

➡

Vitamin	Sources	Functions	Deficiency diseases	Prevention
Vitamin B₃ Nicotinic acid (Niacin) A vitamin that is stable with regard to light, heat and oxidation.	Meat, chicken, fish, peanuts and brewer's yeast and the husks of grains. Nicotinic acid may be synthesised from the amino acid tryptophan and so adequate amounts of animal protein are also necessary to ensure sufficient nicotinic acid.	• Together with thiamine and riboflavin it plays a part in tissue respiration. • It is also involved in the metabolism of amino acids. • Assists body to break down glucose. • Important in the energy-producing chemical reactions in cells and in the formation of fat.	*Pellagra:* Common in the tropics and subtropics and occurs mainly among maize-eating people. A characteristic dermatitis appears on parts of the body that are exposed to light; there are disturbances of the gastrointestinal tract, including diarrhoea, and mental changes occur; at first there is depression, followed later by confusion and eventually dementia. Classically, pellagra is described as the disease of the four Ds, dermatitis, diarrhoea, dementia and debilitation.	• Nutrition education should stress the importance of using unrefined maize meal, and less emphasis should be put on the sale of white maize meal. • Maize meal should be enriched. Because it is the staple diet of millions of people in southern Africa, many of whom cannot afford variety in their diet, we should ensure that it contains sufficient quantities of the necessary vitamins and mineral salts.
Pantothenic acid This is a co-enzyme B-vitamin that is needed for the proper utilisation of carbohydrates and fats.	It is present in most foods but yeast, liver, eggs, pork, organ meat and grains are rich sources.	Plays a role in the synthesis of fatty acids.	Loss of appetite, indigestion, neuritis. A burning sensation in the feet.	Create public awareness by giving health education to maintain and promote dietary health, and prevent disease by utilising nutrients optimally; preserve nutrients during cooking and food preparation.

➡

322

Vitamin	Sources	Functions	Deficiency diseases	Prevention
Vitamin B$_6$ Nicotinic acid (Niacin) A vitamin that is stable with regard to light, heat and oxidation.	It is found in meat, poultry, fish, egg yolk, peas, beans, soya beans, yeast, wheat germ and wholegrain cereals, and in liver.	It forms part of the enzyme systems concerned with the metabolism of amino acids and fats, including the synthesis of non-essential amino acids and molecules.	*Infants:* anaemia, vomiting, weakness and convulsions. *Children:* irritability and convulsions. *Adults:* seborrhoeic dermatitis around eyes and eyebrows, a smooth red tongue, nausea, vomiting, irritability, mental confusion.	Educate to maintain and promote dietary health, and prevent disease by utilising nutrients optimally. Preserve nutrients during cooking and food preparation, eg prevent unnecessary exposure of food to light.
Vitamin B$_9$ Folic acid (Folate) Known as the anti-anaemic factor. Destroyed by heat and moisture.	It is present in liver and other organ meat, eg kidney. Yeast and leafy green vegetables.	• Helps to convert carbohydrates into glucose that is used to produce energy. • It is necessary for the formation of normal red blood cells. • Works with vitamin B$_9$ to control blood levels of homocysteine, which is associated with heart disease.	Deficiency is evident within a short time. Alcoholism, inflammatory bowel disease and coeliac disease cause folic acid deficiency. Megaloblastic anaemia. Other conditions include poor growth, smooth red inflamed tongue, gingivitis, anorexia, gastrointestinal disturbances and a macrocytic anaemia in which the red blood cells are large and pale. Deficiency at conception and during early pregnancy is linked to incidence of spina bifida.	Health education to create awareness of risk factors that lead to loss of the vitamin, eg excessive alcohol is detrimental to the absorption of folic acid. Motivation of pregnant mothers to attend antenatal classes for risk assessment and folic acid supplementation to prevent birth defects, eg spina bifida and neural tube defects. Nutrient preservation to preserve vitamin B$_9$ as it is destroyed by heat and moisture. Fortification of food products to substitute the vitamin.

➡

Vitamin	Sources	Functions	Deficiency diseases	Prevention
Vitamin B$_{12}$ (Cobalamin) This vitamin contains cobalt and phosphorus in its molecule.	Only animal products, eg meat, poultry, fish, eggs and milk contain vitamin B$_{12}$. Fermented liquors.	• Necessary for the production and maturation of red blood cells. • Maintains nervous system functioning. • Required for formation and maintenance of myelin, the fatty substance that surrounds and protects some nerves. • Intrinsic factor in the stomach is necessary for the absorption of vitamin B$_{12}$.	Deficiency is not often due to a dietary lack, except in strict vegans. Usually the result of failure of absorption in persons who have undergone gastrectomy, or who have an abnormality of the gastric mucous membrane. The anaemia that results in this latter case is known as pernicious anaemia. Nutrititional anaemias are the most common deficiency diseases, excluding protein-energy malnutrition. Many nutrients are necessary for the formation and maturation of red blood cells, and if one or more of these are missing a nutritional anaemia results. Iron, copper, protein, folic acid and vitamin B$_{12}$ are all essential for the maintenance of haemoglobin levels. Deficiency causes irreversible neurological damage, eg peripheral neuropathy and/ or subacute spinal cord degeneration.	Health education promoting annual health check-ups to maintain optimal health status.

Storage of vitamins in the body

Vitamins A, E and K are readily stored in the body in adequate amounts. Vitamins B$_1$, B$_2$, C and D are retained by the body in moderate amounts. The major body reserves of vitamins are accumulated late in fetal life. A premature infant is therefore disadvantaged, as it has far less of a vitamin reserve to draw upon.

When preparing food, it is important to keep in mind that heat causes a considerable reduction in the vitamin content of foods. The best method to enhance vitamin intake is to eat fruit and vegetables fresh and uncooked.

Mineral salts

Mineral salts are inorganic substances required by the body in minute amounts. Minerals are divided into macrominerals and trace elements because they are needed in different amounts in the body to sustain normal physiological functioning.

Table 17.4 classifies mineral salts and provides sources, functions and deficiencies of various mineral elements.

Table 17.4 Classification of mineral salts

Mineral salt	Sources	Functions	Deficiencies
Calcium	Milk, cheese, dark green vegetables, dried beans	Development of healthy bones and teeth Blood clotting Cardiac muscle contraction Transmission of nerve impulses Neutralisation of acidity in body Clearing toxins	Stunted growth Malformations of bones and teeth Increased excitability of nerves Tetanus
Phosphorus	Milk and milk products. Fish, poultry, meat, liver and brain, nuts and whole grains	Together with calcium it forms bones and teeth Helps to maintain normal acid-base balance Forms part of DNA and RNA Necessary for oxidation of fats, carbohydrates and protein	
Magnesium	Leafy green vegetables, nuts, soya beans, whole grains, pulses	Plays a role in the formation of bones Assists in the transmission of nerve impulses Needed for normal muscle contraction such as peristalsis	Tremors and convulsions

➡

Mineral salt	Sources	Functions	Deficiencies
Sodium	Fish, meat, cheese, eggs, any salted food	Necessary for maintenance of normal osmotic pressure and fluid balance	Muscular weakness and muscle cramps; more often due to excessive loss than inadequate dietary intake
Potassium	Instant coffee, whole-wheat cereals, orange juice	Necessary for normal fluid balance	Disorientation, muscular weakness, cardiac arrhythmias
Sulphur	Eggs, vegetables, wheat germ, Brussels sprouts, garlic, onions	Forms part of the molecule of some B-group vitamins and amino acids Is a constituent of keratin	Exacerbates acne, arthritis, convulsions, memory loss
Iron	Liver, meat, dried fruit, leafy green vegetables, legumes, egg yolk	Necessary for the formation of haemoglobin	Iron deficiency (anaemia)
Cobalt	Liver, kidney, meat, poultry, fish, milk	Biosynthesis of vitamin B_{12} family of coenzymes	Pernicious anaemia
Copper	Liver, kidney, nuts, shellfish, eggs, whole grains	Necessary for the formation of red blood cells Forms part of certain enzymes	Anaemia
Iodine	Water, seafood, vegetables, iodised table salt	Necessary for the formation of thyroxin	Endemic or simple goitre (enlargement of the thyroid gland)

Water

Water is a vital constituent of every tissue in the body and, with the exception of oxygen, the substance most essential to life.

Functions of water in the body

- Water is an important regulator of body processes.
- Water provides the fluid medium essential for the chemical processes that take place in every cell in the body.
- Water is responsible for transporting food substances and oxygen (O_2) to the cells, and carbon dioxide (CO_2) and waste products away from cells. These substances can be carried to and from the cells only when they are in solution.

- Water plays an important part in the regulation of body temperature. It distributes heat throughout the body and cools the body surface when it evaporates as sweat.
- It forms the fluid part of the blood, the lymph and the secretions and excretions of the body.
- Water assists the digestion and absorption of food.

Sources of water in food products

We obtain water from the liquids we drink and the food we eat. Some foods such as broths, soups and fresh salads made with fruits such as strawberries, watermelon and oranges, contain a high percentage of water. All types of food, even bread, yield some water when oxidised:

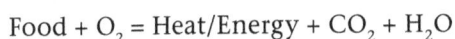

Food + O_2 = Heat/Energy + CO_2 + H_2O

Requirements for water

Fluid balances must be maintained, which means that fluid intake must be equal to the fluid lost from the body through the kidneys, lungs and skin. In a healthy adult under normal circumstances the amount of water lost in this way is about 3 000 ml a day, and to replace this we require at least six glasses of liquid a day in addition to any water which we may receive in our food. Under abnormal conditions such as high environmental temperatures or strenuous exercise this amount must be increased.

Food safety

Nutrition, food safety and food security are inseparably linked. Safe food supplies support national economies, trade and tourism, contribute to food security, and underpin sustainable development (WHO, 2020). On the other hand, unsafe food creates a vicious cycle of disease and malnutrition, particularly in infants, young children, the elderly and the sick. As the world's population grows, industrialisation of agriculture and animal production intensifies to meet the increasing demand for food. Climate change also impacts food safety. The International Forum on Food Safety and Trade held in Geneva in 2019 reiterated the importance of food safety and of making food safety a public priority to achieve the Sustainable Development Goals (SDGs) (WHO, 2020).

The principles of food safety aim to prevent food from becoming contaminated and causing food poisoning. The following aspects are considered to be the pillars of food safety:

- *Cleaning and sanitising*: the first step in creating a food safety system
- *Personal hygiene*: hand washing is critical to prevent cross-contamination

- *Food storage*: correct storage of perishable foods (cold storage) and dry goods to ensure that food quality is maintained
- *Temperature control:* to prevent the growth of bacteria
- *Food handling*: relates to best practices of handling food during storage and preparation.

Foodborne disease

Foodborne disease is any illness that results from the consumption of food contaminated with pathogenic bacteria, viruses or parasites. Foodborne diseases are an important cause of morbidity and mortality worldwide and impede socioeconomic development, contributing to further strain on healthcare systems, national economies, tourism and trade. Foodborne diseases can cause short-term symptoms, such as nausea, vomiting and diarrhoea, as well as longer-term illnesses, such as cancer, kidney or liver failure and brain and neural disorders. These diseases may be more serious in children, pregnant women, elderly people and those who have a weakened immune system. Children who survive some of the more serious foodborne diseases may suffer from delayed physical and mental development, impairing their quality of life permanently.

Food contamination refers to the presence of harmful chemicals and microorganisms in food. Foodborne diseases usually originate from toxins caused by bacteria, viruses, parasites or chemical substances entering the body through contaminated food or water. An estimated 600 million people, that is one in almost ten people, in the world, fall ill after consuming contaminated food (WHO, 2020). We will look at several biological contaminants and chemical substances that contribute to food contamination.

Biological contaminants

Food provides the ideal medium for the growth and multiplication of bacteria, and a number of infections, including food poisoning, may be transmitted by contaminated food. Bacterial food poisoning is a term used to refer to certain toxaemias and infections that result from the bacterial contamination of food. *Salmonella, Campylobacter,* and *enterohaemorrhagic Escherichia coli (E. coli)* are among the most common foodborne pathogens and affect millions of people annually (WHO, 2020). Examples of foods involved in outbreaks of salmonellosis are eggs and poultry. Foodborne cases with Campylobacter are mainly caused by raw milk, raw or undercooked poultry and contaminated water. Contamination of food with enterohaemorrhagic *E. coli* may be found in unpasteurised milk, undercooked meat and unwashed fruits and vegetables (WHO, 2020). We will have a look at the following biological contaminants responsible for foodborne disease:

Staphylococci

This acute toxaemia follows the ingestion of food that has been infected by a food handler suffering from a staphylococcal infection such as from a septic lesion on the face, hands or fingers. Although heat destroys the microorganism, the staphylococcus produces a heat-stable toxin that is not destroyed by cooking. Vomiting starts a few hours after the infected food has been eaten and is followed later by abdominal pain and diarrhoea. The person usually recovers within a few hours and the condition is usually not serious.

Salmonella food poisoning

This is an infection caused by eating food that has been contaminated with the organism. The reservoirs of infection may be chickens, rats, mice, cattle or other animals that are suffering from salmonella infections, or that are carriers of the bacteria. Human carriers can also infect food. The incubation period is longer than that of staphylococcal food poisoning, and diarrhoea, abdominal pain and pyrexia start about 12 to 24 hours after eating the infected food. Vomiting is not as marked as it is in staphylococcal food poisoning.

Botulism

This is a severe, and often fatal, type of poisoning caused by eating food that contains *Clostridium botulinum*, an anaerobic, sporing bacterium that produces a powerful exotoxin that affects the central nervous system. It gives rise to muscular paralysis, visual disturbances, difficulty in swallowing, respiratory failure and cardiac arrest. Canned fish and canned vegetables are the foods most frequently responsible for botulism. Cooking the food will not destroy the toxins although it will kill the organism.

Parasitic infection of food

A number of parasites undergo part of their development in an animal, and humans become infected by eating the undercooked flesh of such animals.

Trichinosis

This disease results from eating contaminated pork. The cysts of the parasite, which is a nematode or worm, are present in the muscles of the infected animal, and if the contaminated meat is not cooked well before it is eaten, the viable larvae are swallowed and live in the small intestine for about six weeks. They then migrate to the muscles and organs of the body and form cysts.

Tapeworms

Two types of tapeworm are important in South Africa. These are *Taenia saginata*, which is present in cattle, and *T. solium*, which is present in pigs. Both occur as cysts in the muscles of the animals, which are the intermediate hosts. Each cyst contains the head of a future tapeworm, which is known as a scolex. Humans are the true, or definitive, hosts of the parasite and become infested by eating meat containing the cysts. When these cysts are swallowed, the gastric juices dissolve the outer wall and the worm is set free. In the small intestine the head of the parasite attaches itself to the wall of the intestine by means of its suckers and/or hooks, and flat white segments, which are known as proglottides, start developing.

T. saginata grows to a length of 5 to 10 metres and *T. solium* to between 2 and 4 metres. After about three months, the terminal segments are mature and contain fertile ova. These are passed out of the body in the faeces of an infested person. In areas where there is no sanitation, the soil and water become contaminated, and animals grazing on such pastures or eating food that contains the ova of these worms swallow the ova. The larvae are set free in the animal's intestines and carried to the muscles where they become encysted. Such meat is known as 'measly' meat because of the appearance of the cysts.

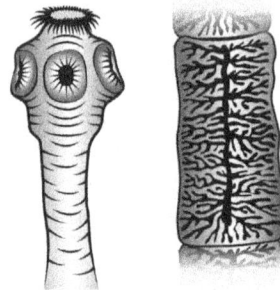

Scolex and proglottides of tapeworm

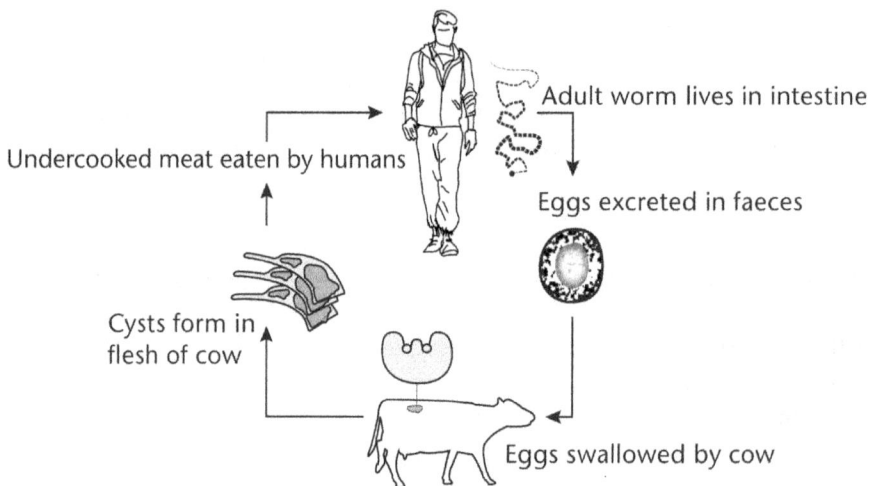

Adult worm lives in intestine

Undercooked meat eaten by humans

Eggs excreted in faeces

Cysts form in flesh of cow

Eggs swallowed by cow

Figure 17.1 Cysticercosis

When a human ingests the ova of *T. solium*, it results in a condition known as cysticercosis. After ingestion of the ova the larvae are set free in the intestines and are subsequently carried by the blood to the muscles of the body, and to organs such as the brain and liver where they form cysts.

The prevention of tapeworm infestation

Early diagnosis and treatment of all people suffering from tapeworm infestation is essential. Hand washing with soap and water before and after handling or preparing food and when in close contact with farm animals or pets will prevent tapeworm infestation. Treatment must be accompanied by health education informing the members of a community of the dangers associated with human and animal waste. Special precautions must be taken after flooding to prevent land contamination where animals graze and feed. The use of safe sanitary facilities is essential to prevent the spread of tapeworm. Animal carcasses containing tapeworm cysts must be destroyed. Tapeworm eggs and larvae in beef and pork can be destroyed by cooking the meat at high temperatures.

Chemical contaminants

Chemical hazards are a main cause of food contamination and foodborne disease outbreaks. Chemical contamination can occur because of naturally occurring toxins and environmental pollutants (WHO, 2020). Sources of chemical contaminants can originate from the soil or environment, disinfection by-products, air, water and packaging material. The following sources of chemical contaminants are outlined:

- **Naturally occurring toxins:** Several bacteria, viruses, and parasites inhabit the surfaces of the raw food naturally. Staple foods like corn or cereals can contain high levels of aflatoxin and ochratoxin, produced naturally by mould on grains. A long-term exposure can affect the immune system and normal development and may cause certain cancers.

- **Persistent organic pollutants (POPs):** These are compounds such as dioxins and polychlorinated biphenyls that accumulate in animal food chains through by-products of industrial processes and waste incineration. Dioxins, as an example of POPs, are highly toxic and can cause reproductive and developmental problems, damage the immune system, interfere with hormones and cause cancer.

- **Heavy metals:** Contamination by heavy metal in food occurs mainly through pollution of air, water and soil. Heavy metals such as lead, cadmium and mercury cause neurological and kidney damage.

- **Food processing contaminants:** During preparation food undergoes a long chain of processing with several potential sources of chemical invasion of contaminants. If foods are in direct contact with packaging materials, it can result in chemical contamination caused by the migration of certain substances in plastic materials, ink, recycled fibres and foaming agents into foods. Certain toxic chemical reactions can occur during food processing, canning or fermentation. Transportation of food can also lay the foundation for contamination of food, especially under poor sanitary conditions. Foods may be intentionally adulterated when some chemicals are mixed deliberately during the food preparation process to improve the shelf life of a food product.

The regulation of food safety

With the support of the WHO, the FAO Conference established the Codex Alimentarius to create an international food standards programme in 1961 (Food and Agriculture Organization of the United Nations, 2016). The Codex Alimentarius is a collection of standards, codes of practice, guidelines and other recommendations relative to food (Food and Agriculture Organization of the United Nations, 2016). South Africa is a member of Codex and the Department of Health implements the Codex food standards in South Africa. The responsibility for food safety and quality legislation in South Africa is a joint function of the following three departments, with specific responsibilities to oversee best practice food standards in our country:

- *The Department of Agriculture, Forestry and Fisheries (DWAFF)* regulates safety and quality of agriculture and animal products in terms of several acts of parliament, such as the Meat Safety Act 40 of 2000, the Agricultural Product Standards Act 119 of 1990 and the Fertilisers, Farm Feeds, Agricultural Remedies and Stock Remedies Act 36 of 1947.

- *The National Department of Health* regulates matters regarding the hygiene of foodstuffs addressed by the National Health Act 61 of 2003 we well as the safety of all foodstuffs in terms of the Foodstuffs, Cosmetics and Disinfectant Act 54 of 1972 (FCD Act) and the hygiene requirements at ports and airports as stipulated in the International Health Regulations Act 28 of 1974.

- *The Department of Trade and Industry* works closely with the South African Bureau of Standards (SABS) and it executes standards and controls on canned meat and frozen and canned fishery products through the Standards Act 29 of 1993.

Promoting food hygiene

In this section, we will look at strategies to enhance food hygiene at home and discuss various strategies to preserve food in order to avoid the growth and multiplication of foodborne pathogens.

Strategies to promote food hygiene at home

Research widely demonstrates that the home setting is the first place in which foodborne diseases develop due to poor personal and/or environmental hygiene, with an increased risk of infection. The following safety precautions should be followed at home when working, preparing and storing food:

- Practice good personal hygiene. Effective hand washing is extremely important to help prevent the spread of pathogens from the hands to the food, as well as from contaminated work surfaces and equipment. People handling food should be educated to wash their hands with soap and running water for at least one to two minutes at the following times:
  - when entering the food-handling area or kitchen, eg after a break or going to the toilet
  - before preparing food
  - after touching raw food, such as meat/poultry and eggs
  - after handling food waste or emptying a bin
  - after cleaning
  - after the person has blown his or her nose.
- Dry hands thoroughly with a clean towel after washing them because bacteria can spread more easily in wet or damp conditions.
- Use clean water when washing, mixing and cooking food.
- Clean utensils and cooking equipment, especially cutting boards, counter tops and blenders properly before preparing food. A meat chopping board, if not cleaned properly, can become a growth medium for bacteria and mould, especially if the surface is worn-out and on the edges. Use different utensils for preparing vegetables and raw meat to prevent food poisoning. Keep dry grains and powdered food away from wet food and liquids because it attracts mould easily, causing illness, allergies and food poisoning.
- Cook food at the required temperature to prevent Salmonella and Escherichia coli (*E. coli*) infections caused by raw foods such as eggs and meat. Foods such as pork, chicken and beef and all processed meats like sausages should be cooked longer because certain bacteria and parasites can survive low cooking temperatures of short duration.
- Keep foods that need to be kept cold in the fridge. Raw meats and dairy products need to be stored at 4 °C or lower to reduce bacterial growth. Frozen foods must be stored at temperatures of about –18 °C and not be allowed to thaw. If they do, they must be used immediately and not be refrozen. Canned food should be stored in a cool place and not be 'blown'. A blown tin contains gases formed by the decomposition of the food. Store dried foods in airtight containers or where they cannot be destroyed by insects.

- Separate raw foods and foods that are ready to eat. Raw food such as meat, chicken and fish host more bacteria and should be refrigerated or frozen in separate sealed containers to avoid cross-contamination of bacteria.
- Keep rodents and insects such as cockroaches and flies under control. Clean the kitchen and mop the floor each time after preparing food. Keep kitchen surfaces, cupboards, dark fridge corners and shelves clean and free of food residue to prevent the transfer of pathogens from one surface to another.
- Wash fruit and vegetables with water, salt or vinegar to remove contaminants such as soil, insects, chemical residues and any contamination that occurred during the food-handling chain.

Food preservation

The world's food supplies could be increased by about 30 per cent if the loss that occurs during storage could be prevented. Preservation of food is necessary to prevent wastage and to facilitate the distribution of food. For example, fresh milk cannot be widely distributed but dried milk can, as it will keep almost indefinitely. One of the major problems in developing countries is the lack of food technology that would make it possible to preserve food in times of plenty for use in the 'hungry seasons'.

If we wish to preserve food, we must prevent putrefactive bacteria from gaining entry to it, and we must destroy any bacteria that are already present. To do this, we can use methods such as:
- cold
- heat
- irradiation
- the addition of certain chemicals
- the addition of sugar
- drying
- smoking.

Cold

This method includes cooling, chilling and freezing.
- **Cooling**: Foodstuffs are cooled rapidly to below 7 °C and kept at that temperature. Cooling will not destroy bacteria but will prevent their growth and multiplication. Cooling is used for any food that may have to be kept for a few days before it is eaten. A refrigerator is the most efficient method of keeping food cool, but if this is not available, fairly simple and effective cool boxes can be constructed and used for this purpose.
- **Chilling**: This method is used for the large-scale preservation of foodstuffs such as meat. It is also used extensively for fruit. The fruit is picked before it

is ripe and stored. When the temperature of the fruit is raised, the ripening process continues.

- **Freezing**: These foodstuffs are quick-frozen and kept at a temperature of below –8 °C. This method is used extensively today for the preservation of a wide variety of foodstuffs such as meat, fish, vegetables, cakes, cooked foods, etc. It has many advantages:
  - Food can be frozen immediately after harvesting or preparation, while it is still fresh.
  - No preservatives need to be added to the food.
  - Frozen vegetables need minimal cooking, therefore vitamins are not lost.
  - Many foods are partially cooked before they are frozen, which saves on preparation time and labour.
  - There is little, if any, change in the flavour of the food.
  - Frozen food does not have to be thawed before preparation.

Heat

Two methods are used: pasteurisation and sterilisation.

- **Pasteurisation**: This is used in the preservation of milk, beer, wine and fruit juices. Pasteurisation involves heating the product to a specific temperature, for a specific period of time in order to kill bacteria.
- **Sterilisation**: This implies the destruction of all microorganisms. Food that has been sterilised and properly sealed will keep indefinitely if correctly stored. The food is subjected to temperatures above boiling point. If a temperature of only 100 °C is used, then the time the food is exposed to the heat is increased. Different foodstuffs require different methods of sterilisation to preserve the taste and appearance. Fruits may be effectively sterilised by boiling as they contain large amounts of acid, which assists in sterilisation. Foods containing large amounts of sugar, such as canned fruits, are also effectively sterilised by boiling as the boiling point of sugar is far higher than 100 °C. Canned fruits are therefore sterile.

Irradiation

Food irradiation is a processing technique that exposes food to electron beams, X-rays or gamma rays. The process produces a similar effect to pasteurisation, cooking or other forms of heat treatment, but with less effect on the appearance and texture. Foods must be irradiated in authorised food-irradiation facilities that are subjected to strict safety inspections. Irradiation is used to kill bacteria that cause food poisoning, such as salmonella, campylobacter and E. coli. This method delays the ripening of fruit and helps stop vegetables, such as potatoes and onions, from sprouting.

The addition of chemicals

Three common chemicals used in food preservation are salt, benzoic acid and sulphur dioxide.

Salt (sodium chloride)

Meat, such as biltong and cured ham, is preserved by either dry or wet salting. In dry salting, salt and various other substances and flavorings are mixed in the correct proportions and rubbed into the meat daily. This draws the fluid out of the meat, and the brine that is formed during the process is allowed to drain away. In wet salting the meat is submerged in brine for the required time. This is also known as pickling the meat.

Benzoic acid and sulphur dioxide

Chemicals such as benzoic acid or sulphur dioxide may be added to certain foodstuffs to preserve them, but the addition of chemicals to foods is strictly controlled by law, and any substances that are added must be stated on the labels.

The addition of sugar

As sugar boils at a higher temperature than water, it is added to certain foods, such as fruits, to facilitate their preservation, for example in jam or crystallised fruit.

Drying

When food is dried, a large proportion of the moisture is removed, which prevents the growth and multiplication of bacteria but not necessarily kill them. Parasitic ova are also not destroyed by this method.

Drying may be used to preserve meat, fish, fruit, vegetables and milk. Dried food will keep for long periods if stored correctly.

Smoking

Foods to be smoked are hung in sealed chambers and exposed to wood smoke for the required time. The foodstuff becomes impregnated with formaldehyde and creosote, and the surface becomes dry. The formaldehyde subsequently evaporates but the creosote remains. This process does not destroy parasitic ova.

Milk

Milk forms an important part of the diet of most people, particularly infants and young children. In fact, milk alone is sufficient to ensure the normal growth and development of the infant for the first few months of life. This is possible because it contains all the necessary food constituents, except iron and cellulose. The infant has sufficient stores of iron for some months after birth and does not require cellulose in early infancy, so these deficiencies do not present a problem.

Contamination of milk

Milk can become infected at any point from the cow to the consumer, and unfortunately when pathogens gain entry to milk, they grow and multiply rapidly as the milk provides everything that the bacteria require. Theoretically, almost any infection can be transmitted by contaminated milk.

Infections may be transmitted by milk in a number of ways:

- Conditions in which the pathogen is present in the milk because the animal was suffering from an infection include:
  - non-pulmonary tuberculosis if the cow was suffering from tuberculosis
  - streptococcal throat infections if the cow was suffering from mastitis, which is a streptococcal infection of the udder
  - sore throat with the formation of vesicles if the cow was suffering from the viral infection known as foot and mouth disease
  - diphtheria if there were diphtheric ulcers present on the animal's teats
  - brucellosis (undulant fever) if the cow was suffering from brucellosis or abortus fever.
- The causative organisms of typhoid and paratyphoid fever, cholera, tuberculosis and diphtheria may be present in milk if the milker suffers from or is a carrier of these infections. This is particularly likely to occur when standards of personal hygiene are poor.
- When standards of environmental hygiene are poor, and stables and their surroundings are dirty, unhygienic and lack the facilities for the adequate disposal of refuse and excreta from the cows, pathogens may easily enter the milk.
- Flies may also contaminate the milk.
- Utensils that have not been cleaned properly and/or polluted water may be responsible for the presence of harmful microorganisms in milk.

Pasteurised milk

This is a process whereby all pathogenic microorganisms are destroyed by heat. Pasteurisation will not alter the taste or appearance of the milk. In South Africa, pasteurisation is no longer compulsory for milk used for human consumption.

One of three methods may be used to pasteurise milk:

1. The low-temperature, longer-time (LTLT) method. The milk is heated to 63°C and kept at the temperature for 30 seconds.

2. The high-temperature, short-time (HTST) method. The milk is heated at 72°C for 15 seconds. This method is commonly used in milk pasteurisation.

3. The ultra-high temperature (UHT) method. The milk is heated to between 138 °C and 150 °C for 2 to 6 or more seconds and then rapidly cooled down to 7 °C. This milk is aseptically packaged and can be kept on the shelf for up to three months. Once opened, it must be refrigerated like fresh milk.

The preservation of milk

Milk can be preserved to last longer. There are two methods for preserving milk: drying and evaporation.

Dried milk

This is milk, either full-cream or skimmed, from which 95 per cent of the water has been removed by evaporation, leaving a whitish powder that contains the milk solids. If mixed as directed on the label, usually one part milk powder to seven parts water, a fluid with the same composition as fresh milk will be obtained. The standards to which dried milk must conform have been laid down by the Dairy Products and Imitation Dairy Products Regulations (R. 260 of 2015).

The advantages of dried milk are that:
- it keeps almost indefinitely if sealed in airtight containers
- it has a uniform composition
- the curd formed is more flocculent and more easily digested than that of fresh cow's milk
- it does not contain any bacteria.

Dried milk powder can be recommended for infant feeding but the importance of vitamin supplementation in addition to milk powder must be encouraged.

Condensed or evaporated milk

This is milk from which about half the water has been removed by a process of slow evaporation. It may be sweetened or unsweetened.

Sweetened condensed milk has sugar added to it. Nothing may be added to evaporated milk (except sugar in the case of sweetened condensed milk). Sweetened condensed milk must not be used for infant feeding as it has a very high sugar content without the required nutrients and could result in an obese and 'flabby' baby. It is necessary to supply the infant with additional vitamins if it is being fed on evaporated milk.

Food security

Food security implies physical, social and economic access to sufficient, safe and nutritious food at all times to meet dietary and food preferences for an active and healthy life. This definition has the following interrelated components:

- **Food availability:** This means effective and continuous food supply at national and household level. Food availability is affected by output market conditions, as well as production capabilities of the agricultural sector.
- **Food access (effective demand):** The ability of a nation and its households to acquire sufficient food on a sustainable basis. It addresses issues of purchasing power and consumption behaviour.
- **Reliability of food:** Utilisation and consumption of safe and nutritious food.
- **Food distribution:** Equitable provision of food to points of demand at the right time and place. The time aspect of food security relates to the fact that a country might be food-secure at national level, but still have regional pockets of food insecurity at various periods of the agricultural cycle.

About 20 per cent of South African households are estimated to have inadequate or severely inadequate access to food (Chakona & Shackleton, 2019). Food insecurity in South Africa is closely linked to socioeconomic status, as indicated by income, employment status and food expenditure. The high level of poverty makes it difficult for many South African households to purchase enough food to feed the entire household. The following strategies have been implemented by the South African government to enhance income of poor households:

- Social grants to improve poverty and food security
- Child support grants and school food programmes to decrease the incidence of stunting and underweight in children
- The Integrated Food Security Programme aiming to eradicate hunger and nutrition deficits among lower-income households

Since the implementation of the above-mentioned initiatives by the national government, statistics suggest a decline in the percentage of food insecure people (Chakona & Shackleton, 2019).

According to a study conducted in the Eastern Cape, South Africa (Selepi et al, 2015), the following factors contribute to food insecurity in rural areas of South Africa:

- Low-income households experience financial constraints and opt for less nutritious food, consuming it mainly for its energy value
- Single-headed households led by women may not have stable and reliable employment to provide adequate and nutritious food on a daily basis
- Inadequate household assets and equipment, such as not having electric stoves and proper food storage facilities like refrigeration

- In the past, rural households produced most of the food for consumption purposes, but recent studies have shown an increase in dependence on market purchases of rural households where up to 90 per cent of the food supplies are being purchased instead of being produced.

An uncertain food supply, challenges with food quantity and quality, lacking money to buy food, skipping meals and ongoing hunger are all elements of being food insecure (Selepi et al, 2015). The community nurse should motivate and empower communities at risk by equipping them with the knowledge and skills to grow their own food gardens. Community gardening should be promoted to enhance food security, to increase financial savings and to gain additional profits when selling vegetables to the local community.

Conclusion

Two important factors have been highlighted in this chapter: eating a nutritional and balanced diet, and the correct storage and preservation of food. By following the basic guidelines outlined in this chapter, you will be equipped to serve the community which you support, by providing health education on how to make healthy eating habits part of their daily living and what strategies to implement to ensure that foodborne diseases are prevented.

Self-assessment

1. Describe the functions of food in the human body.
2. Explain the three broad groups of conditions related to malnutrition.
3. Discuss community-specific factors that influence food choices and food consumption.
4. Identify the five pillars of food safety.
5. Food contamination refers to the presence of harmful chemicals and microorganisms in food. Justify this statement by discussing the contaminants associated with food poisoning.
6. Develop a health education talk to young women about food hygiene at home.

Bibliography

Aidara-Kane, A., Tritscher, A. & Miyagishima, K. 2016. The WHO and its role as an international organization influencing global food policy. Available: https://www.researchgate.net/publication/306357249_The_WHO_and_Its_Role_as_an_International_Organization_Influencing_Global_Food_Policy (Accessed 17 September 2020).

Aryal, S. 2020. Carbohydrates: definition, structure, types, examples, functions. Microbe notes. Available: https://microbenotes.com/carbohydrates-structure-properties-classification-and-functions/ (Accessed 29 September 2020).

Bari, L. & Yeasmin, S. 2018. Foodborne diseases and responsible agents. Available: https://www.researchgate.net/publication/324931587_Foodborne_Diseases_and_Responsible_Agents (Accessed 22 September 2020).

Bjarnadottir, A. 2019. Seven nutrient deficiencies that are incredibly common. Healthline. Available: https://www.healthline.com/nutrition/7-common-nutrient-deficiencies (Accessed 22 September 2020).

Chakona, G. & Shackleton, C.M. 2019. Food insecurity in South Africa: To what extent can social grants and consumption of wild foods eradicate hunger? Elsevier. Available: https://www.sciencedirect.com/science/article/pii/S2452292917302734 (Accessed 26 September 2020).

ChemPages NeTorials. Biomolecules: carbohydrates - polysaccharides. Available: https://www2.chem.wisc.edu/deptfiles/genchem/netorial/modules/biomolecules/modules/carbs/carb6.htm (Accessed 22 September 2020).

Clarke, M. 2014. *Vlok's Community Health*. 6th edition. Cape Town: Juta.

Cleveland Clinic. 2019. Triglycerides and heart health. Available: https://my.clevelandclinic.org/health/articles/17583-triglycerides--heart-health (Accessed 22 September 2020).

Department of Agriculture. 2002. The Integrated Food Security of South Africa. Pretoria: Government Printers.

Department of Agriculture, Forestry and Fisheries. 2017. Dairy products and imitation dairy products regulations (R. 260 of 27 March 2015). Available: https://www.nda.agric.za/doaDev/sideMenu/foodSafety/doc/localImportRegulations/Circular%201%20of%202016%20-%20Interpretation%20of%20the%20Dairy%20and%20Imitation%20Dairy%20Regulations%20-%20Revised%209%20Nov%20'17.pdf (Accessed 26 September 2020).

Du Toit, D.C. 2011. *Food Security*. Directorate Economic Services: Department of Agriculture, Forestry and Fisheries (DAFF).

Foil, L.D. & Gorham, J.R. 2000. Mechanical transmission of disease agents by arthropods. In: Eldridge, B.F. & Edman, J.D. (eds). *Medical Entomology*. Dordrecht: Springer. Available: https://link.springer.com/chapter/10.1007%2F978-94-011-6472-6_12#citeas (Accessed 17 September 2020).

Food Advisory Consumer Service (FATS). nd. Regulation of food safety and quality in South Africa. Available: https://foodfacts.org.za/regulation-of-food-safety-and-quality-in-south-africa/ (Accessed 17 September 2020).

Food and Agriculture Organization (FAO). 2016. Understanding Codex. Available: http://www.fao.org/3/a-i5667e.pdf (Accessed 26 September 2020).

Food and Agriculture Organization (FAO). 2019. The future of food safety: The first FAO/WHO/AU international food safety conference, Geneva. Available: http://www.fao.org/3/CA3225EN/ca3225en.pdf (Accessed 26 September 2020).

Food Facts. nd. Regulation of food safety and quality in South Africa. Food advisory consumer service. Available: https://foodfacts.org.za/regulation-of-food-safety-and-quality-in-south-africa/ (Accessed 26 September 2020).

Grandjean, P. & Bellager, M. 2017. Calculation of the disease burden associated with environmental chemical exposures: application of toxicological information in health economic estimation. Available: https://ehjournal.biomedcentral.com/articles/10.1186/s12940-017-0340-3 (Accessed 17 September 2020).

Grumezescu, A.M. & Holban, A.M. 2018. Food safety and preservation: Modern biological approaches to improving consumer health. Available: https://www.sciencedirect.com/book/9780128149560/food-safety-and-preservation (Accessed 23 September 2020).

Hygiene Food Safety.com. 2020. Why is food hygiene important? Available: https://hygienefoodsafety.org/why-is-food-hygiene-important/ (Accessed 17 September 2020).

Johnson, J. 2018. What is the difference between animal and plant proteins? Medical News Today. Available: https://www.medicalnewstoday.com/articles/322827 (Accessed 17 September 2020).

Langiano, E., Ferrara, M., Lanni, L., Viscardi, V., Abbatecola, A.M. & De Vito, E. 2012. Food safety at home: Knowledge and practices of consumers. *Z Gesundh Wiss*. Available: https://www.ncbi.nlm.nih.gov/pmc/articles/PMC3268974/ (Accessed 17 September 2020).

Mastovska, K. 2013. Modern analysis of chemical contaminants in food. Available: https://www.foodsafetymagazine.com/magazine-archive1/februarymarch-2013/modern-analysis-of-chemical-contaminants-in-food/ (Accessed 17 September 2020).

McCarthy, C. 2018. Common food additives and chemicals harmful to children. Harvard Health Publishing, Harvard Medical School. Available: https://www.health.harvard.edu/blog/common-food-additives-and-chemicals-harmful-to-children-2018072414326 (Accessed 26 September 2020).

Media Lane Community College. 2018. Types of carbohydrates. Available: https://media.lanecc.edu/users/powellt/FN225OER/Carbohydrates/FN225Carbohydrates2.html (Accessed 21 September 2020).

Medic8.com. nd. The food groups. Available: https://www.medic8.com/healthguide/articles/foodgroups.html (Accessed 17 September 2020).

Nutrients Review.com. 2016. Raffinose, stachyose and verbascose. Available: https://www.nutrientsreview.com/carbs/soluble-fiber-raffinose-stachyose-verbascose.html (Accessed 29 September 2020).

Rather, I.A., Koh, W.Y., Paek, W.L. & Lim, J. 2017. The sources of chemical contaminants in food and their health implication. Available: https://www.ncbi.nlm.nih.gov/pmc/articles/PMC5699236/ (Accessed 26 September 2020.

Selepe, B.M., Mtyingizane, S.S. & Masuku, M.M. 2015. Factors contributing to household food insecurity in Mhlontlo area, Eastern Cape, South Africa. *African Journal of Hospitality, Tourism and Leisure* Volume 4 (1). Available: http://www.ajhtl.com/uploads/7/1/6/3/7163688/article45vol4(1)_jan-june2015.pdf (Accessed 26 September 2020).

UNICEF. nd. 2010. *Facts for Life* (journal). Available: www.unicef.factsforlife (Accessed 22 September 2020).

United Nations. 2015. Zero hunger challenge. Available: https://www.un.org/sustainabledevelopment/blog/2015/06/three-years-into-the-zero-hunger-challenge-its-time-to-accelerate-action-and-commitment-to-end-hunger-in-our-lifetimes/ (Accessed 22 September 2020).

University of the Free State (UFS). nd. UFS support services: Learning at our university home / food gardening projects. Available: https://www.ufs.ac.za/supportservices/departments/service-learning-at-our-university-home/links-for-community-projects/food-garden-projects (Accessed 26 September 2020).

Wallace, T.C., Bailey, R.L., Burton-Freeman, B., Chen, C.O., Crowe-White, K.M., Drewnowski, A., Hooshmand, S., Johnson, E., Lewis, R., Murray R., Shapses, S.A. & Wang, D.D. 2019. Fruits, vegetables, and health: A comprehensive narrative, umbrella review of the science and recommendations for enhanced public policy to improve intake. Available: https://www.tandfonline.com/doi/full/10.1080/10408398.2019.163 2258 (Accessed 17 September 2020).

Waugh, A. & Grant, A. 2010. *Ross and Wilson anatomy and physiology in health and illness.* 11th edition. Edinburgh: Churchill Livingstone.

Wikipedia. nd. Food contaminant. Available: https://en.wikipedia.org/wiki/Food_contaminant (Accessed 17 September 2020).

World Health Organization (WHO). 2001. WHO world water day report. Available: https://www.who.int/water_sanitation_health/takingcharge.html (Accessed 26 September 2020).

World Health Organization (WHO). 2020a. Food safety. Available: https://www.who.int/news-room/fact-sheets/detail/food-safety (Accessed 26 September 2020).

World Health Organization (WHO). 2020b. Malnutrition Available: https://www.who.int/news-room/fact-sheets/detail/malnutrition (Accessed 17 September 2020).

Your Dictionary. nd. Nutrition definition. Available: https://www.yourdictionary.com/nutrition (Accessed 17 September 2020).

Index

Page numbers in *italics* refer to tables and figures

10 Point Plan 54–55

A

abortion *see* termination of pregnancy (TOP)
abuse
    alcohol 226, 232, 235
    child 230–237, *234–235*
    substance 235, 254
    trauma 104–105
access to health services *37, 52*
accident(s)
    definition 207
    types of 208–210
acid rain 267, 268
acid-fast bacilli 119–120
acme stage of communicable diseases 142
acquired immunity 126, *126*
acute confusional states 203
acute diseases 83
adipose 221
administrative support 51
adolescent health 195–196
Adult Basic Education and Training (ABET) 8
advocacy for health 64–65
aerosol-generating procedures (AGP) 121
aetiology
    arthritis 89
    cancer 93
    cerebrovascular accident (CVA) 100–101
    description 83, 221
    diabetes mellitus 103
    ischaemic heart disease 97–98
    obstructive pulmonary disease (COPD) 102
    rheumatic heart disease 99–100
affective psychoses 242
affordability 53
aflatoxins 95
African Sustainable Development Association (A-SDA) 259
Africare 258

age
    cancer *92*, 93
    ischaemic heart disease 97
    standardised cancer incidence rates *92*
ageing process 199, 200–201
ageism 204
agent, communicable diseases 141
agriculture 281
AIDS (acquired immune deficiency syndrome) *see* HIV and Aids
air
    conditioning 273
    elements of 265, *265–266*
    pollution 266–269, *270*
    quality 265–266, 267
airborne transmission 263
airbricks 272
alcohol
    abuse 226, 232, 235
    consumption 225–227
    disinfectant 115
    drowning and drinking 216
    harmful use of 84, 85, *86*
    preventative measures 226
    psychological conditions 226
    social problems 226
    tobacco *see* tobacco smoking
alcoholics 225
Alma Ata Declaration 44
amniocentesis 172, 179
amoebic dysentery 119, 123, *158*
analytic studies 81
Ancylostoma duodenale 156
animal protein 315
animal-derived sources of fat 318
Anopheles mosquito 123–124
anorexia nervosa 181
anoxia 221
anthrax 118, *143, 145*, 275
antibiotics 116
antimalarial medication 162
antimicrobial stewardship 131, 137
antiretroviral (ARV) treatment 161, 183, 185
antiseptics 115
anxiety 203

appropriate health service provision 5–6, 53
aquifer 287
arboviruses 122
arenavirus *153*
argo 266, *266*
'Arrive Alive' campaign 104
arthritis 89–90
artificial culture media 113
artificial heating 279
artificial lighting 277–278
artificial ventilation 272
ascaris lumbricoides *157*
asset management for water management 293
athlete's foot 122, *155*
autosomal-dominant inheritance 174–175, *175*
autosomal-recessive inheritance 175–176, *176*
auxiliary nurses 59

B
baby clinics 193–194
bacillary dysenteries 119, 125
Bacille Calmette-Guerin vaccine *127*
Bacillus anthracis 111, *117*, *118*
Bacillus cereus 119
bacteria 111, 117–120, *117*
bacterial contamination of food 328–320
Batho Pele 36, *37*
BCG (bacille Calmette-Guerin) *127*, 128
behaviour therapy 246
behavioural problems 7
benzoic acid in food preservation 336
best practices
    food standards 332
    questions to help determine 74–75
    statistical research to help determine 80
bilharzia *159*
biological contaminants of food 328–331
biological determinants in food choices and preparation 309
biological factors
    ageing process 200
    cancer 93
biomass fuels 264

biomedical model of health 2
birth
    defects *15*, 166, 171, 179, 270, 323
    registration 77
body and tissue-building foods *310*
boiling of water to purify 297
Bordetella pertussis 119, *147*
borehole latrines 302
boreholes 287
botulism 329
'Breaking New Ground' (BNG) 275
breastfeeding
    advantages 194
    prevention of mother-to-child transmission (PMTCT) of HIV 183, 184–185
    well baby clinics 194
Brucella 119
brucellosis 119, *143*, 275, 337
bubonic plague 119, 154
bucket system 302–303
building(s)
    maintenance 274
    planning 274
    regulations and standards 273, 274
    sites for housing 273–274
built environment 282
bulimia nervosa 181
bundles of care 136
buoyancy ventilation 271
burden of disease 10, 46, 89–105, 256
burns 210–214, *211*

C
calcium *325*
cancer 7, *12*, 13, *14*, 90–96, *270*
Cancer Association of South Africa (CANSA) 90, 96
Candida albicans 122, 155, *156*
Candida auris 122, 155, *156*
candles 277
caps 190
carbohydrates 311–313, *311–312*
carbon dioxide 266, *266*, 279
carcinomas 7, 92, 93, *93*, 94, 96, 222, 223, 225, 313
cardiovascular diseases 13, 85, 89, *270*
    see also cerebrovascular accident (CVA); hypertension; ischaemic heart disease; rheumatic heart disease

carriers of microorganisms 125, 139
case studies as teaching method 68
catchment
    definition 287
    management 292
catheter-associated urinary tract
    infection (CAUTI) 136
cell division 168–169
cellulose 313
central line-associated bloodstream
    infections (CLABSIs) 136
centralised chronic medicine
    dispensing and distribution
    (CCMDD) 54
centrosome 110
cerebrovascular accident (CVA) 100–
    101
chancroid 150
chemical burns 213
chemical closets 302
chemical contaminants of food
    331–332
chemical methods to destroy
    pathogenic microorganisms 115
chemicals, cancer 94
chemotherapeutic agents 115
childhood illnesses 195
child(ren)
    abuse
        hotline 236
        long-term consequences 231
        recognising and preventing
            230
        reporting 236–237
        risk factors 235–236
        types of 231–233
        warning signs 233, 234–235
    effect of air pollution on 270
    health services see maternal and
        child health services
    mortality 16, 28, 46, 127
    neglect 232, 234, 235–236
    rights of 34
    spacing 187–188
    support grants 339
chilling of food 334
chlamydia trachomatis infection 151
choking 216–217
cholera 111, 119, 149, 281, 283, 295, 337
chromosomal abnormalities 172–173,
    173
chromosomal syndromes 171,
    172, 173

chromosomes 166–167, 167–168
chronic diseases 83, 203
chronic mental states 240, 242
chronic obstructive pulmonary disease
    (COPD) 102
cities and communities, sustainable 255
cleaning and sanitising of food 327
climate action 255
climate change 279–283
clinical support services 56, 57
Clostridium botulism 118
Clostridium difficile 119
Clostridium perfringens 119
Clostridium tetani 111, 118
cobalt 326
Codex Alimentarius 332
coitus interruptus or withdrawal as
    contraception method 189
cold
    to destroy pathogenic
        microorganisms 114
    food preservation 334–335
colonies of microorganisms 113
commensal 107
communicable diseases see also specific
    diseases
    in Africa 144, 144–154
    bite of an infected (or carrier)
        interim host 152–155
    challenges 14
    description 139, 140–141
    epidemiology of 141–144
    major 159–163
    mode of spread 144–152
    parasitic diseases 155–159
    prevention and control 142–144,
        143
    sustainable development and
        256–257
    triad of host factors in 141–142, 141
community(ies)
    -associated infection (CAI) 131,
        132, 137
    gardening 340
    health 41, 48, 49, 81, 193, 195,
        245, 316
    health workers (CHWs) 48, 49,
        51, 59
    involvement 11, 16, 28, 41, 45, 65,
        99, 155, 249, 258, 259, 260
    mental health programmes
        243–246
    sustainable 255
complete (or first-class) proteins 314

comprehensive approach to
    health 1, 4, 44, 66
comprehensive healthcare system
    42–44
condensed milk 338
condoms 189–190
conduction 279
congenital abnormalities 165–166, 174
    see also birth: defects
consanguinity 176
conservancy method of disposing of
    human excreta 302–303
conservation 287
Conserve Africa 258
Constitution of the Republic of South
    Africa, 1996 33–35, 52–53, 264
consultation 37
consumption, responsible 255
contact tracing and management 140,
    143
contaminated water 294–295
contraception 187, 188–192, 191, 197
controlled tipping of refuse 299–300
convalescence stage in communicable
    diseases 140, 142
convection 279
Convention on the Rights of Children 51
cooling of food 334
copper 326
copying skills 4
coronary artery disease 89, 96–98, 270
coronaviridae 122
Corynebacterium diphtheriae 119
counselling
    genetic 178–180
    preconception care and 174
    well baby clinics 193
counsellors 50
courtesy 37
COVID-19 (coronavirus) 29, 79, 80,
    116, 120–122, 121, 122, 137, 145,
    227, 256
Crimean-Congo fever 153
crude rates 76, 181, 182
cultural practices 2, 7
culture
    cancer 94
    health and 4, 7
    obesity 228
'culture-borne' diseases 222
curative health services 33
customer impact 37

D
daily exercise 87
darkness as supportive environment
    for microorganisms 111
data
    definition 73
    demographic 76–77
    epidemiology 75
    health 77–78
death see also mortality
    major causes of 13
    principle causes of 13
    rates 76–77
    registration 77
deep water 290
dementia 203, 226, 241, 242, 243, 322
demographic data 76–77
demography 15–16
demonstration as teaching
    method 67
Dengue fever 153
Department of Agriculture, Forestry
    and Fisheries (DWAFF) 332
Department of Trade and
    Industry 332
Depo-Provera 191
depression 203
dermatomycoses 122
descriptive studies 81
development
    health and 10–11, 26
    health systems 32–33
    policies 32–33
diabetes mellitus 13, 98,
    102–104
diagnosis, early 142
diaphragms 190
dietary cholesterol 317
dietary factors and
    obesity 229
diphtheria 119, 125, 126, 127, 128,
    128, 129, 143, 337
disability-adjusted life years (DALYs) 89
disabilities, limitation of 43
disaccharides 312
disease(s) see also specific diseases
    international classification 79
    notification of 142–143, 143
    presence or absence of affecting
        ageing process 200
    profiles 11–15
    tobacco smoking 222–224
    water-related 295–297

disinfectants *38*, 112, 115
disinfection of water to purify 298
disorders of the intellect 240
dissolved impurities in water 294
distillation of water to purify 297
district clinical specialist teams (DCST)
    46, 47–48, 54
District Health Authority (DHA) 36
District Health System (DHS) 35–36,
    41–42
domestic accidents *see* home accidents
domestic fires 267
domestic violence 235, 237
dominant genes *171*
Down syndrome (Trisomy 21) 172
dried milk 338
drink driving 227
drinking water, purification of 296–
    298
droplet transmission 263
drowning 215–216
drug(s)
    abuse 232, 235, 240
    addiction 239
    effects of on brain 239
    psychotropic 245
dry-earth closets 302
dry heat to destroy pathogenic
    microorganisms 113
dry household refuse 299–300
drying
    to destroy pathogenic
        microorganisms 114
    of food 336
dysentry 117, 119, 123, 125, *158*

E
ears, objects in 219
Earth Summit 19, 288
eating for health 87
ebola *148*, *152*
economic determinants in food
    choices and preparation 309
economic development 249
economic factors
    cancer 94
    health status and 2
economic growth 250, 255
ectomorph 221
education
    alcohol 226
    communicable diseases 144

definition of health education 66
health determinant *4*, 8
mental health 244
methods of teaching 67–68
obesity and 228–229
organisations promoting health
    69–70
outcomes of 67
planning of health education
    session 69
prenatal care 183–184
principles for success in 70–71
promotion of health 66
quality 254
teaching aids and media 68
well baby clinics 193
educators 8, 70
Edwards' syndrome *173*
effectiveness 53
efficiency 53
elderly
    decreasing importance of
        traditional age roles 204
    demographics 197–198
    falls 209
    family and 201
    health of 197–204
    legislation 198
    loss of respect for 204
    problems of 202–204
    process of ageing 199–201
    services for 198–199
electric lighting 278
electrical burns 213
electro-convulsive therapy 245
emergency card for poison treatment
    215
emergency medical treatment 34, 218
emotional child abuse 232, *234*
emotions, trouble regulating 231
employment and working
    conditions *4*
empowerment 67, 251, 260
endemic disease 140
endomorph 221
endotoxins 112
energy
    affordable clean 254
    sun's 278
    as supportive environment for
        microorganisms 110
enrolled nurses 59
Entamoeba histolytica 122–123,
    122, *158*

Enterobius vermicularis 157
Enterococcus faecalis 118
enteroviruses 122
environment
    communicable diseases 141
    manipulation of during mental
       illness treatment 246
environmental conditions
    cancer 94–95
    health status 2
    WHO function to enhance 28
environmental factors 8
environmental healthcare 45
environmental hygiene 144, 298–299
environmental rights 264
environmental sustainability
    climate change 279–283
    definition 264
    health effects of air pollution
       and inadequate ventilation
       269–270
    housing 273–276
    lighting and heating 276–279
    sustainable development goals
       (SDGs) 265–269
    ventilation 271–273
epidemic
    definition 73, 140
    -prone diseases 26
epidemiological research methods 81
epidemiology
    of communicable diseases 141–
       144
    data collected 75
    description 73, 74
    in healthcare practice 74–75
equality, gender 254
equity 26, 35, 36, *39*, 45, 52, 53, 60, 65
erythema 140
Escherichia coli 119
ethnicity or race, cancer 94
evaporated milk 338
evidence, harnessing 27
executive authority 34–35
Executive Council of World Health
    Organization (WHO) 24
exercise, lack of 98
exotoxin 111, 329
Expanded Programme of
    Immunisation (EPI (SA)) 126
experimental methods 81
exposure to pollutants 267–268
external parasites 155

external ventilation 272
eyes, objects in 219

F
falls 209–210, *210*
family
    elderly and 201, 204
    planning 187–188
fans 273
fats 316–318
feelings of being 'worthless' or
    'damaged' 231
fellowships 28
fibre 313
filoviridae *148, 152*
filtration
    to destroy pathogenic
       microorganisms 114
    of water to purify 297, *298*
financial problems of elderly 203
fire burns 213–214
fire hazards 223
fish-derived sources of fat 318
flagella 112
flaviviridae *150*
flavivirus *153*
floor safety tips 210
folic acid 174, 178, *323*
fomites 107, 125, 142, 143, *153, 157,*
    263
food
    access (effective demand) 339
    availability 339
    choices and preparation 309
    contamination 328–332
    distribution 339
    groups and classifications 310–
       327, *310*
    handling 328
    insecurity in rural areas 339–340
    irradiation 335
    poisoning 118, 119, *143, 149*, 327,
       328, 329, 333
    preservation 334–336
    production 77, 253, 257, 281, 283
    safety 332
    security 339–340
    standards 332
    storage 328
    temperature 328
Food and Agricultural Organization
    (FAO) 20
foodborne disease 328

foreign-body accidents 209
freezing of food 335
fructose *311*
fungi 122, 155–156, *155–156*

G

galactose *311*
games as teaching method 68
gas lamps 278
gastrointestinal diseases 119
gender
    cancer *91–92*, 93
    equality 254
    health determinant *4*
    ischaemic heart disease 97
gene defects 173–174
general practitioner (GP) contracting
    54
genes 170–171
genetic counselling 178–180
genetics
    ageing process 200
    cancer 93
    cell division 168–169
    chromosomal abnormalities
        172–173, *173*
    chromosomes 166–167, *167–168*
    gene defects 173–174
    genes 170–171
    health determinant *4*
    inheritance patterns 174–177
    ischaemic heart disease 97
    meiosis 169, *169*
    obesity 228
    referring people who may be at
        risk 178–180
    sex determination 169–170, *170*
genital herpes *151*
genital warts *151*
genotype 165
geological or geochemical factors 8
geriatrics 198, 202
German measles *see* rubella
gerontology 198
giardiasis *159*
Global Action Plan for the Prevention
    and Control of NCDs 2013–2020
    84, 85
Global Burden of Disease (GBD) 89
Global Jobs Pact of the International
    Labour Organization 255
Global Malaria Programme 162
Global Vaccine Action Plan 127

global warming *see* climate change
glucose *311*
going green 280–281
Golgi apparatus 110
gonorrhoea *151*
good health and well-being 182, 254
government departments 69, 332
government structure 34–35
grains *310*
gram stains 112
gram-negative bacilli 119
gram-negative cocci 118
gram-positive bacilli 118–119
gram-positive cocci 118
granuloma inguinale *151*
grass roots 18
greenhouse gases (GHGs) 279
greywater 293–294
groundwater 290
group discussions 67
guilt of sexual abuse 233

H

haematopoietic system *270*
Haemophilus ducreyi 150
haemophilus influenza type B *127, 128*
halogens 115
hand hygiene 133–134, *134, 135*, 143,
    156, 332
Hansen's disease 120, 143, *146*, 296
health
    appropriate service provision 5–6
    attaining and maintaining 2, 4–9
    data 77–78
    definition 2–4, 25
    departments *40*
    determinants *3, 4*, 10, 27, 281,
        309
    development and 10–11, 26
    education *see* education
    emergencies 26
    impact of climate change on
        282–283
    inequity in 5
    information 6
Health for All 4–5, 9, *9*, 10, 11, 16, 43,
    44, 45, 60, 61, 64
health services
    accessibility 6
    adequate 6
    determinants of health and *4*
    legislation 5

WHO function to establish
national 28
health systems 27, 32–33 *see* also
National Health Insurance (NHI)
healthcare systems 42–46, 53–54
healthcare-associated infection (HAI)
131, 132, 133, 137
heart disease
ischaemic 12, 13, 79, 96–99, 223
rheumatic 99–100
heat
accidents 209 *see also* burns
to destroy pathogenic
microorganisms 113–114
heating 276, 278, 279
heavy metals 331
helminthic infections 156, *156–157*
hepadnavirus *150*
hepatitis A 128, *143*, *149*
hepatitis B 95, 128, 132, *150*
hepatitis C *150*
herd (or community) immunity 126
heredity 165
herpes genitalis *151*
herpesvirus *151*
heterozygotes 171
HIV and Aids
challenges 13
communicable diseases 160–161
dementia due to 241, 243
education and 8
home-based community care 11
mode of spread *150*
mother-to-child transmission
183, 184–185
policy and strategy 37
prevention 160–161
stages of 161
statistics 160
status 160
holistic approach 1, 2, 4–5, 44
home accidents
burns 210–214, *211*
choking 216–217
definition of
accident 207
injury 207
demographics 208
description 208
drowning 215–216
elderly 202
groups at risk 208
objects in ear, nose and eye 219
poisoning 214–215, *214–215*

suffocation 217–218
types of 208–210
home-based care 11, 90, 161
homeostasis 181
homozygotes 171
hookworm *156*
Hospice Association of South Africa
83, 96
host, communicable diseases 141
household
recycling 280–281
refuse 299–303
housing 255, 273–275
Human Development Index (HDI) 249
human excreta
disposal of 301–303
treatment of wastewater in
sewerage system 300
human papillomavirus *151*
human rights 34
humanitarian
meaning 18
programmes and agencies 21
hydrogen ion concentration as
supportive environment for
microorganisms 111
hypertension 96, 98, 101, 103, 200,
270
hypnotherapy 246

I
ideal clinic realisation and
maintenance model (ICRM) 54
immune system *270*
immunisation 143, 194
immunity 107, 125–126
impact accidents 208, 209
incidence rates 78–79
incineration 113, 299, 331
income, health determinant *4*
incomplete (second-class) proteins 314
incontinence 181
incubation period 142
industrial disposal of refuse 299–300
industrial emissions 267–268
industrial waste disposal 303
industry
air pollution 267
sustainable development goals
(SDGs) 255
inequality, reducing 255
infant mortality 11, 15, 16, 76, 182

infected animals 122, *154, 295*
infection(s)
    antimicrobial stewardship 137
    bundle of care 136
    chain of 133, *133*
    cycle of malnutrition and *109*
    definition 107
    droplet infection or inhalation
      144–149
    hand hygiene and 133–134, *134,*
      135
    outbreaks 137
    prevention and control 135–136
    reservoirs of 124–125
    risk factors for healthcare
      associated infections 133
    routes of 133
    surveillance 132
    transmission of 124–125
influenza *32, 144*
informal settlements 255, 267
information
    Batho Pele *37*
    definition 73
    harnessing 27
    health 6
infrastructure
    projects 54
    sustainable development goals
      (SDGs) 255
ingestion/inhalation accidents 209
inheritance patterns 174–177
injectable long-acting contraceptives
    and implants 191, *191*
injury(ies)
    definition of 207
    main causes of *209*
innate immunity 126
innovation *37,* 255
insect vectors 144
insurance *see* National Health
    Insurance (NHI)
Integrated Food Security Programme
    339
integrated management of childhood
    illnesses (IMCI) 195
integrated school health programme
    (ISHP) 46, 51, 54
integumentary system *270*
International Classification of Diseases
    (ICD) 79
International Council for Local
    Environmental Initiatives (ICLEI)
    250

International Labour Organization
    (ILO) 19
intersectoral approach
    to health *9,* 16
    sustainable development 250,
      252, 259–260
interventions
    cerebrovascular accident (CVA)
      101
    obstructive pulmonary disease
      (COPD) 102
intimate partner violence (IPV)
    237–238, *239*
intra-family stressors 204
intra-uterine devices (IUDs) 191–192
iodine *326*
iron *326*
iron deficiency 315, *326*
irradiation of food 335
ischaemic heart disease 12, 13, 79,
    96–99, 223
isolation period 140, 143

J
Johannesburg Declaration on
    Sustainable Development 10
Joint United Nations Programme on
    HIV and AIDS (UNAIDS) 21
justice
    security and 25
    sustainable development goals
      (SDGs) 256

K
karyotypes 167
keratosis 83
kerosene 278
Klebsiella granulomatis 151
Klinefelter syndrome *173*
kwashiorkor 315–316
kyphosis 181

L
laboratory examination of
    microorganisms 112–113
lack of support and child abuse 236
lactose *312*
Lassa fever *153*
learning, obesity 228–229
Legionella pneumophila 119, *146*
Legionnaires' disease 119, *145*
legislation 5, 32, *38–39,* 39–40

legislatures 32, 35
leprosy 120, *143*, *146*, 296
lessons or lectures as teaching
    methods 67
leukoplakia 83
life
    basics of 264
    below water 255
    expectancy 13, 46, 53, 200, 204,
        223, 227, 249
    on land 255
lifestyle diseases 14, 84, 257
lighting 276–277
literacy 5, 8, 9, *9*, 249
living characteristics of
    microorganisms 110–112
local government 35
lockjaw *see* tetanus
low-cost housing 274–275
lowland surface water 289

M

M. lepromatosis 120
macule 140
magnesium 294, 297, 314, *325*
malaise 83
malaria *12*, *15*, 111, 115, 123, *123*, 152,
    161–162, 282, 283
malnutrition 13, *14*, 108, *109*, 257,
    308, 315
maltose *312*
marasmus 315–316
Marburg *148*
mass-media education and information
    68
maternal and child health services
    breastfeeding and prevention of
        mother-to-child transmission
        of HIV 185
    integrated management of
        childhood illnesses (IMCI) 195
    postnatal care 186–187
    prenatal care 183–185
    services for delivery 186
    sexually transmitted infection
        management 192
    weaning 195
    well baby clinics 193–194
maternal mortality 46, 49, 76, 182,
    254
measles *128*
measles vaccine 129, *238*
mechanical transmission 307

mechanical ventilation 272–273
medical practitioners 50, 59, 186, 245
medical supervision at baby clinics 194
medical technology 204
meiosis 169, *169*, 172
meningitis *15*, 118, 125, 242, *270*
meningococcal meningitis 125
men's health *91–92*, 197
mental conditions 239–243
mental health 239–246
mental illness, untreated 235
microbes *see* microorganisms
microbiology 108
microdeletions 173
micronutrient-related malnutrition
    282
microorganisms
    artificial culture media 113
    capsules 112
    classification of 117–124
    colonies of 113
    definition 107
    destroying pathogenic 113–116
    flagella 112
    immunisation 126–127, *127–128*
    immunity 125–126
    laboratory examination 112–113
    living characteristics 110–112
    non-pathogenic 108
    pathogenic 108, 113–116
    portals of entry 116–117, *116*
    reproduction 111
    reservoirs of infection 124–125
    single-cell *110*
    spore formation 112
    supportive environment 110–111
    toxin production 111–112
    vaccine administration 128–130
migration 282
milk and milk products
    contamination 337
    food group *310*
    as part of diet 336–337
    pasteurisation 337–338
    preservation of 338
mineral salts 325, *325–326*
mitochondria 110
mitosis 168
moist heat to destroy pathogenic
    microorganisms 113
moisture as supportive environment
    for microorganisms 111
monograph 18, 28

monosaccharides (simple sugars) *311*
morbidity 1, 6, 8, 77, 208
mortality 1, 6, 8, 11–12, *12, 14,* 15–16, *15,* 28, 76, 77, 182, 254
mother-to-child HIV transmission prevention 183, 184–185
motivation, ageing process 201
multidisciplinary teams (MDT) 51, 58–59
multifactorial inheritance 177
multinational agency(ies) 18, 29
mumps *146*
muscular relaxation 246
mutations 173–174
Mycobacterium leprae 120, *146*
Mycobacterium tuberculosis 111, 114, 119, 145, 163
mycoses 122

N
N95 respirator 121
Nairovirus *153*
National Adolescent-friendly Clinic Initiative 196
National Assembly 34
National Core Standards (NCS) 56–59
National Council of Provinces 34
National Department of Health 332
national drug policy 37
National Health Act 61 of 2003 39–40
National Health Insurance (NHI) 52–53
national housing subsidy scheme 275
natural light 276–278
naturally occurring toxins 331
neglect, child 232, *234,* 235–236
Neisseria gonorrhoeae 118, *151*
Neisseria meningitidis 118
neuroses 243
New Partnership for Africa's Development (NEPAD) 258
NHI pilot districts 53–54
nitrogen *265,* 266
Nokero ('No Kerosene') N200 LED light 278
non-communicable diseases (NCDs) *see also specific diseases*
    caring for patients with chronic 87–89
    description 84–85
    major cause of death 13, 84

medical/nursing needs 87
    prevention and control 85–87
    role of nurse 88, *88*
    sustainable development and 257
non-governmental organisations 70
non-pathogenic microorganisms 108
North–South cooperation 256
nose, objects in 219
nosocomial infections 132
notification of diseases 142–143, *143*
nucleus 110
numerical abnormalities 172
Nur-Isterate 191
nursing auxiliaries 50
nursing care
    arthritis 90
    cancer 96
    chronic non-communicable diseases (NCDs) 87
    diabetes mellitus 103–104
    ischaemic heart disease 99
    non-communicable diseases 88, *88*
    rheumatic heart disease 100
    trauma 105
nutrients 311–327 *see also specific nutrients*
nutrition, description 308
nutritional status 144

O
obesity 98, 103, 200, 227–230, 307, 308, 317
objects in ear, nose and eye 219
observational methods 81
occupational health 28, 59
occupations and cancer 94
Office of Health Standards Compliance (OHSC) 57–58
oil lamps 278
oligosaccharides *312*
openness *37*
oral contraceptives 190–191
organic mental states 240, 242
osteomalacia 7, *319*
Ottawa Charter 65
outbreaks 137
outreach teams *see* ward-based primary healthcare outreach teams (WBPHCOTS)
overcrowding 275–276

overnutrition 228, 317
overweight 101, 227, 229, 230, 308, 317
oxidising agents 115
oxygen 110–111, *265*, 266

P
pantothenic acid *322*
papule 140
paramyxovirus *146*
parasitic diseases 155–159
parasitic infection of food 329–331
parasuicide 181
paratyphoid fever 119, 295
parenting skills 235
Parliament 34
partnership enhancement 27
partnerships for sustainable development goals (SDGs) 256
pasteurisation
    description 308
    of food 335
    of milk 113, 337–338
Patau syndrome *173*
pathogenic microorganisms 108, 113–116
pathogenic protozoa 111
pathological conditions 227
patient(s)
    rights of 38, *38*, 56, *57*
    safety 56
Patients' Rights Charter 38, *38*
peace, sustainable development goals (SDGs) 256
pentavalent vaccine *127*
performance improvement 27
persistent organic pollutants (POPs) 331
personal behaviour *4*
personal hygiene 144, 327, 333
personal protective equipment (PPE) 121
personality
    ageing process 201
    disorders 243
    ischaemic heart disease 97
pertussis *see* whooping cough
pH as supportive environment for microorganisms 111
pharmaceutical advances 204
pharmacists 59

pharmacy assistants 50
PHC nurse practitioners 50, 58
PHC outreach teams *see* ward-based primary healthcare outreach teams (WBPHCOTS)
phenotype 165
phosphorus *325*
physical child abuse 232, *234*
physical determinants in food choices and preparation 309
physical environment *4*
physical factors and health 2
physical inactivity 84, 85, 86, *86*, 229
physical methods used to destroy pathogenic microorganisms 113–116
physical problems of elderly 202–203
picornavirus *149*
plant protein 315
plant-derived sources of fat 318
plasmodium falciparum 123–124, *123*, *152*
plasmodium parasites 161
pneumococcal diseases *127*, *128*
poison, definition 207
poisoning
    food 118, 119, *143*, *149*, 327, 328, 329, 333
    home accidents 214–215, *214–215*
policy(ies)
    definition 32
    development of 32–33
    in SADC 60–61
    South African 35–42
polio 14, *127–128*, 142, 148, *148*
poliomyelitis 122, 125, 128, 129, 143, 148
political factors in health service provision 5, 7, 257
pollution
    air 266–269
    definition 288
    water 291–292
Pontiac fever 119
population growth 77
portals of entry for microorganisms 116–117, *116*
postnatal care 186–187
potassium *326*
poverty
    alleviation 21, 27, 250, 258, 296
    description of 251

environmental links to 141, 156, *252*
food security 339
migration 282
rural areas 6
socio-economic factors 7
sustainable development 10, 11, 253, 258, 259
water and 296
Prader Willi syndrome 173
precision/personalised medicine 177–178
preconception care and counselling 174
pregnancy, tobacco smoking 223
premature deaths 84, 85
prenatal care 183–185
pressurised steam to destroy pathogenic microorganisms 114
prevalence rates 78–79
preventative health services 33
preventative measures
  alcohol 226
  arthritis 90
  burns 211–212
  cancer 95–96
  cerebrovascular accident (CVA) 101
  choking 217
  diabetes mellitus 103
  drowning 216
  falls 210
  health in general 222
  ischaemic heart disease 98
  mental illness 243–245
  obesity 229–230
  objects in ear, nose and eye 219
  obstructive pulmonary disease (COPD) 102
  poisoning 214
  rheumatic heart disease 100
  suffocation 217–218
  trauma 104–105
preventative medicine 64, 66, 71
prevention
  of mother-to-child transmission (PMTCT) 183, 184–185
  primary 42–43, 66, 86–87, 95, 98, 100, 102, 243–244
  secondary 43, 66, 87, 95–96, 98, 100, 245
  tertiary 66, 87, 96, 245
primary healthcare (PHC)
  basic principles for organisation 45
  core principles 45
  description 44–46
  elements to achieve goals 45
  model *47*
  re-engineering (rPHC) 46–50
  service offered 45–46
primary prevention 42–43, 66, 86–87, 95, 98, 100, 101, 102, 243
prodromal stage in communicable diseases 142
production
  food 77, 253, 257, 281, 283
  responsible 255
professional nurses 58–59
professional organisations 70
programmes, community mental health 243–246
healthier populations 26
promotion of health
  conferences 64–65
  description 26, 65
  education and 66
  mental illness and 244
  primary prevention 87
promotive health services 33, 42–43
promulgation 32
protective foods *310*
protein 314–316
protein-energy malnutrition 315–316
protoplasm 110
protozoa 122–124, 158, *158–159*
provincial governments 35
provincial health departments 41
psychoanalysis 246
psychological determinants in food choices and preparation 309
psychological factors
  ageing process 201
  obesity 228
psychological methods of mental illness treatment 246
psychological problems of elderly 203
psychoses 242
psychosocial
  definition 1
  –environmental model of health 2, *3*
  factors and health 2
  needs of patients with chronic non-communicable diseases (NCDs) 87
psychosomatic illnesses 243
psycho-surgery 246

psychotherapy 179, 226, 246
psychotropic drugs 245
public health 4, 6, 24, 26, 32, 64, 65, 256
pulmonary tuberculosis *145*
pulverisation of refuse 300
purification 288

Q
quality
    of care 56, 193
    of life of patients with chronic non-communicable diseases (NCDs) 88
quarantine 140

R
radiation 279
raffinose *312*
rainfall pattern changes 280, 281, 282, 294
rainwater conservation 294
rape 104–105, 237–238, *239*
Rare Diseases South Africa (RDSA) 179
rate(s)
    crude death rate 76
    definition 73
    incidence 78–79
    of mortality *see* mortality
    of natural increase 77
    prevalence 78–79
recessive genes *171*
recommended dietary/daily allowance (RDA) 308
Reconstruction and Development Programme (RDP) 11
recycling
    description 264
    household 280–281
    refuse 280–281, 300
    water 293–294
redress *37*
refined carbohydrates 313
refuse
    household 280–281, 299–303
    industrial disposal of 299–300
registration, births and deaths 77
regulation, definition 32
rehabilitation 44, 46, 99, 101, 105, 203
remission 84
renewable solar lights 278
reproduction of microorganisms 111

Republic of South Africa 33
research 27
resources, adequate 6
respiratory diseases
    air pollution and inadequate ventilation *270*
    major cause of death 13
respiratory illness 267
retrovirus HIV-1, HIV-2 *150*
reward *37*
rheumatic heart disease 99–100
rheumatoid arthritis 89–90
rhinovirus 122
rhythm method of contraception 188–189
ribosomes 110
rickettsiae 120, 157, *158*
Rift Valley Fever *154*
ringworm 122, *155*
role play 68
Roll Back Malaria (RBM) 162
rotavirus *127*
roundworm *157*
rubella 129–130, *146*

S
safe period as contraception method 188–189
salmonella food poisoning 329
Salmonella typhi *149*
salmonellae 119
salt (sodium chloride) in food preservation 336
sanitation 254, 257, 300–301
saprophytes 108
SARS-CoV-1 *144*
SARS-CoV-2 *see* COVID-19 (coronavirus)
saturated fats 316
scarlet fever *147*
schizophrenia 173, 242, 245
school health 46, 51, 54
scientific approach to medicine 2
secondary prevention 43, 66, 87, 95–96, 98, 100, 101, 245
Secretariat of World Health Organization (WHO) 24
security
    food 339–340
    fostering health 26
    and justice 25

self-destructive behaviours
    alcohol consumption 225–227
    child abuse 230–237, *234–235*
    drug addiction 239
    intimate partner violence (IPV)
       and rape 237–238, *239*
    obesity 227–230
    tobacco smoking 222–225
self-determination 44, 64
Severe Acute Respiratory Syndrome
    Coronavirus (SARS-CoV-2) *see*
    COVID-19 (coronavirus)
sewerage system 300, 303
sex determination 169–170, *170*
sexual behaviour, inappropriate 231
sexual child abuse 233, *235*
sexually transmitted infections (STIs)
    13, 192
shame of sexual abuse 233
shigellae 119
shock treatment 245
single-cell microorganism 109–110,
    109
sites for housing 273–274
sleep disturbances 203
sleeping sickness *154*
smoking
    of food 336
    tobacco *see* tobacco smoking
social determinants in food choices
    and preparation 309
social divisions in society 2
social factors
    ageing process 201
    obesity 228
social grants 339
social interaction and integration 201
social problems of elderly 204
social solidarity 53
social status as health determinant *4*
social support networks *4, 239*
social welfare 9
socio-cultural factors, cancer 94
socio-economic factors 6–7
socio-economic level, ageing process
    201
sodium *326*
solar energy 278
solar heating systems 278
South African Social Security Agency
    (SASSA) 203
Southern African Development

Community (SADC) 60–61,
    257–258
South–South cooperation 256
Spanish flu 32
specific immunity 126
spermicides 190
spirochaete 120
sporadic disease 140
spore formation 112
springs 290
stachyose *312*
staff nurses 59
stair safety tips 210
standard(s)
    Batho Pele *37*
    building 274
    definition 32
    food 332
staphylococcal food poisoning 329
staphylococci 118, 329
statistics
    definition 73
    function of WHO 28
    intimate partner violence (IPV)
       238
    use of 79–80
    vital 77
steam to destroy pathogenic
    microorganisms 114
sterilisation
    as contraceptive method 192
    to destroy pathogenic
       microorganisms 115
    of food 335
stock visibility system (SVS) 54
storage of vitamins in body 324–325
streptococci 118, *147*
stress, child abuse and 236
stroke *see* cerebrovascular accident
    (CVA)
strong institutions 256
structural abnormalities 172, 173
sub-economic housing 274
subsoil water 290
substance abuse 235, 254
sucrose *312*
suffocation 217–218
sugar, addition of in food preservation
    336
sulphur *326*
sulphur dioxide in food preservation
    336

sunlight, cancer 94–95
sun's energy 278
supportive environment for
    microorganisms 110–111
surface water 289
surgical site infections (SSIs) 136
surveillance 132
suspended impurities in water 294
sustainability 264 *see also*
    environmental sustainability;
        sustainable development
sustainable cities and communities 255
sustainable development
    communicable diseases and
        256–257
    community participation 260
    core objective 251
    definition 250
    environmental sustainability *see*
        environmental sustainability
    goals (SDGs) 181, 252–256
    intersectoral approach 259–260
    non-communicable diseases and
        257
    organisations involved in 257–259
    in southern Africa 256–257
    triad of health 257
syndromes 165, 171, 172, *173*
syphilis 120, *152*

T
T. solium 157, 330–331
Taenia saginata 157, 330
tapeworms *157*, 325, 330–331, *330*
task-shifting 11
teaching
    aids and media 68, 69
    methods 67–68, 69
technical and official manuscripts 28
temperature as supportive environment
    for microorganisms 111
teratogens 174, 178
terminal disinfection 140
termination of pregnancy (TOP) 179,
    192
tertiary prevention 43–44, 66, 87, 96,
    245
tetanus 111, 116, 118, 127, *127*, 128,
    128, 129, *143*, *183*, 325
tetanus neonatorum 7, *143*
tetanus toxoids 129
therapeutic, definition 64

thermal buoyancy-driven ventilation
    271
threadworm *157*
thrush 155, *156*
tick-bite fever 120, *158*
tissue-building foods *310*
tobacco, cancer 94
tobacco smoking
    advice to give up 224–225
    ageing process 200
    and diseases 222–224
    fire hazard 223
    forms of tobacco use 222
    and ischaemic heart disease 98,
        223
    legislation 224
    life expectancy 223
    origins 222
    perpetuation 223–224
    during pregnancy 223
tobacco use 84, 85, 86, *86*, 93
TORCH viruses 178
toxin production by microorganisms
    111–112
Toxoplasma gondi 124
toxoplasmosis *159*
traditional healers *39*, 59
training programmes 28
trait 165
trans fats 316–317
translocations 173
transparency *37*
trauma 84, 104–105, 207
Treponema pallida 120, *152*
triangular cooperation 256
trichinosis 329
Trichomonas vaginalis 152
trichomoniasis *152*
Trisomy 21 172
trust, lack of in child abuse victims 231
Trypanosoma 124, *154*
trypanosomiasis 124, *154*
Tsetse fly *154*
tuberculosis (TB) 13, 127, *145*, 163
Turner syndrome *173*
typhoid fever 117, 119, *143*, *149*, 295
typhus 120, *143*, *158*

U
ultraviolet germicidal irradiation
    (UVGI) 114
ultraviolet light 114

UN Conference on Sustainable Development 10
undernutrition 254, 282, 308
undulant fever *see* brucellosis
unhealthy diet 84, 85, *86*
Union of South Africa 32–33
United Nations Children's Fund (UNICEF) 20–21
United Nations Development Programme (UNDP) 21
United Nations Environmental Programme (UNEP) 20
United Nations (UN) 19–22
United Nations Women (UN Women) 21–22
universal health coverage (UHC) 26, 52, 254
urinary tract infections 118, 119, 138

V

vaccine administration 128–130
value for money *37*
valvular disease 100
vectors 1, 108, 131, 144
vehicle emissions 267
ventilated improved privy (VIP) toilet 302
ventilation
    description 271
    external 272
    inadequate 269, *270*
    mechanical 272–273
    natural 271–272
    prevention and control of communicable diseases 144
ventilator-associated pneumonia (VAP) 136
vesicles 140, *151*, 337
vibrio 111, *117, 149*
Vibrio cholerae 119
viruses 95, 111, 120, 122, 178
vital statistics 77
vitamins 7, 318, *318–324*, 324–325

W

ward-based primary healthcare outreach teams (WBPHCOTS) 46, 48, *48*, 49, *49–50*, 50–51, 54
waste 288
wastewater treatment 300
water
    asset management 293

basic supply 292
-carriage system of disposing human excretion 303
clean 254, 257
contaminants 294–295
description 288
fluid balances 327
functions of in body 326–327
greywater 293–294
ground- 290–291
metering 293
pollution 291–292
poverty 296
pressure in reticulation systems 293
protection of resources 291
provision goals 292–293
purification of drinking 296–298
quality 292
rainwater conservation 294
-related diseases 295–297
re-use and recycling 293
security 281
sources of in food products 327
surface 289
tariffs 293
treatment of wastewater in sewerage system 300
use 292
vapour *266*
watercourse 288
weaning 195
welfare, description 251
well baby clinics 193–194
well-being 182, 254 *see also* health
wellness *see* health
wells 290–291
White Paper on the Transformation of the Health System 35–36
whooping cough *15*, 119, *127*, 128, 129, *143, 147*
wind-driven cross ventilation 271
windows 271–272, 277
women's health, cancer *91–92*
workload indicator for staffing needs (WISN) 54
World Food Programme (WFP) 21
World Health Assembly (WHA) 23
World Health Organization (WHO) 20, 22–28
World Summit on Sustainable Development (WSSD) 10, 288
worm infestation 156, *156–157*

X
X-linked inheritance 176–177

Y
yellow fever *143, 153*
Yersinia pestis 112, 119, 154

Z
zero hunger 253–254
zoonoses 125
zygotes 169, 170

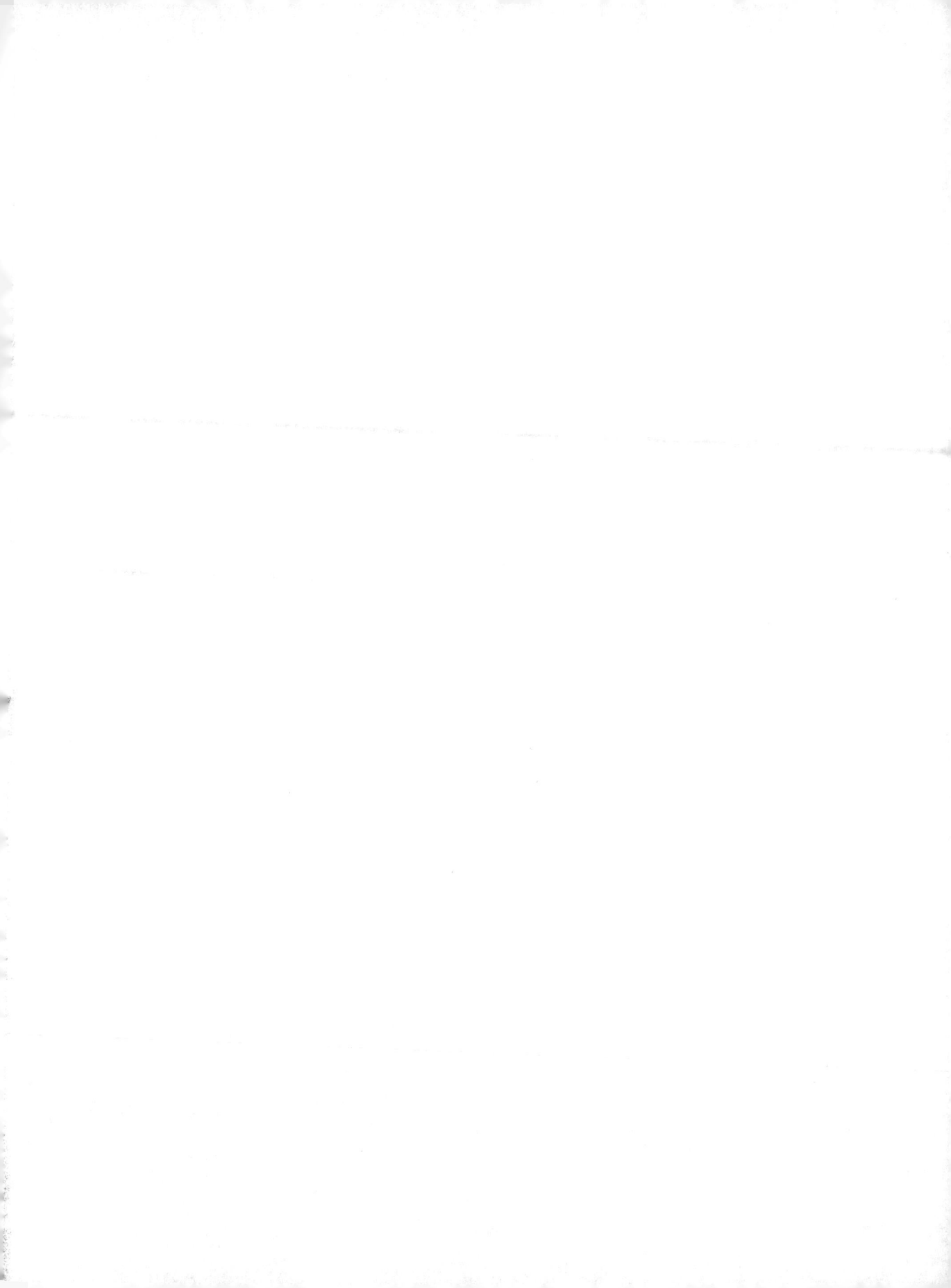